乳腺癌 腺叶疾病

Breast Cancer A Lobar Disease

主　　编　［瑞典］Tibor Tot
主　　译　王　岭　王　廷　樊　菁
副 主 译　张　凌　赵　戈
译　　者　（按姓氏笔画排序）
　　　　　于　铭　王　廷　王　岭
　　　　　巫　姜　李松朋　李南林
　　　　　张　凌　张　瑞　张红梅
　　　　　张聚良　赵　戈　赵娓娓
　　　　　徐玉乔　崔风强　董曦文
　　　　　樊　菁　魏洪亮

西安　北京　广州　上海

图书在版编目(CIP)数据

乳腺癌：腺叶疾病/(瑞典)蒂博尔(Tibor Tot)主编；王岭，王廷，樊菁主译. —西安：世界图书出版西安有限公司，2017.6

书名原文：Breast Cancer：A Lobar Disease

ISBN 978-7-5192-1973-4

Ⅰ.①乳…　Ⅱ.①蒂…　②王…　③王…　④樊…　Ⅲ.①乳腺癌—诊疗—研究　Ⅳ.①K924

中国版本图书馆CIP数据核字(2017)第122774号

Translation from the English language edition：
Breast Cancer. A Lobar Disease
edited by Tibor Tot
Copyright© Springer-Verlag London Ltd. 2011
Springer is part of Springer Science + Business Media
All Rights Reserved

书　　名	**乳腺癌**腺叶疾病 Ruxianai Xianye Jibing
主　　编	[瑞典]Tibor Tot
主　　译	王　岭　王　廷　樊　菁
责任编辑	杨　莉
装帧设计	绝色设计
出版发行	世界图书出版西安有限公司
地　　址	西安市北大街85号
邮　　编	710003
电　　话	029-87214941　87233647(市场营销部) 029-87234767(总编室)
网　　址	http://www.wpcxa.com
邮　　箱	xast@wpcxa.com
经　　销	新华书店
印　　刷	中闻集团西安印务有限公司
开　　本	889mm×1194mm　1/16
印　　张	14.75
字　　数	400千字
版　　次	2017年6月第1版　2017年6月第1次印刷
版权登记	25-2016-0110
国际书号	ISBN 978-7-5192-1973-4
定　　价	130.00元

(版权所有　翻印必究)
(如有印装错误，请与出版社联系)

致 献

献给我生命中的女性：我的妻子Mária、母亲Zsuzsanna、姐姐Jolán以及女儿Boglárka和Emese。

译者前言

乳腺癌是一种严重影响女性健康的疾病，人们和其斗争的历史可以追溯到公元前。随着近代医学的发展，乳腺癌患者的死亡率逐渐下降，可发病率仍然居高不下，在我国甚至逐渐升高。究竟是现代的生活方式使乳腺癌的发病率升高？还是这种疾病的实际病因我们仍不清楚？在本书中，Tot教授提出了自己的观点。阅读这部著作，我们仿佛与不同领域的专家面谈，既探讨具体的专业知识，也了解他们的思辩与心路历程。

如果说我们翻译的《高风险乳腺癌的防治策略》一书是在讲具体操作的"术"，那么，这本著作就是在谈起源的"理"。Tot教授从临床上受人冷落的腺叶结构谈起，将肿瘤干细胞、基因突变等不同的内容巧妙地穿插在一起，娓娓道来，又从X线、超声、内镜等具体检查中寻得有力的支持证据，令人信服。最令人佩服的是，Tot教授并未因意见相左而将相关领域的专家避之门外，相反，他邀请他们参与这本著作，并鼓励其畅所欲言，丝毫不避讳这些专家对自己观点的质疑和争议。这种实事求是的工作态度在Gorden教授撰写的第10章中表现的淋漓至尽。同样，Tot教授这种严谨的治学态度也打动了Gorden等专家，正如Vincent教授所说："（病态腺叶理论）是一个极具挑战性的问题，需要耗费多年时间才能解决。""所以，我们3个人达成了一致意见，接受这个挑战"，Gorden教授如是说。

尽管现在Tot教授的理论并非主流，但是，他的这种特立独行、严谨求证的科学态度值得我们每个人学习！

本书适用于临床肿瘤学专业医生、乳腺专业医生、研究生及科研工作者。参与翻译的各位老师包括科研工作者、临床医生等，专业涉及分子生物学、病理学、超声科、肿瘤外科及内科等，他们活跃在各自的工作岗位上，富于激情，充满理想。在此，衷心感谢各位参与者的倾情付出！特别要感谢王廷副教授和樊菁博士，他们为本书的选题和后期的校对工作付出了大量的时间及精力。感谢世界图书出版西安有限公司杨莉编辑的耐心和大力支持。

本书涉及专业领域广泛，艰难晦涩之处较多，翻译校对过程十分困难，其中涉及工科影像专业的章节数易其稿！限于译者的能力，书中可能存在错误及不当之处，敬请读者不吝指教。

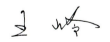

2017年4月于西京医院

序

这几年，不论在哪种场合，当谈及病态腺叶的话题时，我都会很关心听众的反应。对于一种新的理论，听众一般有3种反应：极少一部分人会认为很创新，从而接受它；怀疑论者会质疑它，并竭尽全力证明它是错误的；但是，绝大部分人会说理论是正确的，但不是新理论，他们需要数十年的时间才能理解。

绝大部分人永远是正确的。"病态腺叶理论和生物时钟理论是新的概念，但是这些理论都植根于之前的观察和研究"。但是，"病态腺叶理论和生物时钟理论都与已知的一种解剖结构的癌变有关，这就是乳腺小叶。而且，这个理论也是乳腺癌独特的演进方式和异质性形态的可能答案。这些理论绝非形态学的描述，而是把基因、发育和形态等糅合到一个概念中，去理解在内源性和外源性因素的作用下，乳腺癌发生演变的过程。这不是一张静态的图片，更像是一部持续一生的电影"（Tot，第1章）。"'病态腺叶'的假说从时间和空间的角度提出了乳腺癌发生的问题，并且观察到关键事件在数立方毫米的组织中发生这一观点是靠不住的"（Going，第2章）。通过在Pubmed上检索，就能证明这个概念的原创性。

2004年，在加拿大的Winnipeg举办的第一届乳腺X线替代研讨会上，我第一次提出了这个理论。本书花了1年的时间编撰，在10个不同的章节中列出了支持和反对的证据。流行病学证据支持"……乳腺癌发生过程中的基因突变或表观遗传学异常很可能是有些细胞本质的特征，这些细胞在腺叶形成的过程中经历了不断的分化和快速的生长。而不是起源于终末导管单元，因为在出生前这些单元还未发育出现"（Xue和Michels，第3章）。基因分析显示"……图谱分析显示某些乳腺癌样本中，基因改变呈节段性簇样分布。研究还进一步揭示，围绕肿瘤的组织存在基因的不稳定现象，这个范围远大于单个的终末导管小叶单元"（Smart，et al，第4章）。

现代影像学以其多种多样的检查手段，为乳腺癌复杂多变的形态提供了证据，本书中有详尽的描述。"当我们检测早期或小尺寸乳腺癌时，我们无法保证每个病例的病变都很局限。实际上，无论在乳腺癌发展过程中的任何阶段，多灶和（或）弥散性乳腺癌都构成了乳腺癌的主体"（Tabár, et al, 第7章）。形态学上存在一些证据，即癌灶和癌前病变的分布范围与乳腺的腺叶范围类似，"如果常规病理中广泛使用大切片组织技术，那么，就可以对原位肿瘤的程度和生长模式有更加精确的理解"（Foschini和Eusebi, 第6章）。导管镜也支持形态学数据，它显示"不管是单灶还是多灶性病变，乳腺癌看起来的确存在于单个导管树中"（Dooley, 第9章）。一种特殊的超声检查——导管超声技术，为乳腺癌的小叶本质提供了进一步的证据。这些证据不仅是研究发现的，而是在日常的诊断工作中随处可见。因此，Dominique Amy医生表态说："我们认为'病态腺叶理论'……反映了日常工作中，我们在'活体检查'时的现实状况"（Amy, 第8章）。

这些理论对实际诊断和治疗有一定意义。"20世纪我们以为的治疗肿瘤的灵丹妙药并没有彻底解决问题"。现在的治疗方案中，生物化学、分子生物学、基因组学和宏伟的制药工业占了统治地位，甚至形成了一种观点——每种疾病都有对应的药物治疗。与此类似，过去的100年间，X线等影像学技术得到了发展和提高。现在是时候抛弃过去的治疗方案了，因为这些方案不够精准，即缺乏检测所有肿瘤的能力"（Gordon, 第10章）。除了放射影像学的进步以外，"如果乳腺癌的治疗需要更合理、更微创的方法，导管或小叶系统的导管内入路的知识也非常关键"（Love和Mills, 第5章）。另一方面，数据也"指出手术时必须切除足够范围的组织，以避免局部复发。这同时也提出了问题，是否这就是某些进行了肿瘤'完全切除'的病例又出现局部复发的原因"（Smart, et al, 第4章）。

谈及听众的反应，一位听过我演讲的乳腺外科"大腕"对我说，正确的理论是最重要的，你的有些观点非常有价值。我希望本书能促进读者重新思考那些已有定论的观点，并且开发出新的、更有效率的乳腺癌诊断和治疗方法。

Tibor Tot
Falun, Sweden

原著作者名单

List of Contributors

Dominique Amy, MD

Peter B. Dean, MD, PhD

William C. Dooley, MD

Vincenzo Eusebi, MD, FRC Path

Maria P. Foschini, MD

James J. Going, MB, PhD

Richard Gordon, PhD

Mats Ingvarsson, MD

Sunil R. Lakhani, BSc, MBBS, MD, FRC Path, FRCPA

Nadja Lindhe, MD

Susan M. Love, MD, MBA

Karin B. Michels, ScD, PhD

Dixie J. Mills, MD

Peter T. Simpson, BSc

Chanel E. Smart, BSc, PhD

László K. Tabár, MD, PhD

Tibor Tot, MD, PhD

Ana Cristina Vargas, MD

Fei Xue, MD, MS, ScD

Amy Ming-Fang Yen, PhD

目　录

第 1 章　"病态腺叶"理论 …………………………………………………… (1)
 1.1 前　言 ………………………………………………………………… (1)
 1.2 理论背景 ……………………………………………………………… (2)
 1.3 假说的形成 …………………………………………………………… (5)
 1.4 证据支持 ……………………………………………………………… (6)
 1.5 早期乳腺癌 …………………………………………………………… (9)
 1.6 实际结果与未来观点 ………………………………………………… (12)
 1.7 结　论 ………………………………………………………………… (13)
 参考文献 …………………………………………………………………… (13)

第 2 章　人体乳腺腺叶解剖及其对乳腺癌的重要意义 …………………… (18)
 2.1 介绍：科学研究的客体——人体乳房解剖 ………………………… (18)
 2.2 传统显微镜的局限性 ………………………………………………… (19)
 2.3 乳腺癌前驱病变的演进：克隆性扩增 ……………………………… (21)
 2.4 全乳腺实质可视化的需求 …………………………………………… (22)
 2.5 乳腺腺叶的解剖 ……………………………………………………… (23)
 2.6 乳头及其解剖 ………………………………………………………… (28)
 2.7 病态腺叶产生时细胞间的超级竞争 ………………………………… (31)
 2.8 乳腺腺叶解剖认识提高的前景 ……………………………………… (32)
 2.9 结　语 ………………………………………………………………… (33)
 参考文献 …………………………………………………………………… (34)

第 3 章　乳腺癌可能起源于子宫：子宫内环境对乳腺癌发生的重要性 ………… (38)
 3.1 引　言 ………………………………………………………………… (38)
 3.2 宫内暴露与乳腺癌风险 ……………………………………………… (38)
 3.3 潜在作用机制 ………………………………………………………… (43)
 3.4 结　论 ………………………………………………………………… (47)

参考文献 ··· (47)

第4章　正常及恶性乳腺组织中的基因改变 ··· (54)

　　缩　写 ··· (54)

　　4.1　背　景 ··· (54)

　　4.2　肿瘤的遗传基础 ··· (54)

　　4.3　浸润性乳腺癌的分子分析 ··· (55)

　　4.4　浸润性乳腺癌的分子分类 ··· (56)

　　4.5　浸润前乳腺癌的分子分析 ··· (57)

　　4.6　正常乳腺的分子改变 ··· (59)

　　4.7　病态的间质组织 ··· (62)

　　4.8　假　设 ··· (63)

　　4.9　结论：与临床实践的关系 ··· (63)

　　参考文献 ··· (63)

第5章　乳管灌洗法的作用——一个发人深省的故事 ·· (68)

　　5.1　背　景 ··· (68)

　　5.2　乳头抽吸液（NAF） ··· (68)

　　5.3　导管灌洗（DL） ·· (69)

　　5.4　研究和经验教训 ··· (71)

　　5.5　未来展望 ·· (76)

　　参考文献 ··· (77)

第6章　早期乳腺癌的分布模式 ·· (80)

　　6.1　简　介 ··· (80)

　　6.2　癌细胞的地砖式（mural）播散 ·· (80)

　　6.3　如何定义原位肿瘤？ ··· (82)

　　6.4　单灶、多灶及多中心DCIS ·· (84)

　　6.5　总　结 ··· (85)

　　参考文献 ··· (85)

第7章　多灶性与弥漫性乳腺癌影像学表现的意义 ··· (88)

　　7.1　概　述 ··· (88)

　　7.2　乳腺癌多灶性本质及影像学方法的选择 ··· (93)

　　7.3　单灶性、多灶性及弥漫性乳腺癌的不同影像学表现与长期预后 ···················· (93)

7.4 区分乳腺癌单灶性病变与多灶性病变的现实意义 ………………………………… (150)

7.5 结论：现有的 TNM 分期系统对于恶性肿瘤的评判存在弊端 …………………… (151)

参考文献 …………………………………………………………………………………… (151)

第 8 章　乳腺腺叶超声 ……………………………………………………………………… (153)

8.1 引　言 …………………………………………………………………………………… (153)

8.2 解剖背景 ………………………………………………………………………………… (154)

8.3 乳腺导管超声成像 ……………………………………………………………………… (154)

8.4 腺叶的形态学改变 ……………………………………………………………………… (156)

8.5 乳腺病理学中腺叶的影响 ……………………………………………………………… (157)

8.6 多灶性、多中心性和弥漫性病变 ……………………………………………………… (159)

8.7 外科观点 ………………………………………………………………………………… (159)

8.8 总　结 …………………………………………………………………………………… (160)

参考文献 …………………………………………………………………………………… (161)

第 9 章　乳腺癌病灶在腺叶中的分布：乳管内镜检查及手术 ………………………… (163)

9.1 引　言 …………………………………………………………………………………… (163)

9.2 乳管内镜的早期历史 …………………………………………………………………… (163)

9.3 乳管内镜在乳腺癌应用中的经验教训 ………………………………………………… (164)

9.4 总　结 …………………………………………………………………………………… (165)

参考文献 …………………………………………………………………………………… (165)

第 10 章　从现在起消灭乳腺癌——设想在乳腺癌细胞转移前发现防御、治愈的方法 …………………………………………………………………………………………… (167)

10.1 概　述 ………………………………………………………………………………… (167)

10.2 3D 电子显微镜 ………………………………………………………………………… (167)

10.3 寻找影像 ……………………………………………………………………………… (169)

10.4 ART 的诞生 …………………………………………………………………………… (170)

10.5 追寻诺贝尔奖的青年 ………………………………………………………………… (170)

10.6 降低 CT 剂量 ………………………………………………………………………… (171)

10.7 用更多的方程式取代数据 …………………………………………………………… (172)

10.8 使 ART 算法得到重视 ……………………………………………………………… (173)

10.9 出售 ART 算法并改进 CT 技术 …………………………………………………… (175)

10.10 来自传统断层摄影术的挑战 ………………………………………………………… (177)

10.11 欠定方程 …………………………………………………………………………… (177)
10.12 超空间漫行 …………………………………………………………………………… (179)
10.13 人体 CT 剂量 ………………………………………………………………………… (179)
10.14 聚焦乳腺癌检查 ……………………………………………………………………… (180)
10.15 显像模式结合 ………………………………………………………………………… (181)
10.16 CT 成像中去卷积算法及自适应邻域 ……………………………………………… (181)
10.17 维纳去卷积技术（Wiener Deconvolution）……………………………………… (182)
10.18 纵向图像的配准 ……………………………………………………………………… (183)
10.19 更快更好的 ART 算法 ……………………………………………………………… (185)
10.20 以小乳腺癌为目标进行流行病学推断 ……………………………………………… (185)
10.21 开展各种成像模式之间的竞争 ……………………………………………………… (186)
10.22 未来设想 0：聚焦像素（Foxels）和第七代乳腺筛查 CT 技术 ………………… (188)
10.23 未来设想 1：智能操控 X 射线微束 ………………………………………………… (189)
10.24 未来设想 2：栅门和纠缠光子：乳腺成像如同一盘海战棋 ……………………… (189)
10.25 从现在起消灭乳腺癌！ ……………………………………………………………… (190)
10.26 病态乳腺小叶理论："一个似是而非的论点，一个自相矛盾的议题，一个机智的悖论"
　　（Gilbert，Sullivan，1879）………………………………………………………… (191)
10.27 结　论 ………………………………………………………………………………… (193)
参考文献 ……………………………………………………………………………………… (193)

第 11 章　结语：X 染色体失活和分化波与病变的乳腺腺叶 ………………………… (216)
参考文献 ……………………………………………………………………………………… (220)

"病态腺叶" 理论

第 1 章

Tibor Tot

1.1 前 言

1.1.1 问题的提出

乳腺癌是全世界范围内女性最常见的恶性肿瘤之一，也是发展中国家年轻女性死亡的首要原因。在发展中国家，1/10~1/7的女性一生中将会罹患乳腺癌（Boyle，Ferlay，2005）。1940年以来，乳腺癌的发病率逐年递增。在西方国家，乳腺癌的发病率以每年1%的速度增加（Harris，et al，1992），而死亡率却以每年1%的速度下降，这归因于乳腺钼靶筛查（Smith，et，al，2004；The Swedish Organized Service Screening Evaluation Group 2006）以及新的、更有效的乳腺癌治疗方法的出现，从而有效延长了患者的生存期并提高了其生活质量（Hortobagyi，2005）。预计在2005—2015这10年间，乳腺癌的幸存者人数将增加31%（De Angelis，et al，2009）。近年来，一些发达国家乳腺癌的发病率虽有所下降，但在人口众多的国家，包括中国、印度等国其发病率仍持续升高（Kawamur，Sobue，2005）。根据目前美国的流行病学数据预测，2010—2030年，乳腺癌的发病率将增加30%，65岁以上女性的发病率将增加57%（Smith，et al，

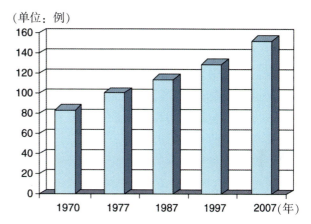

图1.1　瑞典的数据（www.sos.se；2009年5月2日）显示，每10万人中每年的新发乳腺癌数目

2009），即每3或4位女性中，将有1人罹患乳腺癌。乳腺癌的筛查、诊断、治疗不仅增加了医疗系统的负担，也给女性带来了沉重的心理负担（图1.1）。因此，只有了解乳腺癌的自然病程，研发更有效的预防、诊断和治疗措施，才能扭转这种趋势。

1.1.2 内源性和外源性危险因素

尽管乳腺癌的相关危险因素已被大家所熟知，但仍不清楚其确切病因。性别是乳腺癌最大的危险因素，女性的发病率较男性高100倍；年龄也是危险因素之一，随着年龄的增长，乳腺癌的患病风险也会增加。地理因素同样影响乳腺癌的发病率，北美洲、西欧、斯堪的纳维亚、澳大利亚以及新西兰地区的乳腺癌发病率远高于亚非国家（Kawamura，Sobue，2005）。从低发病区迁徙到高发病区

T. Tot
Department of Pathology and Clinical Cytology,
Central Hospital Falun, Falun,
Sweden
e-mail: tibor.tot@ltdalarna.se

的女性，其后代表现出与迁入地区女性相同的乳腺癌发病率，由此表明环境和生活方式是影响乳腺癌发病率的危险因素（Buell，1973）。较高的社会经济地位和高学历也是乳腺癌发病的危险因素（Clarke, et al, 2002）。此外，种族因素在乳腺癌发病中也扮演了重要角色（Harper, et al, 2009）。长期暴露于金属放射源或化学物质的环境中也会增加乳腺癌的患病风险（Wolff, et al, 1996）。出生时情况，包括出生时体重、身高、父母的生育年龄等，同样影响女性成年后患乳腺癌的概率（Xue, Michels, 2007）。性激素相关的因素，包括未生育、晚育、初潮早、绝经晚等，也是重要的高危因素。目前，限制激素替代疗法是包括美国在内的多个国家乳腺癌发病率降低的主要原因，预示着外源性雌激素可促进乳腺癌的发展，而抗雌激素治疗可抑制其发展（Fisher, et al, 1998）。

乳腺癌和（或）卵巢癌家族史也是重要的危险因素，超过27%的乳腺癌患者在疾病的发展过程中，个体遗传基因背景扮演了重要角色（Hiller, et al, 1997）。携带 *BRCA*1和 *BRCA*2突变基因是罹患乳腺癌的高危因素，但这仅能代表部分乳腺癌患者（Ford, et al, 1994; Easton, et al, 1997）。

乳腺的结构对乳房X线片所显示的乳腺密度有影响（Tot, et al, 2000）。乳腺密度与基因、激素、体质（体重、身高）及环境因素相关，激素替代疗法同样会影响乳腺的密度（Tabar, et al, 2007）。

居住在乳腺癌高发地区、携带突变基因以及具备上述高危因素的女性均具有一个共同特征：即高危因素影响了整个机体、机体的所有细胞以及乳腺细胞。另外，乳腺癌往往发生于单侧乳腺的一个象限，提示着这一区域的组织具有高危性，对内源或外源性致癌因素更为敏感。我们的假说是：这些高危的乳腺组织与"病态腺叶"的形成有关，后者在胚胎发育过程中就出现了"错误"。

以上列举的部分高危因素可能出现于胚胎期。如果携带潜在恶性细胞的"病态腺叶"起始于胚胎期，将需要几十年的时间完成恶性转变。我们认为：导致恶性转变的必要步骤是由潜在的恶性细胞及其克隆的遗传基因决定的。位于病态腺叶不同位置的潜在恶性细胞可同步或不同步地完成这一恶性转变。完成恶性转变所需要的时间由内源性和外源性因素决定，例如，长期暴露于放射源的女性，其乳腺癌发病率增加，且常发生于30年或更长时间以后（Little, Boice, 1999）；携带 *BRCA*1和 *BRCA*2突变基因的女性患乳腺癌的初诊年龄要小于未携带突变基因的患者。

以上数据是我们定义"生物时控理论（the theory of biological timing）"这一概念的基础。

1.2 理论背景

1.2.1 解剖学与胚胎学

乳房是具有腺叶结构的腺体器官。典型的乳房腺叶由以下部分组成：一个单独开放于乳头的输乳管，向下分为一系列的分支导管和小导管，终止于成百上千的终末小导管和小叶，后两者构成终末导管小叶单元（terminal ducts and lobules, TDLUs）。腺叶的上皮结构就像一棵具有树枝和树干的大树，TDLUs相当于树叶。上皮与间质成分共同组成了一个尖部为乳头、宽大的基底朝向胸肌的金字塔形结构。除一项研究显示乳房腺叶间具有罕见的联系外（Ohtake, et al, 1995），通常认为乳房腺叶是互不相连的独立结构单元。每个女性一生中乳房腺叶的数目是不变的，但年龄与激素状态会改变腺叶的大小和形态，主要是改变小叶和小导管的数目与大小。

人类乳房发育始于胚胎发育的第4个月，由原始外胚层向外形成乳头芽，即原始乳头。怀孕21~25周乳头芽分化为乳腺芽并伸入间质形成剩余的乳腺组织（Howard, Gustersson,

2000；Jolicoeur，et al，2003）。亦有研究证实，怀孕8周是乳头芽的形成时期（Russo，2004）。腺叶在乳头芽分化为乳腺芽时形成，所有的乳腺芽都可能成为潜在的乳腺腺叶，但其中一部分在胎儿期发生退化。

乳腺导管伴随着乳腺芽的形成而开始发育，最终形成"终末囊"。乳房发育早期表现为双细胞结构特性，在乳腺芽中心区域细胞表达细胞角蛋白（cytokeratins，CKs）19和14，而外周区域细胞（基底细胞）逐渐失去对CK19的表达。腺叶可在出生时存在，但多数情况下，腺叶在出生时非常少或基本没有。

乳房在发育过程中，除乳房组织的薄壁分隔发生变化外，乳头芽和乳腺芽周围的胚胎间充质也发生了重要变化。例如，黏合素C过表达是间充质重构为乳管周围基质的重要标志，因此，细胞黏合素抗体的过表达即代表胚胎期和胎儿期，乳头芽及其分支开始发育（Sakakura，et al，1991）。它是乳腺腺叶内出现分支发育的信号。在一些原位癌细胞间质中，细胞黏合素抗体C过表达意味着成人亦可以出现新的导管，是癌细胞进展的标志（Tabaúr，et al，2004）。

乳房在婴儿离开母体后持续发育，至青春期前，几乎全部由导管组成。青春期时，乳房开始增大，主要是基质细胞发育，但也有部分为导管树和小叶的发育增大（Wellings，et al，1975）。有报道提出乳腺芽可从导管的侧面形成（Rudland，1991）。

在生育期，女性的乳房经历了随月经周期变化而发生的周期性改变。黄体期，导管和腺叶的细胞大量扩增，导致上皮细胞、腺泡数目增加。月经周期时，上皮和肌上皮细胞开始凋亡，逐渐回复至月经前状态（Ramakrishnan，et al，2002）。

在怀孕期间，乳腺的发育，无论腺叶数量还是大小、或是每个腺叶中腺泡的数量均呈全盛状态，包括乳腺导管出芽、次级导管成枝、终末导管形成腺泡等。在哺乳期后，腺泡和导管崩解、上皮和肌上皮细胞凋亡以及小叶间质再生，乳腺逐渐萎缩。然而，哺乳后的经产乳房一般不会回复到怀孕前状态，经产后的女性乳房形态、分子及基因水平也与未产女性存在差异（Russo，Russo，2004）。

在停经时和停经后，乳房腺体出现类似哺乳期后或月经期后的一个退化过程，导致小叶、腺泡、终末导管、段和亚段导管数量减少，而女性一生中乳腺小叶的量基本保持不变。与实质细胞退化伴随发生的是间质细胞发生退化，导致脂肪组织替换了小叶间和导管周的间质（Tot，et al，2002）。

我们认为，初始化、分枝化、小叶化过程是乳腺发育的不同阶段。初始化过程发生于胎儿早期，在此阶段大量初始小叶形成。分枝化发生于胎儿和青春期前，是乳腺导管样结构出现分支。小叶化起始于胎儿乳腺，是青春期和成人期乳腺的特征。恶性转化也瞄准了这些过程，低级别原位癌企图改变正常的小叶化过程，高级别原位癌可能影响分支化过程，小叶形成起始即出现偏差将导致"病态腺叶"的发生（Tot，2005b）。

1.2.2 祖细胞概念

组织的实际形态取决于细胞的更新、丢失和非细胞元素之间的平衡。组织特异性干细胞具有自我更新和分化为成熟细胞的能力。干细胞主要有3种类型：来源于囊胚泡的胚胎干细胞，代表机体所有细胞的起源；生殖干细胞，是男性和女性生殖细胞的起源；躯体干细胞，对正常组织进行更新（Gudjonsson，Magnusson，2005）。已经分化的细胞寿命很短，但干细胞始终保持自我复制能力。干细胞可分化为两个类似的干细胞，或形成两个进一步分化的"祖细胞"，更多的是生成一个干细胞和一个祖细胞。干细胞与祖细胞具有多向分化潜能，可分化为同一器官的不同成熟细胞。干细胞存在的微环境对其分化方向起着至关重要的作用。多数成熟器官均有一小部分具有干细胞特性的细胞（Liu，et al，2008）。

Deome等人在1959年首次提出正常的乳腺组织中存在可以自我更新的多潜能干细胞，他报道称，多次随机移植的乳腺上皮组织可以生成一个完整的乳房腺体。成熟乳房组织腔面细胞和肌上皮细胞似乎起源于同一个干细胞或祖细胞（Boecker, Burger, 2003）。越来越多的证据支持在乳腺中存在3种不同类型的上皮祖细胞：一种是具有产生所有上皮细胞能力的祖细胞，另外两种是具有产生分泌腺泡和分支导管能力的祖细胞（Smith, Boulanger, 2003）。在乳腺胚胎发育阶段，干细胞分化是分步骤进行的（Villadsen, 2005），分化的最后一步出现了两种成熟的细胞，其中腔面细胞表达CK18，肌上皮细胞表达CK14。Villadsen等人（2007年）证实了位于乳腺导管的干细胞只具有繁殖生长和自我更新为导管的能力，小叶中也可能含有祖细胞。Liu等（2008年）证实了具有BRCA1突变基因携带者的乳房发生了类似癌的改变。正常组织中的干细胞或祖细胞可经特殊染色被发现，BRCA1突变基因携带者的腺叶中干细胞或祖细胞含量较健康人群多。Clarke等（2005）报道了乳腺上皮干细胞具有两种亚型，一种表达雌激素受体α和孕激素受体，在月经周期内自我更新；另一种不表达上述受体，更新的是乳腺干细胞。因此乳腺腺叶结构的发育和维持似乎是多种干细胞或祖细胞参与的复杂过程，在某种程度上，导管和小叶的发育是互相独立的。

正常细胞转化为恶性肿瘤所发生的一系列变化需要克服细胞分裂的严密调控。恶性肿瘤代表了一类具有异质性的突变细胞，其基因型和表现型多种多样。原始的肿瘤细胞及其后代具有干细胞的特性，这些肿瘤细胞与组织特异性干细胞一样有永生化的特征，可自我更新和分化、缓慢分化、长期生存（Agelopulos, et al, 2008）。只有一小部分恶性细胞具有这种无限增殖并导致肿瘤生成的潜能，这些细胞被称为肿瘤干细胞。肿瘤中绝大多数细胞是分化好的肿瘤细胞，拥有非常强的增殖潜能，但不是无限增殖。

许多类型的肿瘤中都存在肿瘤干细胞。异种移植的乳腺癌细胞实验中，表达CD44但不表达CD24的细胞被分离出来。这些孤立的细胞不表达上皮类型的标记物，相比其他细胞而言，具有更强的转变为乳腺癌细胞的倾向。这些CD44+或CD24-细胞很可能是乳腺癌干细胞。但这些仅为一小部分乳腺癌的起源，其中包括基底样乳腺癌和与BRCA1基因突变相关的乳腺癌（Honeth, et al, 2008）。在干细胞模型中发现，同一肿瘤的癌细胞可能起源于好几种干细胞，其克隆增殖更多地取决于细胞微环境（Clarke, et al, 2006b; Villadsen, et al, 2007）。

肿瘤干细胞起源是目前肿瘤研究的热点，不同的肿瘤起源不同。肿瘤干细胞可起源于正常组织的干细胞，也可以起源于因突变而获得自我更新能力的祖细胞（Al-Hajj, et al, 2003）。干细胞、祖细胞、肿瘤干细胞均为缓慢分化、长期生存的细胞，因此易受内部和外部有害环境因素的刺激。与成熟细胞比较，这些细胞生存时间长，对导致突变的各种刺激更加敏感。根据肿瘤发生的"多次打击学说"，逐渐积累的突变将引发干细胞或祖细胞转变为肿瘤细胞。首次恶性的基因突变可能出现于胎儿期或受精卵时期，此后需要更长甚至几十年时间的基因突变积累（Baik, et al, 2004）。这一概念在不同的恶性肿瘤中已被提出，也是"病态腺叶"的理论基础。

突变的干细胞可将突变遗传至其子代细胞中，这些突变可在外观正常的小叶导管、腺泡、上皮和肌上皮细胞中被检测到（Lakhani, et al, 1999）。如果基因突变出现于定向祖细胞中，则可能产生正常和突变的嵌合状态，导致恶性转化的遗传变异（Tsai, et al, 1996）。尽管突变细胞可能具有相同的基因变异，但再次突变则不尽相同。因此，额外的基因打击将导致同一部位存在独立的或不同基因型的肿瘤病灶（Agelopoulos, et al, 2008）。我们的观点是，导致病态小叶发生的基因突变发生于小叶初始发育时的干细胞。这一概念及肿瘤干细胞对不同治疗方法具有抵抗性这一现象，为早期乳腺癌提供了理想的治疗靶点。

1.3 假说的形成

1.3.1 "病态腺叶"理论

我们的假说是，乳腺癌是小叶性疾病，即在单个独立的"病态腺叶"中，肿瘤病灶将同步或不同步发展。病态腺叶的特性是由分散于小叶中多个位点的大量具有恶变倾向的突变干细胞或祖细胞所决定的，与那些没有、少量存在或者存在不敏感的潜在恶性细胞的乳腺小叶相比，病态小叶对内源性和外源性的肿瘤刺激更为敏感。

根据前述流行病学数据，在发达国家约1/10的女性一生中会罹患乳腺癌，解剖学数据显示单个乳房中的导管数目最大中位数为27（Going, Moffat, 2004; Going, Mohun, 2006）。我们的结论是：大约500个小叶中有1个出现结构异常（图1.2）。一般情况下，仅存在1个病态腺叶，但也有例外；偶尔，一个女性可能有超过1个的病态腺叶，从而出现多灶性病变或双侧乳腺癌。长期暴露于致癌因素刺激下，一侧乳房的多个腺叶均可能成瘤，但由于大多数女性的生存时间较短，不足以显示出肿瘤；但20世纪以来，随着女性平均寿命的延长，乳腺癌变得更为多见（图1.3）。

1.3.2 生物时控学说

在内源性和外源性的促肿瘤刺激性因素的作用下，潜在的恶性细胞可以发生恶性转化。转化时间由突变基因的数量决定，基因变异通常发生于细胞分化的过程中。如果致癌因素保持一定的强度，病态腺叶中突变干细胞或祖细胞复制的数量和这些细胞以及其子代细胞中的遗传基因的结构决定了发生恶性转化的时间。另外，恶性转化时间也受内源性和外源性促肿瘤刺激性因素的影响。恶性转化可发生于病态腺叶的一处，也可同时或不同时出现于病态腺叶的多处。因此，病态腺叶中潜在恶性细胞的恶性转化具有生物时控性，尽管这一时间控制在所有突变的干

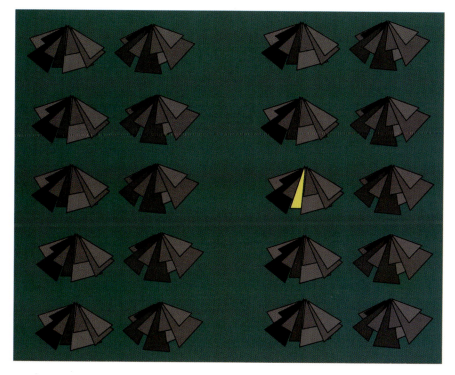

图1.2 病态腺叶出现的示意图。腺叶是金字塔形结构，顶端朝向乳头，基底朝向胸肌筋膜。理论上，每500个腺叶中大概就存在一个异常腺叶

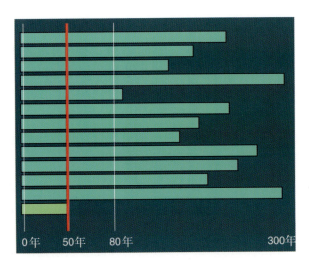

图1.3 不同腺叶的潜在恶性干/祖细胞恶性转化需要的时间。任何腺叶都会在基因突变的累积下出现恶性转化，但是，这个过程所需要的时间可能远远长于女性的生存时间。由于存在大量的突变细胞/易感的细胞，病态腺叶是个例外，完成恶性转化的时间相对短

细胞或祖细胞并不完全一致，这一假说被称为生物时控学说。

总之，乳房腺叶发育于胚胎早期。病态腺叶学说指出，在干细胞或祖细胞发生第一次突变时，病态腺叶结构已经发生异常改变，经过出生后几十年的基因突变积累，才能形成肿瘤。因此，生物时控能力可在很长的一段时间内发挥作用。乳腺癌是一个终身性疾病，可通过消除或破坏完整的病态腺叶来阻断乳腺癌的发生。

1.3.3 相似的概念

"病态腺叶"学说和"生物时控"学说是全新的概念，但在很早以前已经有关于这些概念的观察和研究，能够追溯到1921年Cheatle的报道。Dawson（1933）和Wellings（Wellings, 1975; Cardiff, Wellings, 1999）曾假定大部分乳腺癌起源于乳腺终末导管-小叶单位（TDLUs）。这些不太准确的概念影响了许多乳腺专家。事实上，导管树也能发生乳腺癌这一事实已被多次报道，但被深深掩盖于Dawson等人的假设理论下。James Ewing在1940年发现："在扩张的导管发生的导管原位癌（ductal carcinoma in situ, DCIS），跨越了很多的乳腺节段。"Gallagher和Martin（1969）也报道："人类乳腺癌并非聚集出现，而是一个涉及乳腺上皮的弥漫性疾病。"早期，研究者采用X线技术检测原位癌微钙化点，发现病变局限于一个三角形区域（Lanyi's 三角形原则，Lanyi, 1977）。Teboul通过超声也证实了作为一种恶性弥散性疾病的乳腺癌，影响了整个病变腺叶的所有上皮细胞（Teboul, Halliwell, 1995）。在过去的几十年，根据临床经验，外科医生非常推荐"金字塔概念"，即扇形切除或区段切除，他们发现进行金字塔形的乳腺切除（类似腺叶的形状），其预后远远优于简单的乳房肿瘤切除术。最新版的世界卫生组织（WHO）乳腺肿瘤专著中描述（Tavassoli, Devili, 2003）："呈段状分布的原位导管癌（DCIS），是先沿着TDLU到乳头的方向在一个导管系统内发展，然后再侵入毗邻的分支"。据此，研究者得出结论，肿瘤起源于TDLU并沿着节段的导管侵润，这才将传统的观念与影像学、临床实际观察到的现象合理地统一起来。我们将在本章的最后重点论述这一观点。

孕期子宫内环境是成人后罹患乳腺癌的风险因素，这一的假说也早有研究者提及（Trichopoulos, 1990）。

1.4 证据支持

在日常诊断工作中，放射影像学能够筛查出乳房腺叶样的微钙化灶，导管超声也可

发现类似结果，MRI则表现为区域增强（图1.4A、B），这些影像学结果明确提示了恶性病变发生于腺叶中，影像学将其描述为"节段性分布的病变"。但是，在解剖上仍无法直接观察到，这让研究人员深感疑惑。这种改变是几何形状的（扇形结构），与解剖学的节段（输乳管和腺叶的分支节段）无关，但似乎与解剖学的腺叶（包含一个输乳管的所有结构）相关。随着一种针对乳腺导管系统的较为新型的检查手段——导管内镜的应用，发现了许多新的结果。应用导管内镜我们发现，即便多个病变间相隔较远，绝大多数恶性病变仍局限于单个导管树系统内（Dooley，2003）。

除以上观察结果外，形态学和基因学相关研究也支持乳腺"病态腺叶"的存在。此外，对孕期和围产期因素影响成年后罹患乳腺癌的危险因素进行流行病学调查，其结论也为生物时控学说提供了证据支持。近年来分子基因学相关研究所得结论也与我们的假说不谋而合。

1.4.1 形态学证据

原位癌若位于乳头后，往往仅侵及单个输乳管。这一现象是支持病态腺叶假说的重要证据之一。若观察到的乳腺癌不限于单个腺叶结构，那么将有1个以上的输乳管受到侵犯。Going等研究者通过对1mm厚的乳腺组织切片进行数字影像重建证实了上述理论（James Going，2007）。常规细致检查乳腺癌患者的乳头区域，可发现绝大多数病例中仅有单个输乳管受侵犯，这也显示了疾病按照"病态腺叶"的模式发展。我们在图1.5中以具体患者为例加以说明（图1.5）。

以上结果与Mai等人（2000）的发现非常

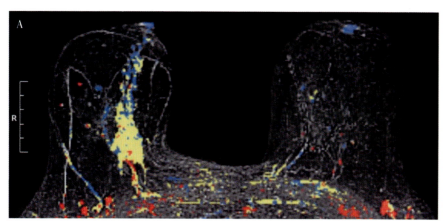

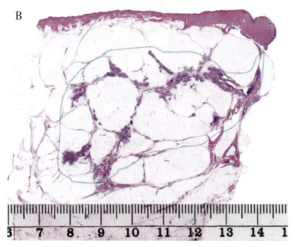

图1.4 A.1例高级别原位癌核磁影像，显示病态腺叶有相应的叶片状增强影（Tabar et al.2008）；B.大组织切片显示广泛的高级别原位癌（伴多灶性浸润），病变范围呈腺叶状

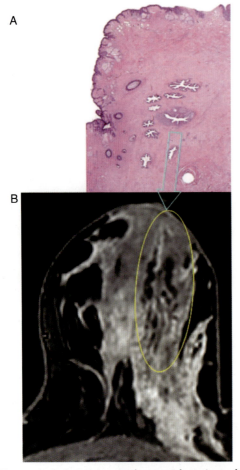

图1.5 A.乳头区的组织切片。B.同部位的MRI表现。原位癌仅侵犯一个输乳管,其他部位是正常的;肿瘤显示出仅侵犯单个导管树的"腺叶模式"

一致,他证实了乳腺导管内癌的形态大致呈一个尖端朝向乳头的金字塔造型。借助3D技术对30例乳腺全切术后的样本进行研究后,Mai发现无论是乳腺癌的原位病灶、侵袭病灶或增生病灶,其中27例患者的病变都仅限于单个输乳管。

Middleton等人(2002)在研究早期多发性癌时发现,在绝大多数患者中此类型的癌代表相同类型肿瘤细胞的克隆增殖,其发表的文章中有一幅图清晰地展示了弥漫性连续性原位癌及2处受侵犯的病灶属于单个乳腺腺叶。但是,他们并未意识到这是疾病的"病态腺叶"模式。

Page与其合作者(2002)提出了"原位导管癌包括单个导管系统",并且该病的多灶性或多中心性与节段性制备病理切片有关。目前,虽然此项研究进一步加深了对乳腺癌病态腺叶本质的认知(单个导管系统是腺叶的主要构成部分),但导管系统中恶性转化的不同模式尚未得知。

1.4.2 遗传学证据

病态腺叶学说指出,乳腺中含有发展为恶性肿瘤潜力的高危组织,其发生恶性转化的时间远早于其他腺叶。在腺叶所有具有恶性潜能的细胞中,能同时进行恶性转化的细胞数量相对较少;初诊为乳腺癌时,更多发现的是仅有很少一部分病态腺叶组织中的细胞发生恶性转化。这项研究结果同时表明,病态腺叶中的恶性细胞部分似乎被高危组织中尚未发生恶性转化的区域所包绕。基于此观点,病态腺叶学说同其他几项研究所提出的乳腺"遗传区"或"癌变区",以及近年来所提出的"癌易感区"是相互吻合的。Slaughter等于1953年在进行口腔鳞状上皮细胞癌的研究中,也提出类似的观点与观察结果(Slaughter, et al, 1953)。回溯近年来的研究成果,有大量的相关论著支持该假说的正确性(Heaphy, et al, 2009)。

原位癌细胞与侵袭性癌细胞具有相似或一致的基因改变,这是由于受侵袭组织的癌肿来源于自原位病变,应用检测原位导管癌杂合缺失的方法(Stratton, et al, 1995),以及比较基因杂交法(Buerger, et al, 1999),这一观点于1990年代得以证实,原位小叶癌也有类似结论。Lakhani等人也证实了在非典型导管过度增生中存在基因杂合缺失。2005年Simpson等在柱状上皮细胞及相关肿瘤侵袭灶中发现了与之一致的改变。原位导管癌、原位小叶癌、非典型性导管过度增生以及柱状上皮细胞改变均被认为是侵袭性肿瘤的前驱病变,因此它们之间可能存在与肿瘤侵袭相关的共同基因改变。

但是,在乳腺癌的样本中,普通导管上皮增

生的细胞也可检测出基因杂合缺失（Lakhani, et al, 1996），这一结果也得到比较基因杂交方法的验证（Jones, et al, 2003）。这些结果在意料之外，这是因为一般认为导管上皮过度增生仅是致癌高危因素而非直接癌前病变。

Deng等研究者（1996）发现包绕在侵袭性癌组织周围的形态学正常的乳腺组织，往往也出现基因杂合缺失，该结论与Meng等人的研究结果一致（2004）。通过单细胞克隆，Lakhani等人证实了组织学正常的乳腺组织同具有侵袭性的癌组织可具有一致的基因改变，无论正常组织与侵袭性癌组织距离近或者远，甚至无恶性形态学证据的乳腺组织也是如此。这种改变不仅在上皮细胞，在肌上皮细胞也可观察到，这提示该种改变可能发生于干细胞或祖细胞。这一重要结论归功于Clarke等（2006a），他们还发现发生基因改变的单个细胞能富集并弥散至由1个以上终末导管小叶单元（TDLU）所组成的区域；这种细胞富集表明了遗传基因改变发生于祖细胞，并能促进乳腺组织的病情进展。换言之，形态学正常的组织中，存在一个基因不稳定区域，该区域围绕于肿瘤组织周围，并且在肿瘤进展前就已存在。对临近原发乳腺癌的"正常"乳腺组织进行DNA甲基化程度检测，可发现这种改变可延伸至距离原发灶超过4cm的区域（Yan, et al, 2006）。这些研究发现与病态腺叶的平均大小是吻合的。

目前认为肿瘤是一种干细胞或祖细胞功能发生异常的疾病。正如上述，若祖细胞发生突变，那么它能够将这种突变传递至所有子细胞，形成一个由正常细胞和突变细胞构成的嵌合细胞网络。发生突变的细胞分散于周围组织中，这也解释了为何这类组织对致癌因子的更敏感（Tsai, et al, 1996; Cariati, Purushotham, 2008）。这一观点是Agelopoulous等人（2008）所提出的"突变祖细胞"概念的基础，而这一观点与我们所提出的病态腺叶及生物时控理论非常类似。

1.4.3 流行病学数据

近年来，流行病学研究所获取的数据同样能够支持病态腺叶理论。Xue和Michels提出：出生体重以及其他新生儿相关的数据与其成年后罹患乳腺癌的风险之间存在有明确的关系（2007）。以上两位研究者认为与成长相关的因素可能会导致胚胎期乳腺内易感干细胞数量的增多，并通过DNA突变的方式启动肿瘤进程。新生儿体重与乳腺摄影成像时的乳腺密度相关（Cerhan, et al, 2005），是乳腺癌发生的高危因素。因此，依据实验数据及流行病学数据，我们认为出生前子宫微环境能够影响个体在成年时期罹患乳腺癌的风险。

综上所述，乳腺组织在女性首次怀孕后才会完全分化。因此，乳腺组织在青年及幼年时期可能对致癌因素更为敏感。乳腺癌发生风险与新生儿体重、身高以及幼年时期体重呈正相关，与受孕年龄及儿童期体重指数呈负相关（Ruder, et al, 2008），这一结论亦支持我们所提出的"乳腺癌的发生是一个长期终生的过程"。

1.5 早期乳腺癌

1.5.1 乳腺癌发展为小叶性疾病的条件

认识乳腺癌的小叶性本质，并将乳腺癌视为小叶性疾病困难重重。仅仅研究侵袭性乳腺癌的一个切片并不能解决问题。尽管如此，在大部分病理实验室中，使用传统的组织病理学切片来诊断乳腺癌仍然是诊断疾病的常规手段，并且受到业内专家的拥护。应用该方法，病理学家们对样本切片进行镜下观察，识别并定位主要病变位置；从手术中获取病变和外科切缘，谨慎地分离出所需要部分并弃去周围组织。周围组织在某种程度上来说，至少部分相当于前文所提及的基因区高危组织，常常包括部分原位和侵袭性癌灶、非典型过度增生灶、上皮细胞单一形态轻度增生（往往被认为是某些侵袭性癌的起源）（Goldstein, et al, 2007）。对原位癌及侵袭癌病灶的正确评估以及对肿瘤进展情况的正确判断，离不开对周围组织的全面筛查检测。采用更加全面的组织学检测方法有助于对上述疾病的重要形态学特征进行评估。

针对大组织切片的组织病理学分析，联合详尽的放射-病理学相关分析，为乳腺癌患者的确诊提供了极大帮助，同时也便捷了对乳腺癌形态学上生长状况的评估（Tot, et al, 2002; Tabár, et al, 2007）。这样的方法同样能让细心的观察者注意到病变在某一个类似腺叶样的空间内的发展趋势。

此外，研究晚期病例将无法认知乳腺癌腺叶的发病本质。因为，对于乳腺癌来说，腺叶是其发生发展的源头，但当其发展至晚期时，体积巨大，更具有侵袭性，因为细胞增殖肿瘤将超出病态腺叶原有的边界。若将病态腺叶作为观察重点，那么乳腺癌即可通过人群大规模的乳腺影像摄影的方法，在早期便能发现。我们将早期乳腺癌定义为单纯的原位癌和侵袭范围不超过15mm厚度的癌。这些患者中，十年生存率超过90%。这类患者在常规人群筛查中大约占全部病患的50%；在我们的筛查诊断患者的数据库中，大约为70%左右（Tot, 2007b）。

1.5.2 早期乳腺癌的形态

本章所表述的两种理论建立于超过3000例的乳腺癌患者大组织标本切片及详细的放射-病理相关性系统分析。以此方法研究早期乳腺癌可帮助我们较好地研究最早期乳腺癌的自然发病过程。

恶性转化可以发生于病态腺叶的任何位置，其发生时机将决定肿瘤病灶的位置。恶性转化的发生可能有多种模式，其中3种形态

模式最为常见（图1.6）。如果病态腺叶中的多数潜在恶性细胞同时转化为恶性克隆，则整个小叶都有可能患癌（包括整个导管树和腺泡）。理论上，这种情况来源于干细胞中突变的累积，这些干细胞可形成整个小叶的所有细胞。因为小叶的体积占乳房2%~23%不等（Going, Moffat, 2004），所以，肿瘤从整个腺叶起源这一模式导致肿瘤初发时瘤体可能就有数厘米大小。这样的患者瘤体大且广泛，含较大量的乳腺组织和肿瘤负荷（当前恶性细胞的数量）。典型的例子就是高级别粉刺样或微乳头原位癌（图1.7A），这些病理类型的病态腺叶最易通过放射影像学检查予以发现。但是，这些肿瘤难以治疗并且预后不佳（Tabár, et al, 2004）。

第二种恶性转化模式发生于部分腺叶，即导管树的部分枝段和分属该枝段的小叶（图1.7B）。肿瘤发展局限于一个病态腺叶，恶性转化同时或逐渐发生于腺叶的节段中。理论上，该种模式是由于多个能产生枝段导管的干/祖细胞发生突变累积而导致的导管树分支发生异常。肿瘤负荷以及肿瘤的侵及范围相对较为局限，往往介于腺叶模式与外周模式之间。

病态腺叶内恶性转化的外周模式是以受侵袭的小叶为特点，往往无节段和输乳管受侵（图1.7C）。小叶可同时或逐步受累。该种模式是由于多个能产生分泌小叶的干/祖细胞

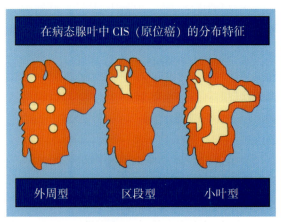

图1.6 原位乳腺癌的3种形态模式示意图

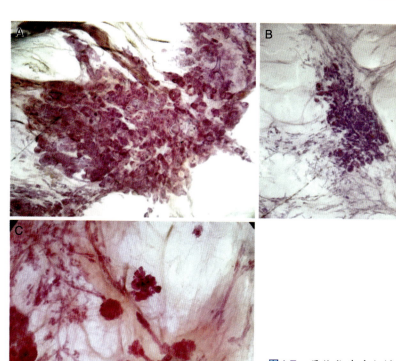

图1.7 原位乳腺癌大样本厚切片（1mm）图像。A.腺叶。B.节段。C.外周模式

发生突变累积，导致在小叶化的过程中出现异常。即使有大量小叶受侵犯，该种模式的瘤负荷通常也比较低，但肿瘤波及范围可能较大，这是由于在同一个病态腺叶内，不同的受侵小叶间相隔距离较大。因此，该种类型的乳腺癌也难以治疗，但预后较为乐观。典型表现为原位小叶癌和低级别的原位导管癌。

在乳腺癌的自然演变过程中，病态腺叶的大小、病态腺叶中突变干细胞和祖细胞的分布范围，以及其恶性转化的生物学时机等都将决定乳腺癌的侵及范围。此外，基因结构（高级别和低级别基因改变）也将影响肿瘤的形态学和分子生物学特征及演变速度。高级别基因突变，其肿瘤进展较低级别基因改变更为迅猛（Wiechmann, Kuerer, 2008）。

在癌症的发展早期，恶性细胞局限于导管和小叶中，导管与小叶将随着恶性细胞及其产物的累积而发生扩张和扭曲。低级别的病变倾向位于终末导管与小叶，而高级别的病变常常累及较大的导管（Tot, Tabár, 2005）。肿瘤发展进程自身也可以维持小叶构造和（或）诱导新小叶及小导管的形成。一些高级别原位癌也能够在受累的病态腺叶中形成新的更大的导管，这一病理过程被称为"癌性新生导管"。这些肿瘤不仅在组织学上可见到更大量的导管，并且表现出上皮-间质转化的早期征象，即导管周细胞黏合素C沉积和淋巴细胞浸润，这一征象被称为传统原位病变与侵袭性病变间的过渡阶段（Tabár, et al, 2007）。

乳腺癌细胞的本质是上皮细胞，但肌上皮细胞层和肿瘤的组织环境同样参与肿瘤的进展。多数乳腺癌的抑癌基因表达于肌上皮细胞，主要发挥原位抑制肿瘤生长的作用（Sager, 1997）。但是恶性细胞及其周围基质细胞进一步突变可能导致上皮-基质平衡失调，从而使肿瘤细胞失去维持肌上皮层的功能，导管和小叶周围基底膜难以维持，使正常的导管周围、小叶内、小叶间的基质发生重构。大量的肿瘤细胞与基质中的重要组分直接接触，并包埋于重构的基质中，它们将改变自己的表型，发生上皮-间质转化。肿瘤细胞也可与前淋巴区域和淋巴管密切接触，侵袭上述组织，并借由乳腺内的淋巴系统进行转移，导致乳腺内的肿瘤发生播散（Asioli, et al, 2008），形成多个具有侵袭性的肿瘤病灶。侵袭性肿瘤进一步播散而超出病态腺叶范围。因此，肿瘤中具有侵袭性的组分可以通过恶性细胞的增殖而进展，不仅在原发灶，在其远隔部位也是如此。新生的癌灶可以合并形成一个更大的具有更复杂形态结构的癌灶。具有侵袭性的新细胞克隆可以通过进一步的突变和去分化，导致同一肿瘤瘤内和瘤外细胞的基因更加具有异质性。从乳腺扩散至淋巴结或其他器官的肿瘤细胞或定向祖细胞，可通过细胞增殖、与靶组织间相互作用而发生转移。由于上述机制，肿瘤将逐渐进展至晚期。

突变的干细胞和祖细胞，与恶性干细胞间具有许多共性。这些可移动的细胞进入外周血液循环中，播散至淋巴结及其他器官内。与乳腺中的恶性细胞相似，这些细胞的恶性转化过程可能需要数年或者数十年的时间。这些迁移的突变祖细胞比乳腺内的突变细胞更早出现恶性转化，这一概念在一定程度上解释了所谓的"原发灶不明癌症"（cancer with unknown primary, CUP；译者注：即隐匿性乳腺癌）。这一转化的发生也可能较乳腺内转化晚数十年。

1.5.3 早期乳腺癌并非"小尺寸癌"

采用大型二维或三维组织切片以及放射-病理相关性系统分析，我们证实原位癌可以局限于小叶、导管或者两者均有，原位癌也可以是单灶性、多灶性或弥漫性（Tot, Tabár, 2005）。我们同样分析了大量的早期和进展期侵袭性乳腺癌样本，发现约1/3为单灶性，包含一个单一的侵袭灶（含或不含原位成分）；1/3为多灶性，1/3包含多个侵袭性位点。一小部分晚期乳腺癌像蜘蛛网一样呈弥漫性生长（Tot 2007c, 2009; Tot, et al, 2009）。图1.8显示2005—2009年我科确诊的907例乳腺癌的病

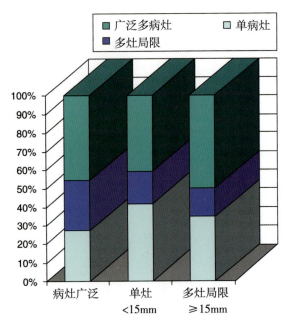

图1.8　907例新诊断乳腺癌（Falun, 2005—2009）病变范围分布示意图

变分布和疾病程度。仅一小部分为单灶性，无论疾病分期（原位或侵袭性）或瘤体大小；40%~50%的患者的瘤体>40mm或更大。早期乳腺癌并非小尺寸癌，相反，大多病例都分布广范且为多病灶。这些结果与大标本组织学的研究结果完全一致（Andersen, et al, 1987; Holland, et al, 1990; Faverly, et al, 2001; Foschini, et al, 2007）。

1.6 实际结果与未来观点

"病态腺叶"理论认为，与其他小叶相比，乳腺的某一个小叶更容易受癌基因的影响而发生恶性转化。这一高风险组织并非单一的TDLU，而是可能有数厘米大小的基因不稳定区域。无论肿瘤大小如何，这一区域包含多个原位和侵袭性病灶，各自相距数厘米远，而且这些病变可能无法通过影像学或在临床检查中检测出来。早期乳腺癌和晚期乳腺癌一样，具有多中心性和广泛性。

仅仅去除恶性组织中可检出的部分而忽视乳腺其余的病态腺叶，将导致原位复发风

险增高。约40%的仅接受保乳手术而没有接受放疗或内分泌治疗的乳腺癌患者，在20年内出现同侧局部复发（Fisher，et al，2002）。最常见的局部复发部位为手术疤痕毗邻区域，这种情况提示：肿瘤复发起源于残余的病态腺叶。根据我们的理论，充分的外科手术切除不仅要切除病变部位，而且要包括高危组织、病态腺叶及周边组织。尽管在活体组织中并不能充分标记出病态腺叶的范围，但与单纯乳房肿块切除（仅切除恶性组织）相比，扇形切除可降低原位复发的风险（切除类似乳腺小叶范围的组织）。如果病变涉及广泛的病态腺叶，则需行乳房全切术。

在发生恶性转变之前切除或破坏病态腺叶可大幅度降低乳腺癌的患病率。在治疗和预防乳腺癌方面，需要开展能有效检出和标记病态腺叶的方法。

1.7 结 论

"病态腺叶"理论和"生物时控"理论将乳腺癌的发生与已存在且非常明确的解剖结构——乳腺小叶联系起来，为乳腺癌的侵袭性和形态异质性提供了一种可能的解释。这些理论并非仅仅是形态学的描述，而是将形态学模型置于一种包含了基因学、发育学、形态学的统一概念，将乳腺癌视为在内源性和外源性因素的影响下随着时间的推移而发生的一个过程，不是照片，更像是伴随一生的电影。

这一概念虽然还处于研究的初期阶段，但我们已然能够列举许多具有前景的实验和重要结论。知识是人类最重要的武器，通过再次审视传统理论，本书将帮助读者更好地理解乳腺癌。这种理解将帮助现在及未来数代人改变当前不断增高的乳腺癌发病趋势，降低21世纪女性罹患乳腺癌的风险。

（张红梅）

参考文献

[1] Agelopoulos K, Buerger H, Brandt B. Allelic imbalance of the egfr gene as key event in breast cancer progression-the concept of committed progenitor cells. Curr Cancer Drug Targets, 2008, 8: 431–445.

[2] Al-Hajj M, Wicha MS, Benito-Hernandez A, et al. Prospective identifcation of tumorigenic breast cancer cells. Proc Natl Acad Sci USA, 2003, 100: 3983–3988.

[3] Andersen JA, Blichert-Toft M, Dyreborg U. In situ carcinomas of the breast. Types, growth pattern, diagnosis and treatment. Eur J Surg Oncol, 1987, 13: 105–111.

[4] Asioli S, Eusebi V, Gaetano L, et al. The prelymphatic pathway, the roots of the lymphatic system in the breast tissue: a 3D study. Virchows Arch, 2008, 453: 401–406.

[5] Baik I, Becker PS, Devito WJ, et al. Stem cells and prenatal origin of breast cancer. Cancer Causes Control, 2004, 15: 517–530.

[6] Boecker W, Burger H. Evidence of progenitor cells of glandular and myoepithelial cell lineages in the human adult female breast epithelium: a new progenitor (adult stem cell) concept. Cell Prolif 36, 2003 (Suppl 1): 73–84.

[7] Boyle P, Ferlay J. Cancer incidence and mortality in Europe 2004. Ann Oncol, 2005, 16 (3): 481–488.

[8] Buell P. Changing incidence in breast cancer in Japanese-American women. J Natl Cancer Inst, 1973, 51: 1479–1483.

[9] Buerger H, Otterbach F, Simon R, et al. Comparative genomic hybridization of ductal carcinoma in situ of the breast-evidence of multiplegenetic pathways. J Pathol, 1999, 187: 396–402.

[10] Cardiff RD, Wellings SR. The comparative pathology of human and mouse mammary glands. J Mammary Gland Biol Neoplasia, 1999, 4: 105–122.

[11] Cariati M, Purushotham AD. Stem cells and breast cancer. Histopathology, 2008, 52: 99–107.

[12] Cerhan JR, Sellers TA, Janney CA, et al. Prenatal and perinatal correlates of adult mammographic breast densities. Cancer Epidemiol Biomarkers Prev, 2005, 14: 1502-1508.

[13] Cheatle GL. Benign and malignant changes in duct epi-thelium of the breast. Br J Cancer, 1921, 8: 306.

[14] Clarke RB. Isolation of characterization of human mam-mary stem cells. Cell Prolif, 2005, 8: 375-386.

[15] Clarke CA, Glaser SL, West DW, et al. Breast cancer incidence and mortality trends in an affuent population: Marin County, California, USA, 1990-1996. Breast Cancer Res, 2002, 4: R13.

[16] Clarke CL, Sandle J, Jones AA, et al. Mapping loss of heterozygosity in normal human breast cells from *BRCA*1/2 carriers. Br J Cancer, 2006a, 95: 515-519.

[17] Clarke MF, Dick JE, Dirks PB, et al. Cancer stem cells-perspectives on current status and future directions. Cancer Res, 2006b, 66: 9339-9344.

[18] Dawson FK. Carcinoma in the mammary lobule and its origin. Edinb Med J, 1933, 40: 57-82.

[19] De Angelis R, Tavilla A, Verdechia A, et al. Breast cancer survivors in the United States: geographic variability and time trends, 2005-2015. Cancer, 2009, 115: 1954-1966.

[20] Deng G, Lu Y, Zlotnikov G, et al. Loss of heterozygosity in normal tissue adjacent to breast carcinoma. Science, 1996, 274: 2057-2059.

[21] Deome KB, Faulkin IJ Jr, Bern HA, et al. Development of mammary tumors from hyperplastic alveolar nodules transplanted into gland-free mammary fat pads of female C3H mice. Cancer Res, 1959, 19: 515-520.

[22] Donnenberg VS, Donnenberg AD. Multiple drug resistance in cancer revisited: the cancer stem cell hypothesis. J Clin Pharmacol, 2005, 45: 872-907.

[23] Dooley WC. Routine operative breast endoscopy during lumpectomy. Ann Surg Oncol, 2003, 10: 38-42.

[24] Easton DF, Steele L, Fields P, et al. Cancer risk in two large breast cancer families linked to BRCA2 on chromosome 13q12-13. Am J Hum Genet, 1997, 61: 120-128.

[25] Ewing J. Neoplastic diseases. A treatise of tumors. 4th edn. Saunders WB: Philadelphia, 1940: p 568.

[26] Faverly DRG, Henricks JHCL, Holland R. Breast carci-noma of limited extent. Frequency, radiologic-pathologic characteristics, and surgical margin requirements. Cancer, 2001, 91: 647-659.

[27] Fisher B, Costantino JP, Wickerham DL, et al. Tamoxifen for prevention of breast cancer: report of the National Surgical Adjuvant Breast and Bowel Project P-1 Study. J Natl Cancer Inst, 1998, 90: 1371-1388.

[28] Fisher B, Anderson S, Bryant J, et al. Twenty-year follow-up of a randomized trial comparing total mastectomy, lumpectomy, and lumpectomy plus irradiation for the treatment of invasive breast cancer. N Engl J Med, 2002, 347: 1233-1241.

[29] Ford D, Easton DF, Bishop DT, et al. Risk of cancer in BRCA1-mutation carriers. Breast Cancer Linkage Consortium. Lancet, 1994, 343: 692-695.

[30] Foschini MP, Flamminio F, Miglio R, et al. The impact of large sections on the study of in situ and invasive duct carcinoma of the breast. Hum Pathol, 2007, 38: 1736-1743.

[31] Gallagher S, Martin JE. Early phases in the development of breast cancer. Cancer, 1969, 24: 1170-1178.

[32] Going JJ, Moffat DF. Escaping from fatland: clinical and biological aspects of human mammary duct anatomy in three dimensions. J Pathol, 2004, 203: 538-544.

[33] Going JJ, Mohun TJ. Human breast duct anatomy, the 'sick lobe' hypothesis and intraductal approaches to breast cancer. Breast Cancer Res Treat, 2006, 97: 285-291.

[34] Goldstein NS, Kestin LJ, Vicini FA. Monomorphic epithelial proliferations. Characterization and evidence suggesting they are the pool of partially transformed lesions from which some invasive carcinomas arise. Am J Clin Pathol, 2007, 128:

1023-1034.

[35] Gudjonsson T, Magnusson MK. Stem cell biology and the pathways of carcinogenesis. APMIS, 2005, 113: 922-929.

[36] Harper S, Lynch J, Meersman SC, et al. Trends in areasocioeconomic and race-ethnic disparities in breast cancer incidence, stage at diagnosis, screening, mortality, and survival among women ages 50 years and over (1987-2005). Cancer Epidemiol Biomarkers Prev, 2009, 18: 121-131.

[37] Harris JR, Lippman ME, Veronesi U, et al. Breast cancer. N Engl J Med, 1992, 327: 319-328.

[38] Heaphy CM, Griffth JK, Bisoff M. Mammary feld cancerization: molecular evidence and clinical importance. Breast Cancer Res Treat, 2009, 118: 229-239.

[39] Hill AD, Doyle JM, McDermott EW, et al. Hereditary breast cancer. Br J Surg, 1997, 84: 1334-1339.

[40] Holland R, Hendricks JH, Vebeek AL, et al. Extent, distribution, and mammo-graphic/histological correlation of breast ductal carcinoma in situ. Lancet, 1990, 335: 519-522.

[41] Honeth G, Bendahl PO, Ringnér M, et al. The CD44+/CD24? phenotype is enriched in basal-like breast tumors. Breast Cancer Res, 2008, 10: R53.

[42] Hortobagyi GN. Trastuzumab in the treatment of breast cancer. N Engl J Med, 2005, 353: 1734-1736.

[43] Howard BA, Gustersson BA. Human breast development. J Mammary Gland Biol Neoplasia, 2000, 5: 119-137.

[44] Jolicoeur F, Gaboury LA, Oligny LL. Basal cells of second trimester fetal breasts: immunohistochemical study of myoepithelial precursors. Pediatr Dev Pathol, 2003, 6: 398-413.

[45] Jones C, Merrett S, Thomas VA, et al. Comparative genomic hybridization analysis of bilateral hyperplasia of usual type of the breast. J Pathol, 2003, 199: 152-156.

[46] Kawamura T, Sobue T. Comparison of breast cancer mortality in fve countries: France, Italy, Japan, the UK and the USA from the WHO mortality database (1960-2000). Jpn J Clin Oncol, 2005, 35: 758-759.

[47] Lakhani SR, Collins N, Sloane JP, et al. Loss of heterozygosity in lobular carcinoma in situ of the breast. Clin Mol Pathol, 1995a, 48: M74-M78.

[48] Lakhani SR, Collins N, Stratton MR, et al. Atypical ductal hyperplasia of the breast: clonal proliferation with loss of heterozygosity on chromosome 16q and 17p. J Clin Pathol, 1995b, 48: 611-615.

[49] Lakhani SR, Slack DN, Hamoudi RA, et al. Detection of allelic imbalance indicates that a proportion of mammary hyperplasia of usual type are clonal, neoplastic proliferations. Lab Invest, 1996, 74: 129-135.

[50] Lakhani SR, Chaggar R, Davies S, et al. Genetic alterations in "normal" luminal and myoepithelial cells of the breast. J Pathol, 1999, 189: 496-503.

[51] Lányi M. Differential diagnosis of microcalcifcations, X-ray flm analysis of 60 intraductal carcinoma, the triangle principle. Radiologe, 1977, 17: 213-216.

[52] Little P, Boice JD Jr. Comparison of breast cancer inci-dence in the Massachusetts tuberculosis fuoroscopy cohort and in the Japanese atomic bomb survivors. Radiat Res, 1999, 151: 218-224.

[53] Liu S, Ginestier C, Charafe-Jauffret E, et al. *BRCA*1 regulates human mammary stem/progenitor cell fate. Proc Natl Acad Sci USA, 2008, 105: 1680-1685.

[54] Mai KT, Yazdi HM, Burns BF, et al. Pattern of distribution of intraductal and infltrating ductal carcinoma: Three-dimensional study using serial coronal giant sections of the breast. Hum Pathol, 2000, 31: 464-474.

[55] Meng ZH, Ben Y, Li Z, et al. Aberrations of breast cancer susceptibility genes occur early in sporadic breast tumors and in acquisition of breast epithelial immortalization. Genes Chromosomes Cancer, 2004, 41: 214-222.

[56] Middleton LP, Vlastos G, Mirza NQ, et al. Multicentric mammary carcinoma, evidence of mono-

[57] Ohtake T, Abe R, Kimijima I, et al. Intraductal extension of primary inva-sive breast carcinoma treated by breast-conservative surgery. Computer graphic three-dimensional reconstruction of the mammary duct-lobular systems. Cancer, 1995, 76: 32-45.

[58] Page DL, Rogers LW, Schuyler PA, et al. The natural history of ductal carcinoma in situ of the breast//Silverstein MJ (ed) Ductal carcinoma of the breast, 2nd. Lippincott Williams & Wilkins, Philadelphia, 2002: pp 17-21.

[59] Ramakrishnan R, Seema AK, Badve S. Morphologic changes in breast tissue with menstrual cycle. Mod Pathol, 2002, 15: 1348-1356.

[60] Reya T, Morrison SJ, Clarke MF, et al. Stem cells, cancer, and cancer stem cells. Nature, 2001, 414: 105-111.

[61] Ruder EH, Dorgan JF, Kranz S, et al. Examining breast cancer growth and lifetime risk factors: early life, childhood and adolescence. Clin Breast Cancer, 2008, 8: 334-342.

[62] Rudland PS. Histochemical organization and cellular composition of ductal buds in developing human breast: evidence of cytochemical intermediates between epithelial and myoepithelial cells. J Histochem Cytochem, 1991, 39: 1471-1484.

[63] Russo J, Russo IH. Molecular basis of breast cancer. Prevention and treatment. Springer, Berlin/Heidelberg/New York/Hong Kong/London/Milan/Paris/Tokio, 2004.

[64] Sager R. Expression genetics in cancer: shifting the focus from DNA to RNA. Proc Natl Acad Sci USA, 1997, 94: 952-955.

[65] Sakakura T, Ishihara A, Yatani R. Tenascin in mammary gland development: from embryogenesis to carcinogenesis. Cancer Treat Res, 1991, 53: 383-400.

[66] Simpson PT, Gale T, Reis-Filho JS, et al. Columnar cell lesions of the breast: the missing link in breast cancer progression? A morphological and molecular analysis. Am J Surg Pathol, 2005, 29: 734-736.

[67] Slaughter DP, Southwick HW, Smejkal W. Field cancerization in oral stratifed squamous epithelium: clinical implications of multicentric origin. Cancer, 1953, 6: 963-968.

[68] Smith GH, Boulanger CA. Mammary epithelial stem cells transplantation and self-renewal analysis. Cell Prolif, 2003, 36 (Suppl 1): 3-15.

[69] Smith RA, Duffy SW, Gabe R, et al. The randomized trials of breast cancer screening: what have we learned? Radiol Clin North Am, 2004, 42: 793-806.

[70] Smith BD, Smith GL, Hurria A, et al. Future of cancer incidence in the United States: burdens upon aging, changing nation. J Clin Oncol, 2009, 27: 1-10.

[71] Stratton MR, Collins N, Lakhani SR, et al. Loss of heterozygosity in ductal carcinoma in situ of the breast. J Pathol, 1995, 175: 195-201.

[72] Tabár L, Chen HT, Yen MFA, et al. Mammographic tumor features can predict long-term outcomes reliably in women with 1-14mm invasive carcinoma. Cancer, 2004, 101: 1745-1759.

[73] Tabár L, Tot T, Dean PB. Breast cancer. Early detection with mammography. Casting type calcifcations: sign of a subtype with deceptive features. Stuttgart: Thieme, 2007.

[74] Tabár L, Tot T, Dean PB. Crushed stone-like calcifcations: the most frequent malignant type. Stuttgart: Thieme, 2008.

[75] Tavassoli FA, Devili P. World Health Organization classifcation of tumors. Pathology & genetics. Tumors of the breast and female genital organs. IARC, Lyon, 2003: p63.

[76] Teboul M, Halliwell M. Atlas of ultrasound and ductal echography of the breast: the introduction of anatomic intelligence into breast imaging. Wiley-Blackwell, UK, 1995: p380.

[77] The Swedish Organized Service Screening Evaluation Group. Reduction in breast cancer mortality from organized service screening with mammography: Further confrmation with expanded data. Cancer Epidemiol Biomarkers Prev, 2006, 15: 45-51.

[78] Tot T. Correlating the ground truth of mammographic histology with the success or failure of imaging.

Technol Cancer Res Treat, 2005a, 4: 23-28.

[79] Tot T. DCIS, cytokeratins, and the theory of the sick lobe. Virchows Arch, 2005b, 447: 1-8.

[80] Tot T. The theory of the sick breast lobe and the possible consequences. Int J Surg Pathol, 2007a, 15: 369-375.

[81] Tot T. How to eradicate breast carcinomas: a hypothetical way of breast cancer prevention based on the theory of the sick lobe// Litchfeld JE (ed) New research in precan-cerous conditions. New York: Nova, 2007b: pp 165-181.

[82] Tot T. The clinical relevance of the distribution of the lesions in 500 consecutive breast cancer cases documented in large-format histological sections. Cancer, 2007c, 110: 2551-2560.

[83] Tot T. The metastatic capacity of multifocal breast carcinomas: extensive tumors versus tumors of limited extent. Hum Pathol, 2009, 40: 199-205.

[84] Tot T, Tabár L. Radiologic-pathologic correlation of ductal carcinoma in situ of the breast using two- and three-dimensional large histologic sections. Semin Breast Dis, 2005, 8: 144-151.

[85] Tot T, Tabár L, Dean PB. The pressing need for better histologic-mammographic correlation of the many variations in normal breast anatomy. Virchows Arch, 2000, 437: 338-344.

[86] Tot T, Tabár L, Dean PB. Practical breast pathology. Stuttgart: Thieme, 2002.

[87] Tot T, Pekár G, Hofmeyer S, et al. The distribution of lesions in 1-14mm invasive breast carcinomas and its relation to metastatic potential. Virchows Arch, 2009, 455: 109-115.

[88] Trichopoulos D. Hypothesis: does breast cancer originate in utero. Lancet, 1990, 335: 939-940.

[89] Tsai YC, Lu Y, Nichols PW, et al. Contiguous patches of normal human mammary epithelium derived from a single stem cell: implications for breast carcinogenesis. Cancer Res, 1996, 56: 402-404.

[90] Villadsen R. In search of stem cell hierarchy in the human breast and its relevance in breast cancer evolution. APMIS, 2005, 113: 903-921.

[91] Villadsen R, Fridriksdottir AJ, Ronnov-Jenssen L, et al. Evidence for stem cell hierarchy in the adult human breast. J Cell Biol, 2007, 177: 87-101.

[92] Wang Y, Yang J, Zheng H, et al. Expression of mutant p53 proteins implicates a lineage relationship between neural stem cells and malignant astrocytic glioma in a murine model. Cancer Cell, 2009, 15: 514-526.

[93] Wellings SR, Jensen HM, Marcum RG. An atlas of subgross pathology of the human breast with special reference to possible precancerous lesions. J Natl Cancer Inst, 1975, 55: 231-273.

[94] Wiechmann L, Kuerer HM. The molecular journey from ductal carcinoma in situ to invasive breast cancer. Cancer, 2008, 112: 2130-2142.

[95] Wolff MS, Collman GW, Barrett JC, et al. Breast cancer and environmental risk factors: epidemiological and experi-mental fndings. Annu Rev Pharmacol Toxicol, 1996, 36: 573-596.

[96] Xue F, Michels KB. Intrauterine factors and risk of breast cancer: a systemic review and meta-analysis of current evidence. Lancet Oncol, 2007, 8: 1088-1100.

[97] Yan PS, Venkataramu C, Ibrahim A, et al. Mapping geographic zones of cancer risk with epigenetic biomarkers in normal breast tissue. Clin Cancer Res, 2006, 12: 6626-6636.

第 2 章 人体乳腺腺叶解剖及其对乳腺癌的重要意义

James J. Going

> 我曾经听一位优秀的解剖学家说:"乳房的结构实在是太复杂了,我对它一无所知。"
> ——Astley Paston Cooper,《论乳房解剖》(Cooper,1840)

> 当一种有效的新方法问世时,它所能处理的问题将迅速成为万众瞩目的焦点,而其他问题就往往被忽视,甚至是遗忘,与其有关的研究也常常会被人嗤之以鼻。
> ——Imre Lakatos,《证明与反驳:数学发现中的逻辑学》(Lakatos,1976)

2.1 介绍:科学研究的客体——人体乳房解剖

一些人相信解剖学曾经历过Lakatos描绘过的命运(Marusi,2008)。然而,尽管分子论在生物学领域已被广泛认同,但仍没有一个"思想流派"(Fleck,1979)可以解释像乳腺癌这类疾病的复杂过程。因为它受到从分子到社会、环境各层次因素的影响,发生的时间跨度可能是1秒钟,也可能是人的一生。本章我们将要探讨乳房组织中被忽视但值得密切关注的结构:腺叶。

乳腺腺叶被忽视的原因包括人类总是不

J. J. Going
Institute of Cancer Science, Glasgow University and Pathology Department, Glasgow Royal Infirmary,
Glasgow, UK
e-mail: going@udcf.gla.ac.uk

注意知识中的漏洞。解剖学家和乳腺解剖学先驱Sir Astley Cooper也有一定的责任:一位严肃的评论家早在20世纪中期就表示过,Cooper已经对乳房的大体解剖做了必要的阐释(Brock,1952),包括其腺叶结构。

Cooper的评论("在乳腺的病态变化得到合理的解释或理解之前,对乳房的自然结构进行说明很有必要";Cooper,1840)无论是在当时的环境下还是现在都是正确的。尽管他的《论乳房解剖》中记录了比20世纪甚至如今的21世纪更多的与人体乳腺腺叶组织结构有关的原始数据,但他并没有对这个课题研究到底。如果他还健在,我猜也会哑然无语。所幸的是,研究人类乳房形态的新工作正在开展(Ramsay, et al, 2005; Going, 2006; Geddes, 2007; Rusby, et al, 2007)。

Cooper作为最后一拨杰出的人体解剖学家中的一员,尽管曾经使用过显微镜,但他并不依赖这种技术(Cooper, 1843)。1920年代Joseph Jackson Lister发明了电子显微镜,但直到组织学相关的理论和实践(Von Gerlach,1848),包括细胞学说(Schleiden, Schwann),Virchow的"所有细胞均来源于先存在的细胞(omnis cellula e cellula)"的观点,Wilhelm His发明的显微镜用薄片切片机,以及改良的染色技术的出现,这些理论和技术均支持细胞是组织结构的基本单位,之后,组织学作为一门学科才开始兴盛起来。

随后发生的20世纪的分子革命,推动了解剖学从同时代的生物科学中迅速发展起来。

研究者们发现，从婴儿期、成年期到老年，无论是正常的乳腺发育，还是疾病的发生，细胞和分子都在乳腺的实质和间质内进行着剧情复杂的表演，这些过程是在多步骤多维度下发生的，其中包括我们关心的结构——腺叶，它的重要性无可比拟。

2.2 传统显微镜的局限性

显微镜十分适用于微观实体，包括局部乳房组织。我们可以十分简单地将整个鼠科动物的乳腺组织用单个固体石蜡固定，但人体乳腺的尺寸过大，因此只观察到极少部分腺体。大型组织切片的出现解决了这个问题，Cheatle（1920）、Eusebi（Foschini, et al, 2006）和Tot（Tot, et al, 2000）等乳腺病理学家均发现了这种技术的优势，但只有极少数专门的实验室才具备进行大型组织切片的条件。

组织学自然也是二维的。三维信息的获取要通过不懈的努力，尤其是较大的研究对象。研究三维解剖和胚胎学的经典连续切片技术早从建立之初起就广为实施。但是，棘手的乳腺腺叶解剖问题鲜少有人关注。有研究者认为太过困难（这个认识是正确的；Osteen, 1995）。也有研究者认为这个问题早已解决（错误的原因是因为有所忽视），或者说是对乳腺癌的特殊意义缺乏认识。近年来，人们已经将乳腺癌视为一种乳腺腺叶性疾病。

2.2.1 乳腺癌的"乳腺腺叶病源"假说

乳腺癌的病因尚未完全清楚。早期的研究者曾在与癌症有关的乳腺组织的导管和腺泡中，发现类似于癌细胞的细胞排成一行（Cheatle, 1906, 1920）。有人解释称，这些细胞是浸润性乳腺癌的前体细胞，这种说法听起来很可信，有时也确实能清楚地观察到这些细胞在导管和腺体结构中入侵邻近的基质。

在Foote和Stewart发表对小叶原位癌（LCIS）的明确描述之前，人们已对类似LCIS的病变有所认识（例如：Cheatle, Cutler 1931:162）。Ewing（1940:563）则描述了"由管道内层细胞来源的管道癌"和"由腺泡上皮细胞来源的腺泡癌"之间的不同。

考虑到乳腺实质中导管和小叶形态上的区别，以及组织起源才是肿瘤分类的原则，导管和小叶上的原位癌分别由导管和小叶的上皮细胞起源，也是导管和小叶浸润癌的前期病变。这个理论简明、整洁，似乎煞有其事，头头是道。然而，像一场大风吹过，1970年代之前的亚肉眼解剖的发展揭露了这个理论的错误。研究强调，肿瘤细胞聚集形成的类导管结构实际是扩大和扭曲的小叶（"unfolded"；Wellings, et al. 1975）。在此基础上，人们普遍相信乳腺癌是由小叶起源，这种看法似乎与"病态腺叶"的观点相左。

John Azzopardi对Wellings及其同事的研究进行了探讨，并著成了《乳腺病理学中的问题》（Azzopardi, 1979）一书。在此书中，他强力支持"乳腺小叶病源"假说。他注意到"这一杰出研究的观察基础是，传统认为导管病源诱发的乳腺疾病大多都是小叶和（或）末端导管病源引起的"。其他的研究者也发表了相应的数据来说明并支持"小叶病源"假说（Ohuchi, et al, 1985; Faverly, et al, 1992），这一假说在没有任何原始数据支撑的情况下，仍能被人频繁引用。从引用的频繁程度上就可以判断出它已被学术界尊为"科学事实"。

小叶病源假说的支持者们提出了一个关键论据：倡导导管原位癌引发乳腺癌的研究者们所认为的导管结构，实际是他们的前辈错认的扩大的小叶。我们很难评估这个观点在多大程度上是正确的。但是，极富洞察力的观察家，如Lenthal Cheatle则完全可以辨认出高度变形的小叶，并在他们的研究中对此进行阐释（例如：Cheatle, 1920:288；图204）。同时，Cheatle也发现了识别变形的导管和小叶的困难之处，并指出使用连续切片技术可以解决这个难题。在同一篇文献中，Cheatle 也列举了某个案例（第290页，图208）。基于大组织切片研究，Sir Lenthal明确提出增生的上皮细胞按腺叶分布，最终形成乳腺癌。

2.2.2 对"腺叶病源"理论的批评

亚肉眼研究并不能得出乳腺癌的病因。

如果我们接受癌细胞是单细胞克隆这个观点的话（Fialkow，1976），那么，我们也应该认为肿块内（不包括间质、炎症性和其他非肿瘤细胞）的所有癌细胞都是体细胞的后代，它们通过多次的（表观）遗传改变获得肿瘤的表现型，我们可能注意到这个观点并没有被广泛接受（Parsons，2008），我们也不会就这个观点展开讨论。

如果癌细胞是单细胞克隆的，那么就可以简单地实现识别乳腺癌起源：即在乳腺实质中，找到某一型特定癌细胞后代细胞的聚集部位，这些细胞可能数年、数十年甚至在临床查体或筛查发现之前就已经存在。可以负责任地说，我们不能在任何一例乳腺癌病例中实现这一点，更不用说检测出乳腺癌的起源了。我想说实际上并不存在所谓的"始作俑者"细胞，这种癌症中所有细胞都可以回溯到某一个细胞的观点并不真实。

2.2.3 谈论癌症的"起源"意味着什么？

当我们思考的越多，就越会发现这个观点晦涩不明。

在标准的模型中，浸润性乳腺癌和其他癌症通常被看做是前期病变克隆化的产物。这些前期病变多种多样，有重度增生、高级别上皮内癌变以及原位癌（其本质与浸润性癌伴随的病变一致；Sinn，2009）。如果确实如此，那么，随着癌细胞开始突破基底膜，原位癌就是整个过程的合理"开端"。

然而，同一个观点也适用于原位癌：许多原位癌起源于不典型增生，后者可能是更早期细胞的后代，或许是正常增生的细胞，或柱状细胞改变；其他方面发生变化的腺叶；表面正常实则异常的实质；完全正常的实质；或者是胎儿体内乳腺形成之前早期的祖细胞；或者是那些携带突变的 *TP53*、*BRCA1*、*CDH1*、*STK11*、*PTEN* 的受精卵，后者已在通向乳腺癌的道路上迈出了重要的一步（Campeau，et al，2008）。

从16世纪中期开始，常见的冰岛 *999del5 BRCA2* 基因突变就被发现有诱发乳腺癌的作用（Thorlacius，et al，1996）。如果许多乳腺癌患者没有遗传这个缺陷基因，那么可能就不会罹患乳腺癌。因此，在什么意义上，我们能够准确地认为这种乳腺癌起源于16世纪或更早时期的断言是错误的呢？

2.2.4 在时间和空间的角度，癌症没有"起始点"

总的来说，癌症并不是在确定的时间和空间开始的。尽管曾经认为可能存在单细胞癌症（one-celled cancer），后来也证明并非如此。只有在无法识别单个的独特细胞，多次传代后才能观察到这种细胞。即使我们通过间接证据推测存在这种细胞，但是，一连串的分子诱因链可以追溯到之前的好几代细胞。我们却没有理由推断，比起其他细胞，子代细胞在发生突变，推动表型转化时更有优势：在推动表型转化时，原代细胞应和子代细胞同等重要。在此基础上讨论癌症的形成过程才更有说服力。

承认这些观点就相当于承认"乳腺癌开始于末端导管小叶单元"的说法，是没有意义的，无论别人同意与否，这个说法都没有说明任何事情。那么，我们也能明白"乳腺癌开始于一个病态腺叶"这个说法同样是没有意义的。这并不是否认，对于个体而言，"病态腺叶（和小叶）"与乳腺癌的演变之间存在密切复杂的关系。

2.2.5 质疑"腺叶假说"的另一个原因

在乳腺癌患者和正常人的乳房中都有很多不正常的乳腺腺叶。Jensen、Rice和Wellings（Jensen，et al，1976）在罹患乳腺癌的乳腺中发现了不典型小叶，中位数15个（第3个四分位数是51，最大值225），在正常乳腺中也有发现，中位数5个（第3个四分位数是11，最大值91）。

如果要用这些发现来支持"腺叶起源"的假说的话，那么，这些腺叶都必须是独立出现的。否则，它们的存在说明存在某种共同的影响因素，这种因素可以影响大范围的乳腺实质，包括导管和腺叶。

我们最多认为，相比乳腺实质的其他部分，外观上，腺叶略早受到了与乳腺癌有关的改变的影响。

一个"乳腺腺叶起源"假说要有单叶肿瘤存在的证据支持，就类似于结肠的异常腺窝灶或是单腺窝腺瘤一样，这二者的存在说明结肠腺窝是始动细胞存在的地方（Preston，et al，2003）。要辨识邻近腺叶都正常且有癌细胞定植的单腺叶，需要在全部组织切片上仔细检查所有邻近的腺叶组织。然而，无论是Wellings等的亚肉眼研究，还是更精细的3D研究（Ohuchi，et al. 1984a、b，1985; Ohuchi，1999; Faverly，et al，1992）都没有做到这一点，尽管后者在几乎每个病例中都发现了多个异常腺叶。即使有研究做到了这一点，仍然不能排除表型显性而突变隐性的区域存在的可能（即腺叶结构正常，但存在基因突变）。

2.3 乳腺癌前驱病变的演进：克隆性扩增

所以，我们应当忘记乳腺癌或者说其假定的前驱病变的"来源"，而去探究乳腺癌的演变过程。在乳腺癌患者的乳房中，形态和基因上异常的实质细胞的空间分布，为我们理解乳腺癌的演变过程提供了明确的信息。

相比于乳腺实质，Barrett食管中癌随时间推移而演变的过程更易被直接观察，这是一个有对比意义的例子。在Barrett食管中，突变的细胞克隆比其他细胞克隆更有选择性优势，能占据10cm以上的食道（Maley，2007）。

如果这个步骤完成的话，一般认为，突变将会经由"选择性清除"而"稳定下来"。倘若这些过程发生在乳房，特别是某个腺叶中，那将会产生一个"病态的腺叶"，它类似于Barrett食管中的那段"病态的食管"。形态明显异常的细胞，如DCIS和LCIS，或多或少能检测到它们定殖在乳腺实质中，包括导管和腺叶（图2.1），有时，DCIS会遍布这个腺叶。

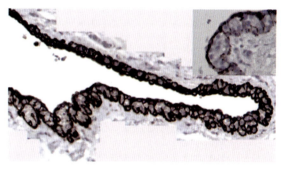

图2.1 恶性上皮细胞在乳腺导管和腺叶的上皮层中广泛浸润。在这条免疫染色的导管中，基底和腔面细胞都是角蛋白5强阳性。在基底和腔面细胞间的空间内，充满了苍白的、中度异型、偶尔空泡化的细胞，它们聚集的方式很独特。本例标本是某患者在乳腺癌术后，对侧乳腺缩乳术时意外发现。这种不典型小叶增生也称为"类Paget样播散"。右上角小图：E-钙黏蛋白表达缺失也是这些细胞的特点

这个过程可连续，亦可间断（Faverly，et al，1992）。但是，在这两种情况下，扩张可能仅局限在异常的细胞克隆存在的腺叶内。这种情况至少在能破坏基底膜的浸润性成分出现之前存在。

当形态学的表型异常不明显时，这样的细胞克隆扩增很难被辨识。然而，这些伴随高恶性转变风险的扩增的细胞克隆也有迹可

循，即在一片基因改变但形态学正常或微异常的细胞中存在原位或浸润性癌。

另一种可能性就是青春期前的乳腺细胞或是胎儿乳房基芽细胞发生突变，这些细胞的克隆原本可以产生成熟的乳腺组织。如果突变导致致癌风险增高，那么，由那个细胞而来的乳腺组织中罹患多病灶乳腺肿瘤的风险就会增高。

有一篇很有远见、但无人关注的文献（Sharpe，1998）提到了乳腺癌的起源，截至2009年10月，该文共被引用5次（不同于主流思想的观念往往被忽视，不受关注）。Sharpe指出，乳腺癌的多灶性可能是异常祖细胞在导管内的播散所致，或者是发育机制所致，在后者，正在发育的乳腺导管树的分支解剖上是互相连通的，某个早期阶段就出现变异的祖细胞的后代细胞通过这些分支播散。第一个解释符合健康的腺叶演变成病态腺叶的说法，第二个则是"病态腺叶"是天生的观点。

这两种看法可能都正确。在5岁之前，人类的乳房对致癌的辐射最敏感的事实符合第二种说法。接触过长崎和广岛原子弹爆炸产生的辐射的女性，乳腺癌的发病率增高。越小年龄（0~4岁）接受辐射的妇女，其相对危险度（ERR）最高（4.6）（Tokunaga, et al，1994）。Land（1995）惊讶地发现，尽管婴幼儿期乳腺上皮的数量很少，但是，那些因为"胸腺肥大"接受放射治疗的女性，其乳腺癌的ERR也相当高（3.6）。因此，婴幼儿期接受电离辐射，增加成年后乳腺癌发病率的关系就得到了明确。同样，诱变剂亚硝基和甲基脲对尚未性成熟的大鼠乳房的致癌作用比性成熟的大鼠更强（Ariazi, et al, 2005）。

乳腺祖细胞由辐射引发的突变可以被后代遗传，甚至不同程度地遍布整个腺叶。单个祖细胞最著名的能力就是可以重构整个啮齿类动物的乳腺（Kordon, Smith, 1998）。这一特点突出显示了单个细胞可以形成更大范围腺体的潜力。

当乳腺实质整个暴露在外界致癌的环境中时，多灶性的肿瘤就可能会出现。在对肿瘤形成有促进作用的环境中，就可能产生多病灶肿瘤，例如某个外部的致癌源或内分泌方面的影响，我们多希望这个过程发生时没有腺体存在。

2.4 全乳腺实质可视化的需求

为了全面研究乳腺实质中乳腺癌形成的演变过程，我们需要研究在完整的乳腺中实现实质组织（腺叶）的可视化，其研究要比3D组织研究的目标大得多。

人们对乳腺癌的发生进行过推测：随着乳腺的发育，乳腺结构渐渐成熟，一小群异常的细胞克隆沿导管播散，或是突变已散布在青春期前的乳房中的（其乳腺芽基的分叉已在出生前形成）某个细胞的后代细胞中，这些诱发多病灶乳腺癌的克隆有可能在某个腺叶上完成了扩增，要证实这个推测需要可视化的能力。

随着乳房的发育，单个导管系统的生长（延长和分支）为某些具有携带突变的细胞克隆的扩增提供了生长优势。尽管这些细胞表型上不一定存在异常，但能在发育中的乳房中占据更多的空间，为后期肿瘤的形成做准备。这就是人们共知的乳腺腺叶的差异化发育（Going, Moffat, 2004）。

在过去的30年中，人们强调乳腺腺叶作为人体乳腺实质的单位，反而忽视了乳腺，这个更大尺度、更大范围的结构，导致相关技术的研究并不成熟。但是，这个领域的发展却是相当有吸引力的。

本章余下部分将探讨目前已知的乳房中央和外围的导管或腺叶解剖；验证腺叶里和腺叶间的接合存在的证据，通过这些接合，上皮内的肿瘤可以实现腺叶间的转移；观察乳腺癌及其祖细胞是否与"病态腺叶"假说一致，以腺叶的形式分布；并思考在我们现有的有关乳腺腺叶解剖的知识中，还需要填补多少知识的漏洞，以及正在研究中的技术的广度，以确保在研究和诊断时能得到形态和分子方面的最优数据。

2.5 乳腺腺叶的解剖

现在很多文章关于乳房解剖的描述非常艺术化，言辞引人入胜，但缺乏事实。

相反，Cooper早期关于乳腺解剖的说明就有原始调查数据支撑。在他的描述中，最突出的特点就是口径大小不一致的导管从中央发散而出，分支，再分支，最后的分支终止于乳腺实质中。尽管研究者都认为乳头处的腺叶很少（Stolier, Wang, 2008），但是，乳腺组织实际上位于乳房的各个部分，而不仅仅只位于外围。不同的腺叶呈现出完全不同的特点（图2.2）。它们的分支在一定程度上互相交叉，但分布没有大面积的重叠。

Moffat和Going曾剖检了一位年轻女尸的乳房，并追踪了所有导管及其分支（Moffat, Going, 1996; Going, Moffat, 2004）。他们试图在完整的人体乳房中获取导管分支的详细信息，这样的研究十分罕见。尽管依靠人力进行类似的这种研究十分费力（Osteen, 1995），但是，到目前为止，研究者已经对开发更便捷的检查流程进行了充分的探索（Going, 2006）。

这些研究揭示了不同导管系统（腺叶）的特点，包括各个方面（图2.3、2.4）：单个腺叶在乳房所占体积可以大到25%，小到1%，甚至更小；外形的多样性（主要有凸面、凹凸面、楔形和V形）；在第一个分支前，中央导管长度的多样性（有长有短）；存在发育不全的腺叶或是萎缩的腺叶，其导管相对较长，深入乳房中央位置，鲜有甚至没有外周分支或是乳腺实质。少数腺叶的导管较长却未分叉，这就说明了当导管分支受抑制时，其主

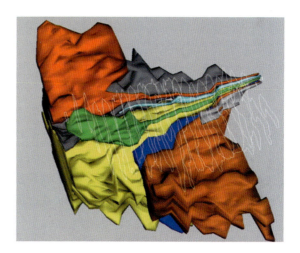

图2.3 乳腺腺叶形态上的变异。一个乳房中7个有代表性的腺叶其大小和分布各不相同。研究者根据一系列亚肉眼切片追踪每一条导管系统。在每一个切片中，导管的分支所在的区域边界复杂，但是尚可分辨。通过"重构"，腺叶可视（Fiala 2005）。前6个腺叶用曲折的表面（Boissonnat Surface）表示，为了避免腺叶遮住图片的中央部分，第7个则是线框框架表示。腺叶间存在着包括大小在内的明显差别；早早分支，并靠近乳头和乳房表层的腺叶（褐色），分支较晚，位于乳房深层的腺叶（橘色，绿色）以及没有分支的腺叶（蓝色）。最后一种是完全没有分支导管存在的未发育完全的腺叶，也是Moffat和Going研究的那个乳房中几个"萎缩腺叶"中最长的一条（1996，2004）

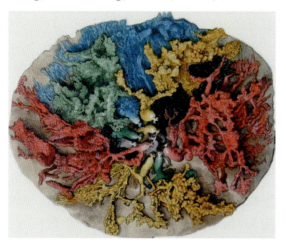

图2.2 《论乳房解剖》*图版VI图3（Cooper, 1840）。用不同颜色的蜡注入到单个腺叶中。相比同一图版的图2，这张图并不常见，前者中乳腺腺叶的分割更一致。这种现象可能表明了一种追求统一性的审美倾向，这解释了已发表的文献中对乳腺腺叶那种艺术化表达的原因，即强调发育和排列的规律性，无视基本的事实

―――――――――
＊：On the Anatomy of the Breast

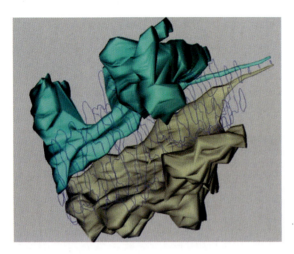

图2.4 乳腺腺叶形态上的变异。II 图2.3中所研究乳房中的另外3个腺叶。绿色的腺叶有两块大的独立的区域，一块靠近乳房表层，一块向深处延伸。所有的腺叶（呈现曲折的表面）被线框结构标示的蓝色部分包围起来。我们可以以此推测蓝色的那个腺叶比其他两个更具生长优势

体仍可以延长（Going, Moffat, 2004）。或许这就表明了人体体内存在一种类似于鼠科动物乳房发育时的非对称性（单轴）分支特点的机制（Davies, 2002）。

研究者发现，一条长长的凸面腺叶包裹着另一个凹面腺叶，这似乎暗示了凸面腺叶比凹面腺叶更具有生长优势（图2.4）。可能是因为"凸面腺叶"比"凹面腺叶"更早开始生长，或者生长速度更快，因而在未经占用的区域中，凹面腺叶的分支导管的生长受到先入为主的凸面腺叶的限制。乳房发育中腺叶间的明显竞争，对于女性乳房扮演着生殖适应性的信号、乳房对称性与患癌风险之间的关系（Møller, et al, 1995）来说，十分有趣（Scutt, et al, 2006）。

2.5.1 腺叶间有交通吗？

一群异常细胞克隆只要还受到基底膜的限制，它们的扩张就会局限在基底膜包裹的上皮层内。就乳腺腺叶而言，只要腺叶间是独立的，这些细胞克隆就是单腺叶存在的。我们暂时忽视这种可能性：理论上，细胞可以从腺叶中爬出进入乳头的上皮层，再通过乳头表层的导管开口进入另一个小叶。

如果腺叶不是相互孤立的，而是由内衬上皮细胞的交通导管连接起来的，那么，这些细胞可以从起源的腺叶上脱离，进入到邻近的腺叶中，再从那里游走到任何一个与之相连的腺叶中；不断重复下去，这样一种细胞克隆就可以扩张进入整个乳腺实质。这个过程就类似于肺炎球菌通过Kohn肺泡间孔，导致大叶性肺炎在整个肺叶的分布。

当采用乳管灌洗或者乳管镜进行乳腺微环境取样时，腺叶间的交通可能也影响结果（Tondre, et al, 2008; Dooley, 2009）；同时，它也可能在哺乳时存在一定的生理意义，例如某个导管堵塞后，乳汁可以通过交通导管绕过堵塞部位到达乳头。这能最大限度地提高泌乳组织的效率，否则，受损的乳管将通过哺乳反馈抑制作用来限制乳汁的分泌（Wilde, et al, 1995），其中的一种抑制作用是通过人类乳腺和鼠类乳腺中5-羟色胺与5HT7受体发挥的（Stull, et al, 2007）。因而，乳腺腺叶间是否存在交通导管是非常重要的问题，但是，目前学术界在这方面仍没有得到满意的答案。

2.5.2 腺叶解剖遇到的挑战

乳腺腺叶仍是研究中一个十分棘手的问题。要完整地界定腺叶，就必须观察到它所有的"枝"（导管）和"叶"（腺小叶）。导管壁很薄，由致密的纤维组织包裹，多次分支，不断向外延伸。一个乳房中有多个腺叶，肉眼检查和显微镜检查都很难定义腺叶的边界。

实际操作中，研究者可以通过注射液体标记物（有颜色的石蜡、树脂、乳胶、尿烷或水银），或是在腺叶被染色和还原之后，通过大量厚的（亚肉眼）切片追踪导管走行来界定腺叶的范围。传统厚度的大体组织切片也许能够提示腺叶的结构，但是，切片间3~5mm的距离不利于进行切片间的导管追踪。

2.5.3 导管注射研究

Cooper是这个领域的前锋（请牢记他是在67岁时才开始研究正常乳房的）。Sir Astley的观点很明确：生理上的交通并没有将独立的导管系统（腺叶）连接起来："正如将不同颜色的标记物注入导管中或是仅注入某一条导管后观察到的那样，乳腺导管间是没有任何联系的"。

"如果每条导管分别被注入多种颜色的标记物，那么，腺体内的颜色不会混合。如果向一条导管小心地注入水银，它也不会跑到其他导管中。这个规则同样适用于其他动物的乳腺。这些动物如野兔、狗、猪的乳腺内导管是分隔的，与腺体内其他导管截然不通。"

"我只见过一次例外，在向一个输乳管（从乳头到腺体内侧）注射时，有两个大的分支彼此交叉，在它们接触的地方，注射液从一个导管进入另一个。这可能是导管破裂所致或是自然结构的变异。对此我画了一幅图（版面Ⅷ图7；图2.5）；因为这个现象在200多次的实验中才发生了一次，所以，这表明这种情况并非广泛存在。"（Cooper，1840）

Cooper的"200多次注射实验"所达到的程度是空前绝后、无人能比的。在这么多次实验中，他采用了一种特别适合探测导管间交通的工具。

在尸体剖检时制作的乳腺亚肉眼切片中，Moffat和Going追踪了所有可识别的导管分支，并未找到任何交通（Going，Mohun，2006）。

乳腺导管造影术的文献中也缺乏进一步证明腺叶间存在罕见交通的证据，即在对一条中央导管注射造影剂后，会有另一条中央导管出现逆行充盈（图2.6）。Love和Barsky的研究并未检测出交通的存在，他们的研究包含了Otto Sartorius（Santa Barbara, California）所操作的乳腺导管造影数据（Love，Barsky，2004）。同样，我本人对那些已发表的经乳头灌洗出现液体逆向流动的证据也不置可否，而且，这种情况可能也并不容易检出。

对乳腺发育过程的思考人们提出了一种理论，即延长的乳腺导管彼此抑制对方的生长，这可能干扰了导管间交通的形成（Faulkin，DeOme，1960）。啮齿类动物（Faulkin，DeOme，1960）和人类（Going，Moffat，2004）的乳腺中导管的分布情况都表明了这种排斥现象的存在（图2.7）。TGFβ有可能是乳腺导管空间分布中关键的负性调节因子（Lee，Davies，2007）。

另一方面，Ohtake等人确实通过亚肉眼研究描述了叶间和叶内导管的交通（Ohtake, et al,1995, 2001）。这个有趣而重要的问题只有在更深层更严谨的形态学研究之后才能得到解决。去记录一个完整乳房中导管分支点和终点的x、y、z坐标（Going，2006），这样的研究经历使我们意识到不管在实验中多么谨慎地避免失误，但这种研究方法仍非常容易弄混分支。一些由Ohtake等人发现的明显的交通很可能只是他们在导管追踪中出错后的结果。

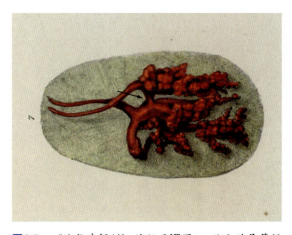

图2.5 《论乳房解剖》的版面Ⅷ图7。独立的导管间极少有的交通（箭头）。Cooper评价这幅图时说道："应把它看成是一般规律以外的少见的意外情况，也就是说，有联系的两条导管是我见过的唯一一个例子。其中注射液是从靠近腺体外周的某个分支中注射的，注射液流向乳头，或许是导管被划破，或者是存在不寻常的交通时，两条导管都充满了注射液"

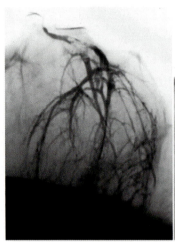
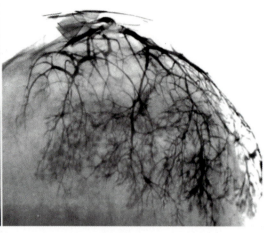

图2.6 一张乳腺造影片中同一个腺叶的两个视图（左边是斜位，右边是头尾位）。这个腺叶范围广泛，占据了乳房体积的一大部分。在头尾位中，腺体组织清晰可见。两个视图中都有明显的充盈缺损，这是由于导管内存在乳头状瘤。请注意中央导管为单条存在，并且其他导管并未出现造影剂的逆行。这张乳腺造影片由Jean Murray医生惠赠（South East Scotland Breast Screening Centre），为提高导管的可见性，图片已经反转。

2.5.4 乳腺癌的前体是以腺叶的模式分布吗？

因乳腺象限和腺叶之间没什么重要关系，所以，只关注疾病在象限间分布的研究让我们对乳腺癌及其前体在腺叶间的分布知之甚少，甚至一无所知。

广泛的导管内癌是局部复发的一个危险因素（Holland, et al, 1990A、B）。对于经常实际操作的乳腺病理学家来说，发现或大或小的、楔型分布的DCIS是司空见惯的事情。其他发表过的研究支持乳腺癌中疾病的分段分布符合腺叶结构这个说法（Johnson, et al, 1995）。分段治疗的提议也似乎行得通，但是，因腺叶假说尚未得到证明，手术操作的难度也曾被人毫不留情地指出（Osteen, 1995）："证明乳腺癌的分段结构需要大量连续的乳腺切片，以保证每条导管和小叶的一致性。而完成这样一项重要的任务可能需要调动不同科室的资源，需要每个参与者的极大耐心。"在同一篇评论中，Osteen还回顾了Holland等人（1990b）进行亚肉眼检测时在82例切除的乳房中发现81处类腺叶区域DCIS病灶的报告，但是，他指出尽管病灶符合分段（腺叶的）分

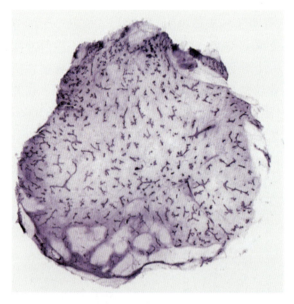

图2.7 经水杨酸甲酯（冬青树油）清洗过的苏木精染色的乳腺亚肉眼切片。切片来自整个乳腺（尸体剖检），冠状面。乳腺实质中各成分之间的距离很远（提示了发育过程中存在排斥现象）

布，然而这种分布模式的理论并未建立，这是由于那个时期腺叶解剖尚处于未知水平。确实，很少有人提出过这样的解剖观点，也只有少数案例验证了这个过程的艰巨。

在同一篇评论中，我们也发现了描述"病态腺叶"存在的痕迹。评论认为："一些

乳腺癌患者的乳腺内含有生物学上被定义为"坏"的部分……在这些例子中，我们产生了新的问题：是否包括不典型乳腺小叶增生、良性上皮细胞的微钙化在内的其他标识，还是基因或是分子生物标志物可以识别治疗中需要扩大切除术或乳腺癌根治术的'坏部分'"。

一份近期的评论调查了有关同侧乳腺中多病灶、多中心病灶的相关文献（Jain, et al, 2009）。

在乳腺小叶肿瘤（ALH/LCIS）中，病灶的分段分布并不是很明显。乳腺小叶肿瘤通常被当做乳腺癌的风险标志，而非乳腺癌的前期病变。它们之间的关系并不十分清晰。但是，2003年由David Page和其同事发表的论文表明，某些患者在诊断为ALH后，再次检测出同侧与对侧乳腺浸润性肿瘤的比率为3:1，这就强烈地暗示了ALH功能不仅仅只是风险标志（Page, et al, 2003）。

2.5.5 邻近癌灶的"正常"乳腺组织存在异常

目前，有大量的证据证明组织学上正常的乳腺组织，可能在基因、表观遗传以及其他的分子分析中表现异常（Ellsworth, et al, 2004A、B; Meeker, et al, 2004; Yan, et al, 2006; Tripathi, et al, 2008; Chen, et al, 2009）。这些数据确实符合"病态腺叶"的观点，但再一次缺少了有关腺叶的解剖数据来支撑，所以无法排除其他可能性。

Chen等人（2009）对来自90例乳腺癌患者的143个组织学上正常或是非不典型良性乳腺组织进行了全基因表达的芯片分析。11个样本的结果表明，其基因表达的特点符合浸润性肿瘤。根据这些数据，作者认为涉及细胞增殖与细胞周期的基因强烈代表了"恶性肿瘤风险"的表达特征。

Ellsworth等发现（Ellsworth, et al, 2004a），乳腺外侧腺体组织形态学正常，但是分子水平异常的比例较高。结合乳腺癌在外侧组织，尤其是外上象限发生率较高的事实，这一发现就格外耐人寻味。详情参照图2.8。

2.5.6 各象限发生乳腺癌的风险不一致

大多数乳腺癌发生在乳腺的外侧象限，尤其是外上象限。这条规律适用于原位癌和浸润性肿瘤。尽管这一现象反映了不少乳腺实质都处于风险中，但是，尚无准确的证据证明。Ellsworth等人（2004a）发现，与内侧象限相比，患乳腺癌的乳房的外侧象限中形态学正常的乳腺组织发生杂合性丢失的趋势较大。他们认为这可能暗示了"区域性癌变"。

外上象限中乳腺实质沿胸大肌的内下边界向外上侧延伸，形成了乳腺腋尾（Spence），这是它的一个明显的独特之处。如果腺叶的发育是一个充满竞争的过程，那么，发育的乳腺中任何占优势的导管都会第一个到达离乳头最远的区域，因此，那个区域中的组织生长能力可能最强。不仅腺叶间分支的深度各不相同（Going, Moffat, 2004），腺叶内不同区域的分支也不一样（Going, 2006）。这是一个可以验证的观点，研究者可以比较腋尾区形态正常的腺体和其他部位的腺体的分子改变，并且观察这些区域的导管范围的不同。

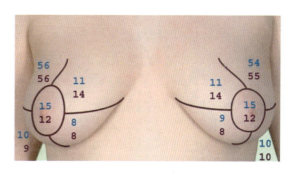

图2.8 原位癌和浸润性癌在双侧乳腺各个象限的位置。数据来源于Perkins等人（2004）。各百分比是根据美国癌症登记处所记录的223 053例浸润性癌（数字标为褐色）以及36 280例原位癌（蓝色数字）的数据而来。原位癌和浸润性癌的分布基本吻合，外上象限是癌症高发的危险地带

说到导管分支的深度与乳腺癌发生风险之间的关系，许多关于乳房大小与患癌风险的研究都有一些结论。尽管结论有些互相矛盾，但是一份大规模研究（Nurses' Health Study Ⅱ）纳入了89 268名护士的健康状况（Kusano, et al, 2006），发现乳房较大的女性患乳腺癌的风险较高，但这种趋势只是存在于那些体重指数<25kg/m²的女性中，因为肥胖这个干扰性因素被排除了。

2.6 乳头及其解剖

前面已经提过乳头中心导管簇的数量之多。这些导管的大小和在乳突顶点的开口都大相径庭。蒙哥马利腺体（Montgomery）是由在乳突侧边或是乳晕处开口的导管组成的，几条导管可能共用一个开口（Rusby, et al, 2007）这点在一定程度上解释了乳头导管簇导管数多，但哺乳时泌乳的导管相对较少的原因。事后再看，乳头处乳腺导管的特点早在旧的出版物上有所暗示；Cooper的图谱集提到了关于共享开口的描述，Cheatle和Cutler（1931）的研究则包含了两条分隔的导管在开口处留下乳汁的显微摄影片。

图2.9展现了乳头导管簇的横切片，展现了导管数目之多和回旋状结构的特点。

图2.10展现了导管内上皮组织/腔面-肌上皮/基底与乳头表面的鳞状角化上皮之间的鳞状-柱状上皮交界。一整条乳头内的导管被DCIS占据，这是不寻常的现象，但没有证据证明这就是Paget病。图片中似乎乳头上皮层抑制了DCIS的扩张，但在Paget病中，病灶在乳头表皮层的定殖现象确实存在。

85%的Paget病中有 *HER2* 基因扩增和过表达现象，这对研究其发病机制有重要作用。由角化细胞产生并释放的调蛋白α是个能动因子，并且Paget细胞表达调蛋白受体Her3和Her4以及它们的辅助受体Her2（Schelfhout, et al, 2000）。调蛋白与Paget细胞表面的受体复

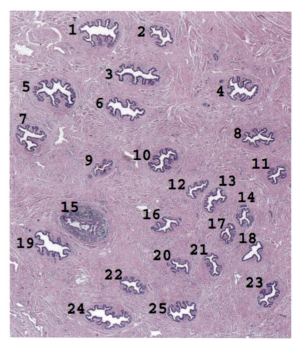

图2.9 乳头上的导管簇切片H和E，低倍显微镜观察。镜下呈现了25条导管，表示存在25个独立的腺叶，并不是所有的腺叶都得到了最好的发育，而且只有一个导管（15）中存在DCIS

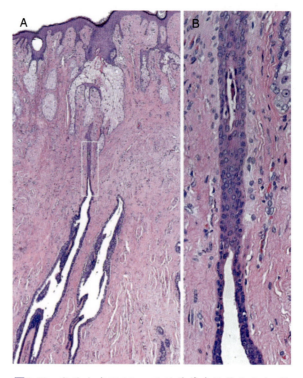

图2.10 乳头上皮下0.5mm处的导管中的鳞状上皮-柱状上皮交界；低倍镜图（A）和高倍镜图（B）。注意此处的导管内空间如此之小

2.6.1 乳头表皮中的透明细胞：Toker 细胞

后来我们意识到了许多乳房中存在一种细胞种群，它们在"病态腺叶"形成的过程中扮演使致瘤化转化风险增大的风险媒介。这些细胞就是Cyril Toker描述的乳头表皮中的"透明细胞"（Toker, 1970），也因此以"Toker细胞"而闻名（图2.12、2.13）。

很明显，类似高级别DCIS的异常细胞能大范围地传播，甚至能传到整个腺叶的导管和腺体组织中。乳腺小叶肿瘤中相对非典型增生程度较低的细胞也有类似行为。没有什么特别的理由解释为何其他易恶变的细胞不存在这样的生物学行为。但是，如果它们没有形态上明显的表型，将会隐藏在乳腺实质的背景里。Toker细胞能代表这样的细胞种群吗？

Toker细胞通常分布在邻近导管出口的乳头表皮细胞中。它们和乳腺腔面上皮细胞一样表达低分子量的细胞角蛋白（细胞角蛋白7、19），曾有人解释说Toker细胞就是乳腺的起源（Marucci, et al, 2002）。尽管在HE切片（10%的病例中）中不太一致，但是免疫组化染色结果（细胞角蛋白）显示它们在乳腺中占了相当大的比例（70%~80%）。从单个稀疏细胞到多个单独细胞和成群的细胞，其数量不尽相同。研究者很有可能把这些细胞认成是Paget细胞了（后者的非典型增生更为剧烈）。

从Toker细胞的分布就可以看出它们在乳头表皮中移动的能力，并且它们的形态学特征，包括细胞凸起呈现出的类片状伪足和线状伪足都支持这一说法（作者未公布的观察结果；图2.13）。尽管Toker细胞清楚明确地表达类固醇激素受体（尽管文献并没有完全赞同这个观点；Garijo, et al, 2009），绝经期后女性乳房中的Toker细胞的数量和绝经期前妇女一样多。Toker细胞偶尔会出现在死亡的角蛋白层中，这表明它们能在本应会失巢凋亡

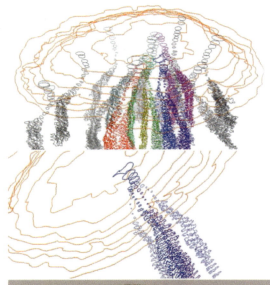

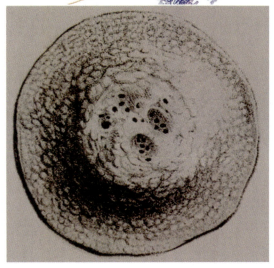

图2.11 乳房切除手术后的乳腺，到达乳头顶点的导管的三维重构图（线框图）。第一张图：可以观察到全部导管。第二张图：四条导管共用一个开口。第三张图：展示了Sir Astley .Cooper描述的开口共享现象。（Cooper, 1840）

合物结合，可能促进了它向乳头上皮层的迁移。因为，正常乳腺导管上皮也表达调蛋白（de Fazio, et al, 2000），所以这个机制也能促进Her2-阳性DCIS在乳腺中的扩张。

图2.11是一副乳腺全切术后乳头局部全部导管的3-D图（尚未公布的），这张图清楚的展示了导管向乳头集中的过程，以及它们公用一个开口的特点。很显然，对这些导管分别进行插管是很困难的。此图与Cooper图册中描述出口的图相当一致。

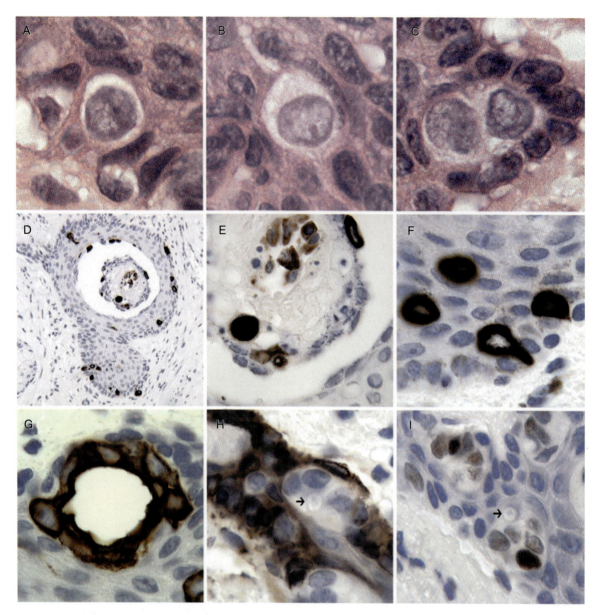

图2.12 乳头表皮中的透明细胞（Toker细胞）。A~C. 苏木精和伊红。A、B. 单个托克细胞与乳腺中或大或小的透明细胞相似；C. 成对的Toker细胞；D~G. CK7免疫染色。D、E. 导管口周围的上皮组织内大量的透明细胞。在角化物填塞充的管腔内也出现了CK7+细胞。F. 细胞多位于基底水平以上，但是向基底层的凸起使得细胞呈现葫芦形。G. 由CK+透明细胞组成的腺泡。H. 相比于周围的角化细胞，透明细胞不表达CK14。图中及I. 图中的箭头标示了内腔的位置。I. Toker细胞的雌激素受体的表达水平不一

的环境中生存下来（图2.12），表现出凋亡抑制。这些都表明Toker细胞的自主性和移动性不仅在可能有关的Paget病中起作用，而且可能与乳腺癌的关系更为密切，尤其是在"病态腺叶"形成过程中可能作为风险载体存在。

很遗憾的是，目前仍没有标记物可以从乳腺上皮中标记出Toker细胞。它们的分子表达谱包括细胞移动、黏附和与移动有关的受体（例如Her3、Her4）等，值得进一步研究。

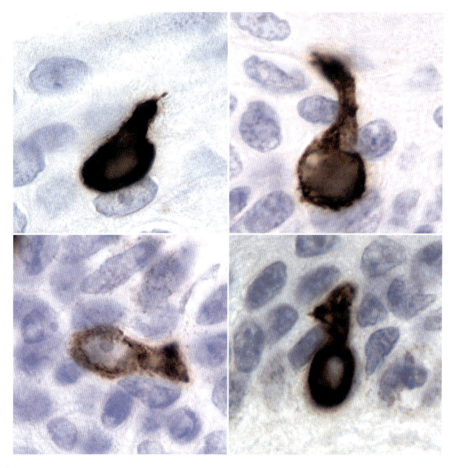

图2.13 用角蛋白7进行免疫组化标记的乳头上皮中的透明细胞（Toker细胞），说明它具有移动性的特点。左上图：这个细胞从线状伪足（"微端丝"）凸起处向外呈类片状伪足式的明显延伸。右上图：一条纺锤状的长凸起。左下和右下图：两个楔型凸起的细胞，其凸起表面呈扁平状，与旁边的角化细胞互相接触

2.7 病态腺叶产生时细胞间的超级竞争

临床上并没有"早期"肿瘤这一说法。数年的时间，细胞经过多轮的克隆扩张（以损害邻近细胞为代价）在组织中建立和巩固突变，在早期突变的基础上累积新的突变，并逐渐增加细胞的数目，为（恶性）肿瘤的最终形成奠定基础。

干细胞紧密地固定在特定的组织巢中，其紧密固定程度的减小都将使竞争性克隆扩张的范围扩大（细胞及其后代修复DNA能力的降低也有利于变异的进一步积累，其中几个机制广为人知）。近期的研究方向已注意到，细胞的竞争和超级竞争可能是一种致癌机制。

细胞竞争现象在果蝇实验中得到了很好的证明（Morata, Ripoll, 1975）。小核糖体基因突变的杂合子细胞能够发育为表型正常的果蝇，而在嵌合体的果蝇中，M/wt细胞将会败给w/wt细胞。同样的现象也会发生在dmyc突变中（(Johnston, et al, 1999），甚至更明显，因为dmyc的过表达产生了胜过野生型细胞的"超级竞争者"细胞（Moreno, Basler, 2004）。超级竞争者细胞的产生也可能是因为Salvador/Warts信号通路异常（Tyler, et al, 2007）。特别重要的一点是，"胜者"细胞群在组织中以损害"败者"细胞为代价进行扩展，然而整个过程没有明显的组织形态学变化，或许Toker细胞就是一种超级竞争细胞。

2.8 乳腺腺叶解剖认识提高的前景

2.8.1 注射研究

将有颜色的或不透射线的液体示踪物、凝胶、树脂、聚合物、液体金属或石蜡（体外和体内）注射到单个导管系统中。这种做法由来已久。这些方法有优点也有缺点。使用合适的液体能很好地显示导管的分支，这无疑就是其中一个优点。但是人类的输乳管十分脆弱，导管外的破裂、渗透现象时有发生；另外，鲜有研究记录过成功注射的导管达到人体内真实的导管数。在文献中很难找到准确计数的导管总数，除了Going的研究。他使用乳房切除术后的乳房标本，制作了乳头基底的乳头导管簇的切片，并通过完整的切片统计了导管数目。他发现中位数为27条导管（范围11~41；Q1 21;,Q3 30）（Going, Moffat, 2004），该数目大于平常在二次文献中引用的数目——11~20条。

由于许多导管系统退化或是发育不全，又缺少准确的数据，这个观点推测的成分很大。但不管怎样，许多注射研究的导管数更少。Khan等人研究了乳头溢液的导管，并成功灌洗了28个乳腺中的39个导管系统（平均每个乳房1.4个）。另一方面，Love and Barsky (2004)对哺乳期女性进行了观察，他们发现乳头开口处排出乳汁的中位导管数为5条；Ramsay等人（2005）发现哺乳期妇女的双侧乳房中，平均每侧有9条导管。最终，这些数据仍不能完全说明问题。某些导管系统的乳腺实质几乎没有功能，可能是退化的系统；有时导管闭合也是另一个因素，导管系统与乳头分离，不能完成泌乳，通过上面提到的机制形成负反馈，从而抑制乳汁的分泌。像这样的主导管或是导管分支的闭合都将对注射研究产生干扰。

2.8.2 导管追踪

乳腺腺叶研究中的另一项主要技术就是导管追踪，即通过一系列染色–还原的厚的（所谓的亚肉眼）切片来研究分支的导管。亚肉眼技术的出现已经有很长的一段历史了，至少可以追溯到Werner Spalteholz的研究中（Spalteholz, 1914）。这种技术被Adolf Dabelow（Dabelow, 1957）和包括Wellings及其同事在内的研究者们广泛使用（Wellings, et al, 1975; Jensen, et al, 1976），而且在发育生物学和实验病理学中被频繁采用。实际上，这一古老的技术仍有新的发展：许多荧光的DNA插入染料与传统的疏水性还原染料如苯甲醇/苯甲酸苄酯、水杨酸甲酯等并不兼容。最近，硫代双乙醇（折射率=1.52）被引进到共聚焦显微镜中，它与DNA染料（Staudt, et al, 2007; Appleton, et al, 2009）兼容，是一种溶于水、毒性低（Reddy, et al, 2005），且折射率高的覆盖介质。这一改进便于镜下观察较厚的标本。改进过的荧光亚肉眼技术将可以运用到乳腺组织中，这项技术的前景是令人激动的。

亚肉眼技术在保证乳腺中所有实质组织均可以被染色和观察上占有较大的优势。但是，作为研究乳腺腺叶解剖的一种方法，尽管它能呈现所有的数据，但其遇到的挑战也是严峻的。在切片和处理的过程中，组织扭曲给辨识带来了很大的问题，即相邻切片的连接点（相似之处）很难被识别，相应的导管追踪也变得困难起来（这些难题在前面探讨Ohtake等人的研究时有所涉及）。

相比于传统大小在15~25mm的小型组织切片，我们能从大的切片中更为直观地观察到相距更远的单位之间的关系。尽管可以构建三维数据，我们仍应该谨慎评估导管的连接情况。如果某个组织块厚达3mm，某导管以10°的角度穿行其中，那么导管横切面将出现超过15mm的侧向移位。这使得我们从来自

3mm厚的组织块的组织切片推断导管连接的情况毫无可信度。

因为包括超声在内的其他成像模式得以运用，传统的X线乳腺导管造影术使用较少，但是MRI（核磁共振成像）乳腺导管造影术在腺叶解剖上仍有十分大的潜力。然而，它也面临着其他导管注射技术都会遇到的挑战，包括造影剂外渗、注射导管数过少以及很难区分不同的导管系统（尽管成功注射过多条导管）。

现在是结合其他新技术来推动乳腺生物学和病理学研究的好时机。分子生物学分析和形态学分析都是有力的分析方法，把两者结合起来就是强有力的分析方法。乳腺癌的复杂性超乎我们的想象。就本身而言，还没有最好的研究方法。"病态腺叶"假说让我们对乳腺癌在时间和空间上的发展提出了疑问，也让我们意识到将注意力集中在几立方毫米之间是远远不够的。当我们了解了这些导管间是如何连接的之后，我们就能够在导管树的不同部分间分析分子事件，从而可以验证那些尚未印证的假说。

我们几乎拥有所有的必须工具：与甲醛相比，对核酸、蛋白质和其他生物分子损伤更小的固定剂；灵敏的专门显示结构的荧光性染料；新的与染料适配的组织还原剂——硫代双乙醇（Staudt, et al, 2007）；用于结构存储、提取、可视化的数据处理技术以及全部的分子生物学技术。

奇怪的是，有一个看起来似乎简单但实际上很难的挑战：制作大量组织结构没有扭曲的厚切片，这是完成切片间导管准确追踪以及腺叶重构的关键。通常，研究者们一直采用长时间甲醛浸泡和琼脂深低温固定办法。Egan还采用了超低温冷冻组织切片方法（Egan, et al, 1969; Egan, 1982）。然而，这两种方法都不是最理想的，也都没有摆脱人工制剂。

真正的挑战是直接在手术台上取走没有固定的乳腺组织——或许是诊断性活检组织、局部扩大切除术后标本或是乳房切除术的组织——在数分钟的时间内将组织切成2~3mm厚的切片。每一个切片都附着在结构稳定的基层上进行理想的固定、染色、组织还原、可视化，收集数据，进行随后的3D分析。随后进行传统的组织学处理、免疫组织化学和其他临床需要的分子分析。完成这些步骤所需的时间，绝不会比我们在传统组织学中花费的更长。我们没有理由认为这是不可能的。这样一项技术能使我们在评估诊断性问题如原位癌和浸润性癌是否切除完整时更加准确。并且，实现这样一项技术也是我们梦寐以求的目标。

2.9 结　语

本章的主题围绕着Astley Cooper的研究开展。此时，我们应该再看一眼Sir Astley的工作，在他著作的版面V的图1（图2.14）中，他阐明了哺乳期乳房中的不同部位腺体的发

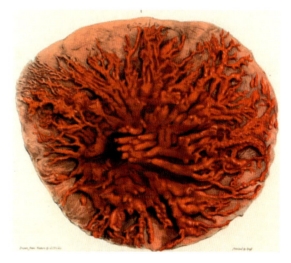

图2.14 《论乳房解剖》版面V图1。Cooper的配文为"哺乳期死亡的女性的乳腺，用红色石蜡注射入输乳管。12条导管被注满，开口处结扎。我们观察到导管在乳腺的底部形成大的储液腔；这些储液腔被认为是无数导管分支联合而成的。导管终止于与分支接触的腺体边缘，少数导管则到达腺泡。"腺泡组织在3~5点和10~11点位置最明显。这可能是第一部提出人体乳腺腺叶间存在明显生物学差异的观点的著作

育程度，他特别关注这一点。这可能是第一部指出人类乳腺不同腺叶间存在不同分化潜能差异的著作。考虑到某些腺叶若不能成功泌乳（并且腺叶分化受损）可能会升高乳腺癌风险，那么这也可能暗示了"病态腺叶"的存在。

1840年，Cooper首次为乳腺组织腺叶结构奠定科学基础，现在在这个后基因组的时代，这个"古老的"项目变得更加重要。看到这一点，我们感到非常欣慰，也深深感觉到理念的传承是多么有趣的一件事情。

参考文献

[1] Appleton PL, Quyn AJ, Swift S, et al. Preparation of wholemount mouse intestine for high-resolution three-dimensional imaging using two-photon microscopy. J Microsc, 2009, 234：196-204.

[2] Ariazi JL, Haag JD, Lindstrom MJ, et al. Mammary glands of sexually immature rats are more susceptible than those of mature rats to the carcinogenic, lethal, and mutagenic effects of N-nitroso-N-methylurea. Mol Carcinog, 2005, 43：155-164.

[3] VAzzopardi JG. Problems in breast pathology. London: W.B. Saunders, 1979.

[4] Brock RC. The life and work of Astley Cooper. Edinburgh: E. & S. Livingstone, 1952.

[5] Campeau PM, Foulkes WD, Tischkowitz MD. Hereditary breast cancer: new genetic developments, new therapeutic avenues. Hum Genet, 2008, 124：31-42.

[6] Cheatle GL. Clinical remarks on the early recognition of cancer of the breast. Br Med J, 1906, 1：1205-1210.

[7] VCheatle GL. Cysts and primary cancer in cysts, of the breast. Br J Surg VIII, 1920：149-166.

[8] Cheatle GL, Cutler M. Tumours of the breast: their pathology, symptoms, diagnosis and treatment. London: Edward Arnold, 1931.

[9] Chen DT, Nasir A, Culhane A, et al. VProliferative genes dominate malignancy-risk gene signature in histologically-normal breast tissue. Breast Cancer Res Treat, 2009. doi：10.1007/s10549-009-0344-y

[10] Cooper AP. On the anatomy of the breast. London: Longman, Orme, Green, Brown and Longmans, 1840.

[11] Cooper BB. The life of Sir Astley Cooper. London: John W. Parker, 1843.

[12] Dabelow A. Die Milchdruse. Berlin: Springer, 1957.

[13] VDavies JA. Do different branching epithelia use a conserved developmental mechanism. Bioessays, 2002, 24：937-948.

[14] Fazio A, Chiew YE, Sini RL, et al. Expression of cerbB receptors, heregulin and oestrogen receptor in human breast cell lines. Int J Cancer, 2000, 87：487-498.

[15] Dooley WC. Breast ductoscopy and the evolution of the intraductal approach to breast cancer. Breast J, 2009, 15 (Suppl 1)：S90-S94.

[16] Egan RL. Multicentric breast carcinomas: clinical-radio-graphic-pathologic whole organ studies and 10-year survival. Cancer, 1982, 49：1123-1130.

[17] Egan RL, Ellis JT, Powell RW. Team approach to the study of diseases of the breast. Cancer, 1969, 23：847-854.

[18] Ellsworth DL, Ellsworth RE, Love B, et al. Outer breast quadrants demonstrate increased levels of genomic instability. Ann Surg Oncol, 2004a, 11：861-868.

[19] Ellsworth DL, Ellsworth RE, Love B, et al. Genomic patterns of allelic imbalance in disease free tissue adjacent to primary breast carcinomas. Breast Cancer Res Treat, 2004b, 88：131-139.

[20] Ewing J. Neoplastic diseases: a treatise on tumours. Philadelphia: WB Saunders, 1940

[21] Faulkin LJ Jr, DeOme KB. Regulation of growth and spacing of gland elements in the mammary fat pad of the C3H mouse. J Natl Cancer Inst, 1960, 24：953-969.

[22] Faverly D, Holland R, Burgers L. An original stereomi-croscopic analysis of the mammary glandular tree. Virchows Arch A Pathol Anat

Histopathol, 1992, 421: 115-119.
[23] Fiala JC. Reconstruct: a free editor for serial section microscopy. J Microsc, 2005, 218: 52-61.
[24] Fialkow PJ. Clonal origin of human tumors. Biochim Biophys Acta, 1976, 458: 283-321.
[25] Fleck L. The genesis and development of a scientific fact. Chicago: University of Chicago Press, 1979.
[26] Foote FWJ, Stewart FW. Lobular carcinoma in situ. A rare form of mammary cancer. Am J Pathol, 1941, 17: 491-496.
[27] Foschini MP, Flamminio F, Miglio R, et al. The impact of large sections and 3D technique on the study of lobular in situ and invasive carcinoma of the breast. Virchows Arch, 2006, 448: 256-261.
[28] Garijo MF, Val D, Val-Bernal JF. An overview of the pale and clear cells of the nipple epidermis. Histol Histopathol, 2009, 24: 367-376.
[29] Geddes DT. Inside the lactating breast: the latest anatomy research. J Midwifery Womens Health, 2007, 52: 556-563.
[30] Going JJ. Ductal-lobar organisation of human breast tissue, its relevance in disease and a research objective: vector mapping of parenchyma in complete breasts (the Astley Cooper project). Breast Cancer Res, 2006, 8: 107.
[31] Going JJ, Moffat DF. Escaping from Flatland: clinical and biological aspects of human mammary duct anatomy in three dimensions. J Pathol, 2004, 203: 538-544.
[32] Going JJ, Mohun TJ. Human breast duct anatomy, the 'sick lobe' hypothesis and intraductal approaches to breast cancer. Breast Cancer Res Treat, 2006, 97: 285-291.
[33] Holland R, Connolly JL, Gelman R, et al. The presence of an extensive intraductal component following a limited excision correlates with prominent residual disease in the remainder of the breast. J Clin Oncol, 1990a, 8: 113-118.
[34] Holland R, Hendriks JH, Vebeek AL, et al. Extent, distribution, and mammo-graphic/histological correlations of breast ductal carcinoma in situ. Lancet, 1990b, 335 (8688): 519-522.
[35] Jain S, Rezo A, Shadbolt B, et al. Synchronous multiple ipsilateral breast cancers: implications for patient management. Pathology, 2009, 41: 57-67.
[36] Jensen HM, Rice JR, Wellings SR. Preneoplastic lesions in the human breast. Science, 1976, 191(4224): 295-297.
[37] Johnson JE, Page DL, Winfeld AC, et al. Recurrent mammary carcinoma after local excision. A segmental problem. Cancer, 1995, 75: 1612-1618.
[38] Johnston LA, Prober DA, Edgar BA, et al. Drosophila myc regulates cellular growth during development. Cell, 1999, 98: 779-790.
[39] Khan SA, Wiley EL, Rodriguez N, et al. Ductal lavage fndings in women with known breast cancer undergoing mastectomy. J Natl Cancer Inst, 2004, 96: 1510-1517.
[40] Kordon EC, Smith GH. An entire functional mammary gland may comprise the progeny from a single cell. Development, 1998, 125: 1921-1930.
[41] Kusano AS, Trichopoulos D, Terry KL, et al. A prospective study of breast size and premenopausal breast cancer incidence. Int J Cancer, 2006, 118: 2031-2034.
[42] Lakatos I. Proofs and refutations. Cambridge: Cambridge University Press, 1976.
[43] Land CE. Studies of cancer and radiation dose among atomic bomb survivors. The example of breast cancer. JAMA, 1995, 274: 402-407.
[44] Lee WC, Davies JA. Epithelial branching: the power of self-loathing. Bioessays, 2007, 29: 205-207.
[45] Love SM, Barsky SH. Anatomy of the nipple and breast ducts revisited. Cancer, 2004, 101: 1947-1957.
[46] Maley CC. Multistage carcinogenesis in Barrett's esophagus. Cancer Lett, 2007, 245: 22-32.
[47] Maley CC, Galipeau PC, Li X, et al. Selectively advantageous mutations and hitchhikers in neoplasms: p16 lesions are selected in Barrett's esophagus. Cancer Res, 2004, 64: 3414-3427.
[48] Marucci G, Betts CM, Golouh R, et al. Toker cells are probably precursors of Paget cell carcinoma: a morphological and ultrastructural description. Virchows Arch, 2002, 441: 117-123.
[49] Marusic A. Jelena Krmpotic Namanic (1921-

2008): conclusion of age of classical anatomy. Croat Med J, 2008, 49: 447-449.

[50] Meeker AK, Hicks JL, Gabrielson E, et al. Telomere shortening occurs in subsets of normal breast epithelium as well as in situ and invasive carcinoma. Am J Pathol, 2004, 164: 925-935.

[51] Moffat DF, Going JJ. Three dimensional anatomy of complete duct systems in human breast: pathological and developmental implications. J Clin Pathol, 1996, 49: 48-52.

[52] Moller A, Soler M, Thornhill R. Breast asymmetry, sexual selection, and human reproductive success. Ethol Sociobiol, 1995, 16: 207-219.

[53] Morata G, Ripoll P. Minutes: mutants of drosophila auton-omously affecting cell division rate. Dev Biol, 1975, 42: 211-221.

[54] Moreno E, Basler K. dMyc transforms cells into super-competitors. Cell, 2004, 117: 117-129.

[55] Ohtake T, Abe R, Kimijima I, et al. Intraductal extension of primary invasive breast carcinoma treated by breast-conservative surgery. Computer graphic three-dimensional reconstruction of the mammary duct-lobular systems. Cancer, 1995, 76: 32-45.

[56] Ohtake T, Kimijima I, Fukushima T, et al. Computer-assisted complete three-dimensional reconstruction of the mammary ductal/lobular systems: implications of ductal anastomoses for breast-conserving surgery. Cancer, 2001, 91: 2263-2272.

[57] Ohuchi N. Breast-conserving surgery for invasive cancer: a principle based on segmental anatomy. Tohoku J Exp Med, 1999, 188: 103-118.

[58] Ohuchi N, Abe R, Kasai M. Possible cancerous change of intraductal papillomas of the breast. A 3-D reconstruction study of 25 cases. Cancer, 1984a, 54: 605-611.

[59] Ohuchi N, Abe R, Takahashi T, et al. Origin and extension of intraductal papillomas of the breast: a three-dimensional reconstruction study. Breast Cancer Res Treat, 1984b, 4: 117-128.

[60] Ohuchi N, Abe R, Takahashi T, et al. Three-dimensional atypical structure in intraductal carcinoma differentiating from papilloma and papillomatosis of the breast. Breast Cancer Res Treat, 1985, 5: 57-65.

[61] Osteen RT. Strategies for breast-conserving surgery. An unresolved dilemma. Cancer, 1995, 75: 1563-1565, discussion 1566-1567.

[62] Page DL, Schuyler PA, Dupont WD, et al. Atypical lobular hyperplasia as a unilateral predictor of breast cancer risk: a retrospective cohort study. Lancet, 2003, 361 (9352): 125-129.

[63] Parsons BL. Many different tumor types have polyclonal tumor origin: evidence and implications. Mutat Res, 2008, 659: 232-247.

[64] Perkins CI, Hotes J, Kohler BA, et al. Association between breast cancer laterality and tumor location, United States, 1994-1998. Cancer Causes Control, 2004, 15: 637-645.

[65] Preston SL, Wong WM, Chan AOO, et al. Bottom-up histogenesis of colorectal adenomas: origin in the monocryptal adenom and initial expansion by crypt fssion. Cancer Res, 2003, 63: 3819-3825.

[66] Ramsay DT, Kent JC, Hartmann RA, et al. Anatomy of the lactating human breast redefned with ultra-sound imaging. J Anat, 2005, 206: 525-534.

[67] Reddy G, Major MA, Leach GJ. Toxicity assessment of thiodiglycol. Int J Toxicol, 2005, 24: 435-442.

[68] Rusby JE, Brachtel EF, Michaelson JS, et al. Breast duct anatomy in the human nipple: three-dimensional patterns and clinical implications. Breast Cancer Res Treat, 2007, 106: 171-179.

[69] Schelfhout VR, Coene ED, Delaey B, et al. Pathogenesis of Paget's disease: epidermal heregulin-alpha, motility factor, and the HER receptor family. J Natl Cancer Inst, 2000, 92: 622-628.

[70] Scutt D, Lancaster GA, Manning JT. Breast asymmetry and predisposition to breast cancer. Breast Cancer Res, 2006, 8: R14.

[71] Sharpe CR. A developmental hypothesis to explain the multicentricity of breast cancer. CMAJ, 1998, 159: 55-59.

[72] Sinn HP. Breast cancer precursors: lessons learned from molecular genetics. J Mol Med, 2009, 87:

113-115.

[73] Spalteholz KW. Ueber das Durehsichti- gmachen von Menschlichen und Tierischen Preparaten. S. Hirzel, Stuttgart, 1914.

[74] Staudt T, Lang MC, Medda R, et al. 2¢-thiodieth-anol: a new water soluble mounting medium for high resolution optical microscopy. Microsc Res Tech, 2007, 70: 1-9.

[75] Stolier AJ, Wang J. Terminal duct lobular units are scarce in the nipple: implications for prophylactic nipple-sparing mastectomy: terminal duct lobular units in the nipple. Ann Surg Oncol, 2008, 15: 438-442.

[76] Stull MA, Pai V, Vomachka AJ, et al. Mammary gland homeostasis employs serotonergic regulation of epithelial tight junctions. Proc Natl Acad Sci USA, 2007, 104: 16708–16713.

[77] Thorlacius S, Thorlacius S, Olafsdottir G, et al. A single BRCA2 muta-tion in male and female breast cancer families from Iceland with varied cancer phenotypes. Nat Genet, 1996, 13: 117-119.

[78] Toker C. Clear cells of the nipple epidermis. Cancer, 1970, 25: 601-610.

[79] Tokunaga M, Land CE, Tokuoka S, et al. Incidence of female breast cancer among atomic bomb survivors (1950-1985). Radiat Res, 1994, 138: 209-223.

[80] Tondre J, Nejad M, Casano A, et al. Technical enhancements to breast ductal lavage. Ann Surg Oncol, 2008, 15: 2734-2738.

[81] Tot T, Tabar L, Dean PB. The pressing need for better histologic-mammographic correlation of the many variations in normal breast anatomy. Virchows Arch, 2000, 437: 338-344.

[82] Tripathi A, King C, de la Morenas A, et al. Gene expression abnormalities in histologically normal breast epithelium of breast cancer patients. Int J Cancer, 2008, 122: 1557-1566.

[83] Tyler DM, Li W, Zhuo N, Pellock B, et al. Genes affecting cell competition in Drosophila. Genetics, 2007, 175: 643-657.

[84] von Gerlach J. Handbuch der allgemeinen and speciellen Gewebelehre des menschlichen Korpers fur Aerzte und Studirende. Mainz: Janitsch, 1848.

[85] Wellings SR, Jensen HM, Marcum RG. An atlas of subgross pathology of the human breast with special reference to possible precancerous lesions. J Natl Cancer Inst, 1975, 55: 231-273.

[86] Wilde CJ, Addey CV, Boddy LM, et al. Autocrine regulation of milk secretion by a protein in milk. Biochem J, 1995, 305: 51-58.

[87] Yan PS, Venkataramu C, Ibrahim A, et al. Mapping geographic zones of cancer risk with epigenetic biomarkers in normal breast tissue. Clin Cancer Res, 2006, 12: 6626-6636.

[88] Yang CP, Weiss NS, Band PR, et al. History of lactation and breast cancer risk. Am J Epidemiol, 1993, 138: 1050-1056.

第3章 乳腺癌可能起源于子宫：子宫内环境对乳腺癌发生的重要性

Fei Xue, Karin B. Michels

3.1 引 言

乳腺癌是全球女性最常见的癌症，死亡率仅次于肺癌，高居因癌死亡的第二位（美国癌症协会，2009）。乳腺癌的发病率在不同国家相差4~5倍，欧洲和北美最高，亚洲最低（Ferlay, et al, 2001）。自1930年代开始，其发病率不断攀升，1980年代更是上升迅速（White, et al, 1990; Devesa, et al, 1994）。2001—2003年乳腺癌在美国的发病率相对稳定，并从2013年开始下降，在某种程度上可能是因为激素替代疗法的使用量减少（Howe, et al, 2006）。据预测，2010年将有207 090名妇女会罹患浸润性乳腺癌，39 840名妇女将死于该病（美国癌症协会，2010）。

经过几十年的研究，一级亲属患乳腺癌的家族史、良性乳腺疾病、乳腺密度、内源激素水平、较小的初潮年龄、产次、初产年龄、绝经年龄、绝经后激素的使用、电离辐射、绝经后过高或过低的体重指数等一系列因素已经被确立为乳腺癌的危险因素（Adami, et al, 2002）。尽管如此，只有少量比例的乳腺癌病例是源于公认的危险因素（Madigan, et al, 1995），而关于乳腺癌病因的流行病学研究将关注点更多地集中在女性生育期间上。本章从另一个角度出发，回顾了子宫内暴露影响乳腺癌发生发展的证据，并讨论了可能的潜在机制，包括妊娠期类固醇激素、生长因子水平的变化以及它们对胎儿期的乳腺干细胞的影响等。

3.2 宫内暴露与乳腺癌风险

在早期的动物实验中，通过子宫壁将致癌剂（溶于橄榄油的二苯蒽）直接注射入23只雌性孕鼠的羊水中，其中有19例（82.6%）生育的后代患上了原发性肺癌（Law, 1940）。其他动物的研究也表明，当怀孕的动物被暴露于38种化学致癌物质中的任何一种时，其后代更容易患肿瘤（Tomatis, 1979）。与来自动物的研究结果一样，接触过致癌物如乙烯雌酚（DES）的女性，其后代患阴道腺癌的风险增加（Greenwald, et al, 1971）。此外，宫内接触电离辐射被认为与小儿白血病以及其他儿童肿瘤有关（Macmahon, 1962）。

基于早期动物和人类研究获取的证据，Trichopoulos推测胎儿在子宫内暴露于高浓度内源性雌激素后可能会诱发乳腺癌，围产期因素同子宫内雌激素暴露具有同样的作用（Trichopoulos, 1990a、b）。随后，大量的流行病学研究已经进行了各种潜在宫内接触的因素检测，包括出生体重和其他出生时的检测数据、

F. Xue
Obstetrics and Gynecology Epidemiology Division,
Department of Obstetrics, Gynecology and Reproductive
Biology, Brigham and Women's Hospital, Harvard Medical
School, Boston, MA, USA and
Department of Epidemiology,
Harvard School of Public Health,
Boston, MA, USA
e-mail：n2fei@channing.harvard.edu

分娩年龄、孕周、双胞胎、辐射以及其他妊娠并发症和产妇特点（Xue，Michels，2007a）。

3.2.1 出生体重

出生时体重作为宫内接触胰岛素类生长因子（IGF）-I（Bennett，et al，1983；Reece，et al，1994），IGF-II（Bennett，et al，1983；Reece，et al，1994；Baldwin，et al，1993；Hill，1990）和雌激素（Petridou，et al，1990；Liehr，2000）的潜在标记，是乳腺癌相关研究中讨论最多的宫内因素。超过30篇文献共同指出：相对低出生体重者，高出生体重者罹患乳腺癌的风险将增加15%~25%（Michels，Xue，2006；Xue，Michels，2007A；Park，et al，2008；Xu，et al，2009），其标准阈值通常分别为：>4 000g为高出生体重和<2 500g为低出生体重。近期，关于乳腺癌与出生体重的关系的一项合并了29项研究的分析，共纳入21 825例乳腺癌患者，结果表明相对于3000~3499g的出生体重，那些体重≥4000g的出生者患乳腺癌的风险更高。相对危险度（RR）=1.12，95%CI 1.00~1.25（Dos Silva，et al，2008）。将乳腺癌病例根据绝经状态进行独立评估时，绝经前患乳腺癌的概率高于绝经后（Michels，Xue，2006）。这种关联在不同的研究设计（病例对照或队列）、不同的出生体重评估方法（出生记录、自我报告、由母亲报告等），以及不同的国家均存在。此外，出生体重和乳腺癌的风险之间的关联不受其他已测量的宫内因素影响，如孕周、出生长度、产妇先兆子痫或子痫、妊娠年龄、出生顺序、父母吸烟、或者多胎妊娠等（Michels，Xue，2006）。

3.2.2 分娩时母亲的年龄

高龄产妇血清中雌激素水平较高，可能使胎儿暴露于这种高水平的激素中（Petridou，et al，1990；Panagiotopoulou，et al，1990）。至少有16项研究已经表明产妇分娩年龄对其女儿患乳腺癌风险有着潜在影响（Xue，et al，2006；Park，et al，2008；Nichols，et al，2008）。大多数研究表明，无论绝经与否，母亲分娩年龄越大，女儿患乳腺癌的概率越高（Xue，Michels，2007 a；Par，et al，2008）。一项meta分析表明，女儿患乳腺癌的风险随母亲分娩年龄的增高而显著增加，最高达13%，这种关联性在队列研究和病例对照研究中同时存在。研究中，高龄产妇的的分界点为近30岁至约40岁。以上分析结果在绝经前乳腺癌和绝经后乳腺癌中没有显著差异（Xue，Michels，2007a）。一些研究将父亲年龄和出生顺序作为潜在的混杂因素，这两者都可能与产妇年龄相关。以父亲年龄进行调整后，结果出现变化：在一些研究(Le Marchand，et al，1988；Zhang，et al，1995；Hemminki，Kyyronen，1999；Xue，et al，2006)中，上述关联性减弱，但在其他人（Janerich，et al，1989；Innes，et al，2000；Choi，et al，2005）的研究中仍然保持不变。出生顺序的影响力较小，以出生顺序调整后，产妇年龄与乳腺癌间的关联性在几乎所有相关研究中保持不变（Xue，Michels，2007a）。

3.2.3 分娩时的父亲年龄

高龄父亲的孩子患常染色体显性遗传疾病的可能性高，这与其精子更可能发生碱基置换和染色体结构异常有关（Jung，et al，2003；Glaser，Jabs，2004）。因为精子细胞在出生后继续分裂，卵子细胞保持稳定，所以，随着年龄的增长，相比母系，父系更易出现减数分裂错误（Jung，et al，2003）。此外，生殖细胞响应诱变剂而凋亡的能力和DNA修复活性随着父亲年龄增加而下降（Wei，et al，1993；Brinkworth，2000）。至少有11项研究探讨了父亲年龄高是女儿患乳腺癌的潜在危险因素（Xue，Michels，2007a；Weiss-Salz，et al，2007），这些研究结果共同表明罹患乳腺癌的风险会随着父亲年龄增加而提高将近10%（年龄分界点从30出头到近40岁）。针对绝经前乳腺癌患者的研究表明，其患病率与父亲年龄有着中等强度的关系（Xue, Michels, 2007a; Weiss-Salz, et al, 2007），目前还没有针对绝经后乳腺癌患者的相关研究。不考虑父亲年龄与母亲年龄之间的潜在共线性关系，在将产妇年龄作为一个潜在混杂变量后，8项研究（Le Marchand, et al, 1988; Janerich, et al, 1989; Zhang, et al, 1995; Hemminki, Kyyronen, 1999; Innes, et al, 2000; Hodgson, et al, 2004; Choi, et al, 2005; Xue, et al, 2006）中有2项研究（Janerich, et al, 1989; Choi, et al, 2005）表明父亲年龄与乳腺癌患病率仍然存在显著相关性。类似对产妇分娩年龄的研究，针对父亲年龄的多数研究将出生顺序作为一个潜在的混杂变量考虑，结果显示基本不受影响（Xue, Michels, 2007a）。

3.2.4 出生顺序

初次妊娠期间，孕期雌激素水平高于二次和后几次的妊娠期（Panagiotopoulou, et al, 1990）。雌二醇、雌酮、黄体酮水平也是初次妊娠时最高，在以后的妊娠期逐渐减少（Maccoby, et al, 1979）。因而，相较于以后的胎次，头胎胎儿在子宫内接触预期激素的水平更高。一项meta分析纳入17项已发表的研究，包括15项病例对照研究和2项队列研究，对出生顺序和乳腺癌之间的关联关系进行研究（Park, et al, 2008）。有14项研究将初产与二产或更高产次进行比较，结果表明，其成年后患乳腺癌的风险没有显著差异（全部研究中，合并RR = 0.97, 95%CI 0.91~1.04）。病例对照研究中（OR=0.99, 95%CI 0.94~1.04），仅有1项队列研究表明，初产患乳腺癌的风险更小（OR=0.28, 95%CI 0.21~0.36）。针对更高产次的研究表明，产次在2~4次（包括4次）的患病风险无明显变化（OR=0.97, 95%CI 0.91~1.03），但产次≥5的女性罹患乳腺癌的风险会出现轻微的下降（a marginal reduced risk）（OR=0.88, 95%CI 0.75~1.01）。最近一项病例对照研究显示，选择母乳喂养的女性中，婴儿期母乳喂养状况可能影响出生顺序与乳腺癌之间的关系，因为母乳喂养时，出生顺序与患乳腺癌风险之间呈负相关（Nichols, et al, 2008）。

3.2.5 孕周

孕周也被认为是乳腺癌的风险因素，主要因为孕周长短与下丘脑的发育程度密切相关，从而决定了出生后促性腺激素的水平。事实上，出生后的最初10周，孕周较短的女婴的促性腺激素水平相当高（Tapanainen, et al, 1981），这将造成卵巢过度刺激，进而提高雌激素水平，升高患乳腺癌的发生风险（Ekbom, et al, 1981）。此外，存活下来的早产女婴很可能出现加速的产后发育，这被认为将使她们存在更高的患乳腺癌风险（Forman, et al, 2005）。到目前为止，关于孕周与乳腺癌之间关联性的研究至少有12项（Xue, Michels, 2007a; Park, et al, 2008）。不考虑生物学上的解释，这些研究在关联性的正负方向与显著与否上都有着相当不一致的结论。以往研究对较短孕周的界定为≤32周至<39周，对较长孕周的界定为≥35周至≥42周。基于以上研究的meta分析表明孕周或者早产与乳腺癌没有显著相关性（Xue, Michels, 2007a; Park, et al, 2008）。分开考虑绝经前和绝经后乳腺癌，孕周与乳腺癌的发病率没有显著相关性。队列研究与病例对照研究的方式对结果没有影响。出生体重、出生顺序、乳腺癌家族病史以及其他幼年因素对评估孕周的影响都很小（Xue, Michels, 2007a）。

3.2.6 出生体长

作为较强的体重关联因素，出生长度可能通过相同的潜在机制影响乳腺癌的发病率，如宫内雌激素、IGF-1以及 IGF-II的暴露增加。而出生长度确实被证实与母亲血液中雌激素的水平呈正相关（(Troisi, et al, 2003a; Mucci, et al, 2003）。到目前为止，已发表的关于出生长度与乳腺癌患病率之间的关联性研究的文献至少有8篇。Meta分析表明，相较于较短出生长度（≤44cm至<50cm），较长出生长度（≥49cm与≥53 cm）患乳腺癌的风险将近增加28%（95% CI 11%~48%）（Xue, Michels, 2007a）。此外，最近一项汇总11项发表或未发表的研究，涉及3 612项病例的分析表明，出生长度≥51cm的女性相较于<49cm的女性其乳腺癌的发病率显著增加，可达17%（95%CI 2%~35%）（Dos Silva, et al, 2008）。单独评估绝经前癌症与绝经后癌症的两项研究中，相较于绝经后乳腺癌，出生长度与绝经前乳腺癌更具有相关性（Mc Cormack, et al, 2003；Vatten, et al, 2005）。其他出生大小数据例如体重、头围，是出生长度与乳腺癌患病率的可能混杂因素。然而，这些因素不能完全解释观察到的出生长度与乳腺癌发病率之间的关联性（Mc Cormack, et al, 2003）。

3.2.7 己烯雌酚（DES）

1938—1971年，己烯雌酚（diethylstilbestrol, DES）作为一种合成雌激素，在美国被用于保胎以防止流产或早产。出生前暴露于DES的青春期少女患阴道腺癌的风险增加（Greenwald, et al, 1971）。这一研究表明，癌症可能起源于子宫内。Trichopoulos后来推测，出生前暴露于较高水平的雌激素可能增加出生后患乳腺癌的风险（Trichopoulos, 1990 a、b）。迄今为止，DES和乳腺癌的风险之间的关联性至少在5项研究（Weiss, et al, 1997；Hatch, et al, 1998；Sanderson, et al, 1998；Palmer, et al, 2002；Troisi, et al, 2007）中被探讨，其中的两项研究（Hatch, et al, 1998；Palmer, et al, 2002）有更新的数据报告，其余3项研究中只有1个将产前暴露于DES的女性与没有暴露的女性进行对比，对乳腺癌整体风险（RR=1.40，95%CI 0.86~2.28）和绝经前乳腺癌风险（RR=1.87，95%CI 0.72~4.83）进行了研究（Palmer, et al, 2002）。另一项meta分析合并了其余3项研究，表明产前暴露于DES的女性患绝经后乳腺癌的合并RR为1.37（95%CI 0.86~2.18）（Xue, Michels, 2007a）。对其他早期暴露的变量，包括第一次接触DES的孕周等，作为潜在的混杂因素被调整后，该关联性基本保持不变（Hatch, et al, 1998）。

3.2.8 双胞胎

与单胎妊娠相比，双胞胎可能引起两倍水平的妊娠相关激素，包括雌激素（TambyRaja, Ratnam, 1981；Gonzalez, et al, 1989）、促性腺激素和泌乳素（Thiery, et al, 1977）。此外，异卵双胞胎相比同卵双胞胎可能引起更高水平的妊娠相关激素，因为他们有两个胎盘（Kappel, et al, 1985）。相反，由于多胎妊娠可能因孕期并发症在早期终止妊娠，双胎可能会比单胎妊娠经历更短的宫内激素暴露。尽管现有研究关于孕周和患乳腺癌风险之间的关联性结论并不一致，但是，持续时间较长的宫内妊娠激素暴露可能增加产后患乳腺癌的风险。至少有14项研究调查了双胎妊娠和乳腺癌患病率之间的关联性（Xue, Michels, 2007 a；Park, et al, 2008）。不考虑乳腺癌病例中的绝经状态，这些研究表明，与单胎妊娠相比，双胞胎的患病风险降低约7%（轻微统计学显著）。当分别检验绝经前和绝经后的乳腺癌病例时，其相关性与前述合并分析结果类似（Xue, Michels, 2007a）。有趣的是，将同卵双胞胎和异卵双胞胎进行单独分析时，尽管纳入研究的结果是异质性的，但是，异卵双胞胎成员患乳腺癌的风险轻微增加；同卵双胞胎成员的风险降低（Xue, Michels, 2007a）。这些结果表明，尽管异卵双胞胎早期终止妊娠而减少了激素暴露的持续时间，但是异卵双胞胎的双胎盘诱发的额外孕激素可能抵消了以上作用。较高、超重或年纪大的女性，或非西班牙裔的黑人女性，更有可能怀上异卵双胞胎，这些因素可能也是造成与同卵双胞胎患乳腺癌的风险特征不同的原因（Shipley, et al, 1967；Oleszczuk, et al, 2001；Hamilton, et al, 2006）。不过，确认这些假设需要更多的数据，特别是直接评价双胞胎与乳腺癌患病率关联性的研究——异卵与同卵双胞胎相比（Swerdlow, et al, 1997）或异性与同性双胞胎相比（Swerdlow, et al, 1996）并没有得出任何显著差异之后。

3.2.9 先兆子痫和子痫

先兆子痫和子痫的特征在于妊娠相关的高血压和水肿是否发作。患有先兆子痫或子痫孕妇的血液（Zeisler, et al, 2002）以及尿（Long, et al, 1979）中的雌激素水平比没有这些疾病或症状的孕妇低。此外，先兆子痫和子痫可引起妊娠早期终止，因为它们会增加孕产妇和胎儿的并发症发生率和死亡率，特别是在孕晚期。相较于正常妊娠后出生的女孩，母亲患有先兆子痫或子痫的女孩患乳腺癌的风险预期将会降低，因为她们宫内接触雌激素和其他妊娠期激素的累计量较少。迄今为止，先兆子痫或子痫对乳腺癌发病率影响的研究至少有6项，对它们的meta分析表明，相较于正常妊娠，先兆子痫或子痫孕妇患乳腺癌的风险显著降低（52%），尽管纳入研究的作用评估存在异质性（Xue, Michels, 2007a）。多胎妊娠和孕前产妇的人体测量因素可能是这种关联性的混在因素，但当前这些研究并未考虑这些因素。

3.2.10 其他宫内暴露

除上述宫内因素或已被广泛研究的宫内曝光标记物外，尽管缺乏证据，其他一些因素也被认为是乳腺癌的风险因素。宫内接触电离辐射可能导致后续癌症风险已经因广岛和长崎原子弹爆炸后的影响被广泛认知。与母亲未暴露于核弹辐射的儿童相比，在子宫中受过原子弹爆炸辐射的孩子更可能患各种癌症，特别是小儿癌症（Kato, et al, 1989）。此外，尽管没有宫内数据的报告，但暴露于原子弹爆炸辐射与癌症发病率的相关性在最年幼的群体（在0~5岁暴露于辐射）中是最高的（Land, 1995）。

一些围产期状态与乳腺癌的后续风险的相关性也有研究，但证据仍不足以得出任何确切的结论。新生儿黄疸是子宫内感染或胎儿肝功能受损的潜在标记，上述疾病或症状会增加内源性雌激素水平（Lauritzen, Lehmann, 1966；Robine, et al, 1988）。一项关于新生儿黄疸与成人后患乳腺癌风险的相关性的研究表明，与未患病的婴儿相比，患新生儿黄疸的婴儿患乳腺癌的风险显著增加了1倍（Ekbom, et al, 1997）。母体妊娠期糖尿病也可以通过改变胎盘生长激素水平影响胎儿的生长，这种激素改变可能影响激素底物的数量，同时调节胎盘床的旁分泌功能（McIntyre, et al, 2009）。在一项研究中，产妇妊娠糖尿病被作为女儿患乳腺癌的风险因素进行检测，但没有发现其中的关联性（Mogren, et al, 1999）。有研究表明，怀孕期间孕妇体重增加与其女儿患乳腺癌的风险呈正相关，增重11~15kg相对于增重<7kg，其OR为1.5（95% CI 1.1~2.1）（Sanderson, et al, 1998）。产妇在怀孕期间的生活方式因素，如饮用咖啡和饮酒，与女儿患乳腺癌的风险无相关性（Sanderson, et al, 1998）。

3.2.11 论据概要

以下总结了现有的论据，表明患乳腺癌的风险与一系列宫内暴露因素的关联性，如表3.1所示。

表3.1 宫内暴露因素与乳腺癌患病风险的关联性总结

宫内暴露因素	关联方向	论据力度
高体重	↑	+++
高龄产妇分娩年龄	↑	++
分娩时高龄父亲年龄	↑	++
高产次	∅	+
较长孕周	∅	±
较长的出生长度	↑	++
己烯雌酚（DES）暴露	∅	±
双胞胎关系	↓	+
同卵	↓	+
异卵	↑	+
先兆子痫和子痫	↓	++
其他子宫内因素	↑	++
电离辐射	↑	±
新生儿黄疸	∅	±
妊娠糖尿病	∅	±
孕期母亲体重增加	↑	±
孕妇饮用咖啡	∅	±
孕妇饮用酒精	∅	±

注：↑=乳腺癌风险增加；↓=乳腺癌风险降低；∅无关联；+++=极可能有关；++=关联可能性一般；+=关联可能性小；±=证据不足以支持结论

3.3 潜在作用机制

前述的每种宫内暴露与乳腺癌患病风险的关联性作用机制大多与母体妊娠激素、生长激素、胰岛素样生长因子（IGFs）以及随之引发的乳腺干细胞的异常改变相关。

3.3.1 激素的改变

3.3.1.1 雌激素

子宫内接触过高水平的内源性雌激素是Trichopoulos最初提出假设的基础（1990 a、b）。出生体重、母亲年龄、孕周、出生时身长、双胞胎、先兆子痫和子痫都会影响子宫内的雌激素水平，可能升高将来患乳腺癌的风险。

在妊娠的第4~7周，胎盘替代卵巢成为母体与婴儿血液循环中雌激素的主要来源（Siiteri, MacDonald, 1966；Csapo, et al, 1973）。在妊娠将结束时，母体产生的雌三醇达到了正常排卵期妇女平均每天水平的1 000倍，成为了最重要的妊娠期雌激素（Tulchinsky, et al, 1971），此外，在这期间，雌二醇和雌酮在母体血液中的水平也在上升，从50~100pg/mL上升至30 000pg/mL（Lindberg, et al, 1974）。在胎儿方面，在妊娠的3个月期，90%左右的雌三醇是胎盘通过胎儿血浆中的16α-羟基去氢表雄酮硫酸酯转化而来，50%的雌二醇是由去氢表雄酮硫酸酯（DHEAS）转化而来。这些来自胎盘的类固醇激素大多数（80%~90%）进入了母体循环（Casey, MacDonald, 1992）。因此，胎儿肾上腺分泌的DHEAS水平决定了产妇和胎儿血液循环中的雌激素水平。胎儿和母体激素水平是相关的，雌三醇、雌二醇和雌酮的相关系数分别为0.26、0.27和0.41（Troisi, et al, 2003b）。

由于雌激素刺激生长发育的潜力，其一直被认为是癌症发展的刺激因子。人体内部或外部的致癌物始动了细胞突变，而雌激素会刺激细胞增殖和细胞生长，因此，雌激素增加了有致癌突变基因细胞大量繁殖的概率，从而推动了癌症的发展（Pike, et al, 1993；Platet, et al, 2004）。基于细胞培养的后续研究表明，雌激素代谢物可以与DNA结合，并触发突变；雌激素的代谢产物也可影响去除活性化合物（如4-羟雌甾二醇）的酶的水平，因而可能引发癌症（Zhu, Conney, 1998）。这些数据表明，雌激素也可以是癌症诱发剂（Service, 1998）。

3.3.1.2 胰岛素样生长因子（IGFs）

胰岛素样生长因子（Insulin-like growth factors, IGFs）是7kDa的多肽结构同源胰岛素

原，几乎所有组织都能合成，但主要是由人体肝脏合成（Le Roith，1997；Zapf，et al，1984）。它们是调节细胞生长、分化和转化的重要介质（Le Roith，1997）。在胎儿组织中IGF1和IGF2的基因表达持续整个妊娠期，并在胎儿胎盘生长中起着重要的调节作用（Fowden，2003）。在妊娠期间，IGF-I和IGF-II通过自分泌、旁分泌和内分泌刺激细胞的分裂和分化（Ostlund，et al，2002）。胎儿血清中的IGF-I和IGF-II随孕周增加而增加（Giudice，et al，1995）。

在人类，部分IGF1基因缺失已同胎儿宫内生长严重迟缓联系在一起（Morison，et al，1996）。许多研究表明胎儿血液中的IGF-I水平是一些出生数据的正相关指标，包括出生体重（Gluckman，et al，1983；Osorio，et al，1996；Klauwer，et al，1997），独立于孕周的出生体重（Gluckman，et al，1983；Lassarre，et al，1991），出生长度（Klauwer，et al，1997），重量指数（Osorio，et al，1996）和胎盘重量（Osorio，et al，1996）。Spencer等发现首次超声波测量较小且其后续生长受限的胎儿，其脐血中IGF-I水平明显低于声波测量较小但后续生长正常的胎儿（Spencer，et al，1995）。

关于胎儿血液中的IGF-II水平与出生大小的相关性研究中，IGF-II在宫内发育中起作用的支持性证据较少。Giudice等人的一项研究显示，宫内发育迟缓胎儿的脐带血清中的IGF-II明显更少（Giudice，et al，1995）。Ong等发现胎儿循环中的IGF-II与出生时重量指数（r=0.18）和胎盘重量（r=0.18）呈弱相关（Ong，et al，2000）。Bennett等还发现出生体重与脐带血清中的IGF-II水平存在显著的正相关（Bennett，et al，1983）。然而，其他研究未能证实胎儿的IGF-II水平与出生大小数据的关联性，包括出生体重（Gluckman，Lasserre，et al，1983；Osorio，et al，1996；klauwer，1997），独立于孕周的出生体重（Gluckman，et al，1983），出生身长（klauwer，et al，1997），体重指数（Osorio，et al，1996）以及胎盘重量（Osorio，et al，1996），可能是因为出生时IGF-II水平的测定未能反映妊娠的水平。IGF-II在宫内发育中所起的作用是最大的，出生后它只起辅助作用。

关于血液中IGF-I和IGF-II水平与人类乳腺癌风险之间关联性的研究，结果大多不理想。早期的研究结果显示IGF-I与绝经前乳腺癌之间存在不显著的正相关（Hankinson，Schernhammer，2003）；然而，近期基于更大样本的前瞻性数据研究不支持这一相关性（Kaaks，et al，2002；Schernhammer，et al，2005，2006）。IGF-II在某些研究（Grønbaek，et al，2004）中被认为与绝经前或绝经后乳腺癌的患病风险存在相关性，但在其他研究（Holdaway，et al，1999；Li，et al，2001；Yu，et al，2002；Allen，et al，2005）中未能证实。然而，IGF-I和IGF-II已经被证实可以刺激细胞增殖和抑制多种组织中的细胞死亡（(Pollak，2000)，包括正常和恶性的乳腺组织（Sachdev，Yee，2001）。虽然证据显示成人血液循环中IGF-I和IGF-II水平与随后的患癌风险之间的关联性很小，但是胎儿独特的IGF系统是否会引发或促进胎儿的乳腺组织癌变，这一问题目前还未被探讨。胎儿的IGF系统在好几个方面是不同于成人系统的。胰岛素样生长因子和胰岛素是两个显著调节胎儿生长的因素，特别是在第2个和第3个妊娠3月期，而生长激素只起轻微作用。此外，在妊娠后半期，IGF-II基因比IGF-I基因表达更丰富（Hill，1990），而出生后IGF-I成为了主导，因为生长激素刺激肝脏导致IGF-I的增加。妊娠晚期，胎儿循环IGF-II水平（150~400ng/mL）比IGF-I水平（50~100ng/mL）高出3~4倍（Gluckman，et al，1983；Bennett，et al，1983；Reece，et al，1994）。因此，IGF-II被认为是调节胎儿生长的主要因子（Jones，Clemmons，1995；Allan，et al，2001）。

3.3.1.3 胰岛素

胰岛素能显著促进正常乳腺组织以及乳腺癌细胞的有丝分裂（Belfiore, et al, 1996; Papa, Belfiore, 1996）。乳腺癌组织中胰岛素受体的浓度比正常乳腺组织中高（Papa, et al, 1990），并直接与肿瘤大小（Papa, et al, 1990）、肿瘤分级（Papa, et al, 1990）和死亡率（Mathieu, et al, 1997）相关。对空腹胰岛素的作用和乳腺癌的风险之间的关联性的流行病学研究虽有定论但存在矛盾（Xue, Michels, 2007 b）。然而，更一致的结果表明，乳腺癌与C肽（Xue, Michels, 2007 b）具有关联性，后者通常作为反映胰岛素分泌水平的标记物。

由于胰岛素受体与IGF-1受体的有着结构上的相似性，胰岛素可以结合IGF-1受体（Grassi, Giuliano, 2000）对胎儿的生长发育产生直接影响。此外，胰岛素还可以反向控制胰岛素样生长因子结合蛋白，提高受体的亲和力，从而调节胰岛素样生长因子的生物利用度，以此影响胎儿的生长（Hill, et al, 1998）。流行病学研究表明，胎儿生长的模式可以受母亲饮食和代谢功能（Gluckman, Hanson, 2004）以及母体胰岛素水平（Chiesa, et al, 2008）的影响。

3.3.2 激素变更、乳腺干细胞及癌变

3.3.2.1 类固醇激素、胰岛素样生长因子与乳腺癌的发生发展

干细胞具有通过自我更新而延续的潜能，并且能通过分化产生特殊组织的成熟细胞（Reya, et al,, 2001）。乳腺组织的分化潜能由它而来。在出生时（Russo, Russo, 1987）及一个人成长的几个阶段，包括从在子宫内直至完成首次足月妊娠，乳腺均未充分发育。出生时，当囊泡中出现初乳时，乳腺发育停止（Russo, Russo, 2004）。干细胞进一步分化成为上皮细胞、腺泡细胞和肌上皮细胞。在青春期前，乳腺腺体由导管构成，青春期时经过增殖分化从而出现乳腺小叶（Rudland, et al, 1996），并在第一次足月妊娠及哺乳期后达到分化终点（Russo, Russo, 1987）。

激素水平影响乳腺的生长，雌激素诱导乳腺导管的生长，孕激素促进小叶的生长（Rudland, et al, 1996）。雌激素是腔上皮细胞群体主要的类固醇类促有丝分裂剂，后者也是致癌转化的主要靶标（Anderson, et al, 1998）。雌二醇具有增殖潜力，并能通过结合乳腺上皮细胞中的雌激素受体影响DNA的合成。类固醇激素能调节刺激类和抑制类生长因子、生长因子受体和结合类蛋白的合成（Kenney, Dickson, 1996）。

同样，生长激素、IGF-I和IGF-II还通过影响乳腺组织的增殖、分化和凋亡对乳腺的发育起着重要的调节作用（(Laban, et al, 2003）。胰岛素样生长因子通过影响类固醇受体的磷酸化及其功能，增加或减少类固醇激素的促有丝分裂效应等方式，与雌激素交互影响乳腺的发育（Kenney, Dickson, 1996）。此外，在体内模型中，正常人类乳腺上皮细胞用雌二醇进行处理后，IGF-1受体的基因表达增加；在体外模型中，恶性肿瘤细胞用雌二醇处理后，该基因表达也增加（Clarke, et al, 1997）。

3.3.2.2 乳腺干细胞和乳腺癌

干细胞被认为是癌细胞的来源，因为它们很长一段时间保持静止，因此可以积累突变，在被刺激增殖后最终导致癌症的发生（Sell, et al, 2004）。乳腺干细胞和癌变之间的关系是由Rudland和Barraclough提出的（Rudland, Barraclough, 1988）。类似于胚胎干细胞，至少相当一部分乳腺细胞具有长半衰期，并在乳腺癌的发展中起着重要作用，因为一部分乳腺癌病例在初始诊断和原发肿瘤切除术后10年出现复发（Rosen, et al, 1989）。

从怀孕8~15周起，胎儿乳腺开始发育，可能是由单个胚胎干细胞而来（Kordon, Smith, 1998）。在胎儿期，乳腺细胞是处于部分未分化的状态，可能更具有受到刺激诱发癌症的潜能（Russo, Russo, 1996），特别是当宫内接触高浓度的有利于细胞复制的雌激素和生长因子时（Gluckman, et al, 1983）。Trichopoulos推测宫内接触高浓度的雌激素和胰岛素样生长因子可能有利于乳腺癌干细胞的产生，而这些细胞的数目与乳腺大小直接相关，而乳房体积增大则提高了基因突变的可能性（Trichopoulos, et al, 2005）。Ekbom等称，乳房X线摄影时高密度的乳腺模式（P2或DY）与胎盘的重量存在显著相关性，后者是怀孕期间雌激素的主要生成器官（Ekbom, et al, 1995）。这表明，改变的宫内雌激素暴露可能以通过增加乳腺密度的方式升高患乳腺癌的风险。

3.3.3 当前关于乳腺癌的病理假说

3.3.3.1 多灶性起源

乳腺癌是一种复杂的、具有广泛形态的疾病。基于经典的全器官研究（whole-organ studies），人们早就推测，大多数原位癌和浸润性乳腺癌病例是多灶性、多中心或弥漫性的（Gallager, Martin, 1969; Holland, et al, 1985）。1975年，基于对整个人类乳房的组织学检查，Wellings等推测大多数乳腺结构不良或纤维囊性病变产生于末端导管小叶单元（TDLU）或小叶自身。这些病变包括大汗腺囊肿、硬化性腺病、纤维腺瘤、各种形式的小叶病变（硬化、扩张、分泌过多、增生、非典型或间变性）、原位导管癌和原位小叶癌（Wellings, et al, 1975）。这个推论后来被广泛接受为乳腺癌发展的经典理论：乳腺大多数恶性肿瘤起源于小叶（即末端导管小叶单元）的上皮细胞，并且随着恶性细胞的迁移扩散至乳腺导管和其他小叶。

3.3.3.2 单叶起源

使用常规组织学技术的传统全器官研究往往不能获得重复的结果。近年来，乳腺癌多灶性起源的传统理论面临着更加现代化的诊断技术的挑战，这些现代技术为病变阶段及其分布提供了更透彻的分析。Tot和其同事使用更详细、系统的二维和三维的大组织切片的先进方法，并结合放射影像学的方法，历时20多年研究和分析了5 000多个连续的乳腺癌病例（Tot, 2005）。他们发现，多数原位导管癌沿着管道连续分布数厘米。这样的距离显示了病变的起源不大可能是单独的末端单元，因为这些单元的尺寸一般以毫米计量。此外，恶性细胞从小叶的上皮细胞转移到小叶导管及其他小叶的说法也未得到组织学检查的支持。因此他们推测，原位导管癌和一般情况下的乳腺癌是一种小叶性病变，即同时或异步发生的原位性（和浸润性）乳腺癌灶来自单侧乳房的某一个小叶（Tot, 2005）。如果这个新的假设被证明是正确的，则可能表明我们可以采用新的方法选择性地视觉化、切除或破坏患病腺叶以减少恶性病变的发生发展，从而降低乳腺癌的发病率(Tot, 2007)。

3.3.3.3 宫内危险因素与乳腺癌的单叶起源

乳腺的实质组织从一个单一的上皮外胚层胚芽发展而来。乳腺的胚胎发育包括10个阶段，即脊形成、乳突、乳盘、小叶形成、圆锥、萌芽、内凹、分支、管化、最终囊泡形成。在出生时，乳腺是由非常原始的结构组成，末端称为乳管，其内排列有1或2层上皮细胞和1层肌上皮细胞（Russo, Russo, 2004）。新生乳腺经过增长和分支扩张形成乳芽，末端发育成腺泡。乳芽进一步发展成包含3~5个原始小叶的芽泡，并继续分裂，直至青春期，达到最大数目（Rudland, 1993）。

由于宫内接触潜在的致癌物质已经被认为会诱发和（或）催化出生前乳腺癌的发生

发展，且出生前乳腺干细胞正在历经各种分化，因此，有观点认为癌变也许影响了乳腺干细胞。尽管分支和分枝过程在子宫内已经几乎全部完成，但是，乳腺小叶发育主要发生在青春期后的时期（Tot，et al，2002）。事实上，青春期前很少存在末梢导管小叶单元（Vogel，et al，1981）。因此，影响乳腺癌发生发展的基因突变或表观遗传异常更有可能通过某种细胞传递下去，这种细胞在小叶形成过程中经历了连续的分支和网状分枝，而不是其他某种来自末梢导管小叶单元内的细胞，因为出生前末梢导管小叶单元的主体部分还未发育形成。这些假定与Tot和他同事的"病态腺叶"假说一致（Tot，2005，2007）。

3.4 结 论

流行病学研究结果显示，宫内暴露的标志物，如出生体重、分娩时父母的年龄、出生时身长、接触DES、双胞胎、先兆子痫和子痫，与日后罹患乳腺癌有关。因此，乳腺癌可能起源于子宫内，可能与乳腺干细胞在子宫内受到变化的雌激素和胰岛素样生长因子的作用有关。人类乳腺在出生前发育成为原始的乳腺腺叶结构，但腺小叶形成主要发生在青春期后的时期。因此，与乳腺癌发生发展有关的基因突变或表观遗传异常很有可能是发生在那些小叶形成过程中经历过连续的分支和网状分枝的细胞，而不是来自末梢导管小叶单元内的细胞，因为大部分末梢导管小叶单元在出生前尚未形成。

参考文献

[1] Adami H, Hunter D, Trichopoulos D. Textbook of cancer epidemiology. Oxford University Press: New York, 2002: pp 301-373.

[2] Allan GJ, Flint DJ, Patel K. In sulin-like growth factor axis during embryonic development. Reproduction, 2001, 122: 31-39.

[3] Allen NE, Roddam AW, Allen DS, et al. A prospective study of serum insulin-like growth factor-I (IGF-I), IGF-II, IGF-binding protein-3 and breast cancer risk. Br J Cancer, 2005, 92: 1283-1287.

[4] American Cancer Society. Cancer facts & fgures 2009. American Cancer Society, Atlanta, 2010. http://www.cancer.org/Cancer/BreastCancer/OverviewGuide/breast-cancer-over-view-key-statistics.

[5] Anderson E, Clarke RB, Howell A. Estrogen responsiveness and control of normal human breast proliferation. J Mammary Gland Biol Neoplasia, 1998, 3: 23-35.

[6] Baldwin S, Chung M, Chard T, et al. Insulin-like growth factor-binding protein-1, glucose tolerance and fetal growth in human pregnancy. J Endocrinol, 1993, 136: 319-325.

[7] Belfore A, Frittitta L, Costantino A, et al. Insulin receptors in breast cancer. Ann NY Acad Sci, 1996, 784: 173-188.

[8] Bennett A, Wilson DM, Liu F, et al. Levels of insulin-like growth factors I and II in human cord blood. J Clin Endocrinol Metab, 1983, 57: 609-612.

[9] Brinkworth MH. Paternal transmission of genetic damage: fndings in animals and humans. Int J Androl, 2000, 23: 123-135.

[10] Casey ML, MacDonald PC. Alterations in steroid production by the human placenta// Pasqualini JR, Scholler R (eds) Hormones and fetal pathophysiology. New York: Marcel Dekker, 1992: p251.

[11] Chiesa C, Osborn JF, Haass C, et al. Ghrelin, leptin, IGF-1, IGFBP-3, and insulin concentrations at birth: is there a relationship with fetal growth and neonatal anthropometry. Clin Chem, 2008, 54: 550-558.

[12] Choi JY, Lee KM, Park SK, et al. Association of paternal age at birth and the risk of breast cancer in offspring: a case control study. BMC Cancer, 2005, 5: 143.

[13] Clark PM. Assays for insulin, proinsulin and C-peptide. Ann Clin Biochem, 1999, 36: 541-564.

[14] Clarke RB, Howell A, Anderson E. Type I insulin-like growth factor receptor gene expression in normal human breast tissue treated with oestrogen and progesterone. Br J Cancer, 1997, 75: 251-257.

[15] Csapo AI, Pulkkinen MO, Wiest WG. Effects of luteectomy and progesterone replacement therapy in early pregnant patients. Am J Obstet Gynecol, 1973, 115: 759-765.

[16] Devesa SS, Grauman DJ, Blot WJ. Recent cancer patterns among men and women in the United States: clues for occupational research. J Occup Med 3, 1994, 6: 832-841.

[17] dos Silva IS, De Stavola B, McCormack V. Collaborative Group on Pre-Natal Risk Factors and Subsequent Risk of Breast Cancer. Birth size and breast cancer risk: reanalysis of individual participant data from 32 studies. PLoS Med5, 2008: e193.

[18] Ekbom A, Thurfjell E, Hsieh CC, et al. Perinatal characteristics and adult mammographic patterns. Int J Cancer, 1995, 61: 177-180.

[19] Ekbom A, Hsieh CC, Lipworth L, et al. Intrauterine environment and breast cancer risk in women: a population-based study. J Natl Cancer Inst, 1997, 89: 71-76.

[20] Ekbom A, Erlandsson G, Hsieh C, et al. Risk of breast cancer in prematurely born women. J Natl Cancer Inst, 2000, 92: 840-841.

[21] Ferlay J, Bray F, Pisani P, et al. GLOBOCAN 2000: cancer incidence, mortality and prevalence world-wide. International Agency for Research on Cancer, Lyon, 2001.

[22] Forman MR, Cantwell MM, Ronckers C, et al. Through the looking glass at early-life exposures and breast cancer risk. Cancer Invest, 2005, 23: 609-624.

[23] Fowden AL. The insulin-like growth factors and feto-placental growth. Placenta, 2003, 24: 803-812.

[24] Gallager HS, Martin JE. The study of mammary carcinoma by mammography and whole organ sectioning. Cancer, 1969, 23: 855-873.

[25] Giudice LC, de Zegher F, Gargosky SE, et al. Insulin-like growth factors and their binding proteins in the term and preterm human fetus and neonate with nor-mal and extremes of intrauterine growth. J Clin Endocrinol Metab, 1995, 80: 1548-1555.

[26] Glaser RL, Jabs EW. Dear old dad. Sci Aging Knowledge Environ 2004, 2004: re1

[27] Gluckman PD, Hanson MA. Maternal constraint of fetal growth and its consequences. Semin Fetal Neonatal Med, 2004, 9: 419-425.

[28] Gluckman PD, Johnson-Barrett JJ, Butler JH, et al. Studies of insulin-like growth factor-I and -II by specifc radioligand assays in umbilical cord blood. Clin Endocrinol (Oxf), 1983, 19: 405-413.

[29] Gonzalez MC, Reyes H, Arrese M, et al. Intra-hepatic cholestasis of pregnancy in twin pregnancies. J Hepatol, 1989, 9: 84-90.

[30] Grassi AE, Giuliano MA. The neonate with macrosomia. Clin Obstet Gynecol, 2000, 43: 340-348.

[31] Greenwald P, Barlow JJ, Nasca PC, et al. Vaginal cancer after maternal treatment with synthetic estrogens. N Engl J Med, 1971, 285: 390-392.

[32] Grønbaek H, Flyvbjerg A, Mellemkjaer L, et al. Serum insu-lin-like growth factors, insulin-like growth factor binding proteins, and breast cancer risk in postmenopausal women. Cancer Epidemiol Biomarkers Prev, 2004, 13: 1759-1764.

[33] Hamilton BE, Ventura SJ, Martin JA, et al. Final births for 2004. Health Estats. Hyattsville: National Center for Health Statistics, 2006.

[34] Hankinson SE, Schernhammer ES. Insulin-like growth factor and breast cancer risk: evidence from observational studies. Breast Dis, 2003, 17: 27-40.

[35] Hatch EE, Palmer JR, Titus-Ernstoff L, et al. Cancer risk in women exposed to diethylstilbestrol in utero. JAMA, 1998, 280: 630-634.

[36] Hemminki K, Kyyronen P. Parental age and risk of sporadic and familial cancer in offspring: implications for germ cell mutagenesis. Epidemiology, 1999, 10: 747-751.

[37] Hill DJ. Relative abundance and molecular size of immu-noreactive insulin-like growth factors I and II in human fetal tissues. Early Hum Dev, 1990, 21: 49-58.

[38] Hill DJ, Petrik J, Arany E. Growth factors and

the regulation of fetal growth. Diab Care 21, 1998 (Suppl 2): B60-B69.

[39] Hodgson ME, Newman B, Millikan RC. Birth weight, parental age, birth order and breast cancer risk in African-American and white women: a population-based case-control study. Breast Cancer Res, 2004, 6: R656-R667.

[40] Holdaway IM, Mason BH, Lethaby AE, et al. Serum levels of insulin-like growth factor binding protein-3 in benign and malignant breast disease. Aust N Z J Surg, 1999, 69: 495-500.

[41] Holland R, Velling SH, Mravunac M, et al. Histologic multifocality of Tis, T1-2 breast carcinomas: implications for clinical trials of breast conserving surgery. Cancer, 1985, 56: 979-990.

[42] Howe HL, Wu X, Ries LA, et al. Annual report to the nation on the status of cancer (1975-2003), featuring cancer among U.S. Hispanic/Latino populations. Cancer, 2006, 107: 1711-1742.

[43] Innes K, Byers T, Schymura M. Birth characteristics and subsequent risk for breast cancer in very young women. Am J Epidemiol, 2000, 152: 1121-1128.

[44] Janerich DT, Hayden CL, Thompson WD, et al. Epidemiologic evidence of perinatal infuence in the etiology of adult cancers. J Clin Epidemiol, 1989, 42: 151-157.

[45] Jones JI, Clemmons DR. Insulin-like growth factors and their binding proteins: biological actions. Endocr Rev, 1995, 16: 3-34.

[46] Jung A, Schuppe HC, Schill WB. Are children of older fathers at risk for genetic disorders. Andrologia, 2003, 35: 191-199.

[47] Kaaks R, Lundin E, Rinaldi S, et al. Prospective study of IGF-I, IGF binding proteins, and breast cancer risk, in northern and southern Sweden. Cancer Causes Control, 2002, 13: 307-316.

[48] Kappel B, Hansen K, Moller J, et al. Human placental lactogen and dU-estrogen levels in normal twin pregnancies. Acta Genet Med Gemellol (Roma), 1985, 34: 59-65.

[49] Kato H, Yoshimoto Y, Schull WJ. Risk of cancer among children exposed to atomic bomb radiation in utero: a review. IARC Sci Publ, 1989, 96: 365-374.

[50] Kenney NJ, Dickson RB. Growth factor and sex steroid interactions in breast cancer. J Mammary Gland Biol Neoplasia, 1996, 1: 189-198.

[51] Klauwer D, Blum WF, Hanitsch S, et al. IGF-I, IGF-II, free IGF-I and IGFBP-1, -2 and -3 levels in venous cord blood: relationship to birthweight, length and gestational age in healthy newborns. Acta Paediatr, 1997, 86: 826-833.

[52] Kordon EC, Smith GH. An entire functional mammary gland may comprise the progeny from a single cell. Development, 1998, 125: 1921-1930.

[53] Laban C, Bustin SA, Jenkins PJ. The GH-IGF-I axis and breast cancer. Trends Endocrinol Metab, 2003, 14: 28-34.

[54] Land CE. Studies of cancer and radiation dose among atomic bomb survivors. The example of breast cancer. JAMA, 1995, 274: 402-407.

[55] Lassarre C, Hardouin S, Daffos F, et al. Serum insulin-like growth factors and insulin-like growth factor binding proteins in the human fetus. Relationships with growth in normal subjects and in subjects with intrauterine growth retardation. Pediatr Res, 1991, 29: 219-225.

[56] Lauritzen C, Lehmann WD. The importance of steroid hormones in the pathogenesis of hyperbilirubinemia and neonatal jaundice. Z Kinderheilkd, 1966, 95: 143-154.

[57] Law LW. The production of tumors by injection of a carcinogen into the amniotic fuid of mice. Science, 1940, 91: 96-97.

[58] Le Marchand L, Kolonel LN, Myers BC, et al. Birth characteristics of premenopausal women with breast cancer. Br J Cancer, 1988, 57: 437-439.

[59] Le Roith D. Seminars in medicine of the Beth Israel Deaconess Medical Center. Insulin-like growth factors. N Engl J Med, 1997, 336: 633-640.

[60] Li BD, Khosravi MJ, Berkel HJ, et al. Free insulin-like growth factor-I and breast cancer risk. Int J Cancer, 2001, 91: 736-739.

[61] Liehr JG. Is estradiol a genotoxic mutagenic carcinogen. Endocr Rev, 2000, 21: 40-54.

[62] Lindberg BS, Johansson ED, Nilsson BA. Plasma

levels of nonconjugated oestrone, oestradiol-17b and oestriol during uncomplicated pregnancy. Acta Obstet Gynecol Scand Suppl, 1974, 32: 21-36.

[63] Long PA, Abell DA, Beischer NA. Fetal growth and placental function assessed by urinary estriol excretion before the onset of pre-eclampsia. Am J Obstet Gynecol, 1979, 135: 344-347.

[64] Maccoby EE, Doering CH, Nagy Jacklin C, et al. Concentrations of sex hormones in umbilical-cord blood: their relation to sex and birth order of infants. Child Dev, 1979, 50: 632-642.

[65] Macmahon B. Prenatal x-ray exposure and childhood cancer. J Natl Cancer Inst, 1962, 28: 1173-1191.

[66] Madigan MP, Ziegler RG, Benichou J, et al. Proportion of breast cancer cases in the United States explained by well-established risk factors. J Natl Cancer Inst, 1995, 87: 1681-1685.

[67] Mathieu MC, Clark GM, Allred DC, et al. Insulin receptor expression and clinical outcome in node-negative breast cancer. Proc Assoc Am Physicians, 1997, 109: 565-571.

[68] McCormack VA, dos Santos Silva I, De Stavola BL, et al. Fetal growth and subsequent risk of breast cancer: results from long term follow up of Swedish cohort. BMJ, 2003, 326: 248.

[69] McIntyre HD, Zeck W, Russell A. Placental growth hormone, fetal growth and the IGF axis in normal and diabetic pregnancy. Curr Diab Rev, 2009, 5: 185-189.

[70] Michels KB, Xue F. Role of birthweight in the etiology of breast cancer. Int J Cancer, 2006, 119: 2007-2025.

[71] Mogren I, Damber L, Tavelin B, et al. Characteristics of pregnancy and birth and malignancy in the offspring (Sweden). Cancer Causes Control, 1999, 10: 85-94.

[72] Morison IM, Becroft DM, Taniguchi T, et al. Somatic overgrowth associated with overexpression of insulin-like growth factor II. Nat Med, 1996, 2: 311-316.

[73] Mucci LA, Lagiou P, Tamimi RM, et al. Pregnancy estriol, estradiol, proges-terone and prolactin in relation to birth weight and other birth size variables (United States). Cancer Causes Control, 2003, 14: 311-318.

[74] Nichols HB, Trentham-Dietz A, Sprague BL, et al. Effects of birth order and maternal age on breast cancer risk: modifcation by whether women had been breast-fed. Epidemiology, 2008, 19: 417-423.

[75] Oleszczuk JJ, Cervantes A, Kiely JL, et al. Maternal race/ethnicity and twinning rates in the United States (1989-1991). J Reprod Med, 2001, 46: 550-557.

[76] Ong K, Kratzsch J, Kiess W, et al. Size at birth and cord blood levels of insulin, insulin-like growth factor I (IGF-I), IGF-II, IGF-binding protein-1 (IGFBP-1), IGFBP-3, and the soluble IGF-II/mannose-6-phosphate receptor in term human infants. The ALSPAC Study Team. Avon Longitudinal Study of Pregnancy and Childhood. J Clin Endocrinol Metab, 2000, 85: 4266-4269.

[77] Osorio M, Torres J, Moya F, et al. Insulin-like growth factors (IGFs) and IGF binding proteins-1, -2, and -3 in newborn serum: relationships to fetoplacental growth at term. Early Hum Dev, 1996, 46: 15-26.

[78] Ostlund E, Tally M, Fried G. Transforming growth factor-beta1 in fetal serum correlates with insulin-like growth factor-I and fetal growth. Obstet Gynecol, 2002, 100: 567-573.

[79] Palmer JR, Hatch EE, Rosenberg CL, et al. Risk of breast cancer in women exposed to diethylstilbestrol in utero: preliminary results (United States). Cancer Causes Control, 2002, 13: 753-758.

[80] Panagiotopoulou K, Katsouyanni K, Petridou E, et al. Maternal age, parity, and pregnancy estrogens. Cancer Causes Control 1: 119-124Papa V, Belfore A (1996) Insulin receptors in breast cancer: biological and clinical role. J Endocrinol Invest, 1990, 19: 324-333.

[81] Papa V, Pezzino V, Costantino A, et al. Elevated insulin receptor content in human breast cancer. J Clin Invest, 1990, 86: 1503-1510.

[82] Park SK, Kang D, McGlynn KA, et al. Intrauterine environments and breast cancer risk: meta-

analysis and systematic review. Breast Cancer Res, 2008, 10: R8.
[83] Petridou E, Panagiotopoulou K, Katsouyanni K, et al. Tobacco smoking, pregnancy estrogens, and birth weight. Epidemiology, 1990, 1: 247-250.
[84] Pike MC, Spicer DV, Dahmoush L, et al. Estrogens, progestogens, normal breast cell proliferation, and breast cancer risk. Epidemiol Rev, 1993, 15: 17-35.
[85] Platet N, Cathiard AM, Gleizes M, et al. Estrogens and their receptors in breast cancer progression: a dual role in cancer proliferation and invasion. Crit Rev Oncol Hematol, 2004, 51: 55-67.
[86] Pollak M. Insulin-like growth factor physiology and can-cer risk. Eur J Cancer, 2000, 36: 1224-1228.
[87] Reece EA, Wiznitzer A, Le E, et al. The relation between human fetal growth and fetal blood levels of insulin-like growth factors I and II, their binding proteins and receptors. Obstet Gynecol, 1994, 84: 88-95.
[88] Reya T, Morrison SJ, Clarke MF, et al. Stem cells, cancer, and cancer stem cells. Nature, 2001, 414: 105-111.
[89] Robine N, Relier JP, Le Bars S. Urocytogram, an index of maturity in premature infants. Biol Neonate, 1988, 54: 93-99.
[90] Rosen PR, Groshen S, Saigo PE, et al. A long-term follow-up study of survival in stage I (T1N0M0) and stage II (T1N1M0) breast carcinoma. J Clin Oncol, 1989, 7: 355-366.
[91] Rudland PS. Epithelial stem cells and their possible role in the development of the normal and diseased human breast. Histol Histopathol, 1993, 8: 385-404.
[92] Rudland PS, Barraclough R. Stem cells in mammary gland differentiation and cancer. J Cell Sci Suppl, 1988, 10: 95-114.
[93] Rudland PS, Barraclough R, Fernig DG, et al. Growth and differentiation of the normal mammary gland and its tumors. Biochem Soc Symp, 1996, 63: 1-20.
[94] Russo J, Russo IH. Development of the human mammary gland//Neville MC, Daniel CW (eds) The mammary gland. New York: Plenum, 1987: pp 67-93.
[95] Russo IH, Russo J. Mammary gland neoplasia in long-term rodent studies. Environ Health Perspect, 1996, 104: 938-967.
[96] Russo J, Russo IH. Development of the human breast. Maturitas, 2004, 49: 2-15.
[97] Sachdev D, Yee D. The IGF system and breast cancer. Endocr Relat Cancer, 2001, 8: 197-209.
[98] Sanderson M, Williams MA, Daling JR, et al. Maternal factors and breast cancer risk among young women. Paediatr Perinat Epidemiol, 1998, 12: 397-407.
[99] Schernhammer ES, Holly JM, Pollak MN, et al. Circulating levels of insulin-like growth factors, their binding proteins, and breast cancer risk. Cancer Epidemiol Biomarkers Prev, 2005, 14: 699-704.
[100] Schernhammer ES, Holly JM, Hunter DJ, et al. Insulin-like growth factor-I, its binding proteins (IGFBP-1 and IGFBP-3), and growth hormone and breast cancer risk in The Nurses Health Study II. Endocr Relat Cancer, 2006, 13: 583-592.
[101] Sell S. Stem cell origin of cancer and differentiation therapy. Crit Rev Oncol Hematol, 2004, 51: 1-28.
[102] Service RE. New role for estrogen in cancer. Science, 1998, 279: 1631-1633.
[103] Shipley PW, Wray JA, Hechter HH, et al. Frequency of twinning in California. Its relationship to maternal age, parity and race. Am J Epidemiol, 1967, 85: 147-156.
[104] Siiteri PK, MacDonald PC. Placental estrogen biosynthesis during human pregnancy. J Clin Endocrinol Metab, 1966, 26: 751-761.
[105] Spencer JA, Chang TC, Jones J, et al. Third trimester fetal growth and umbilical venous blood concentrations of IGF-1, IGFBP-1, and growth hormone at term. Arch Dis Child Fetal Neonatal Ed, 1995, 73: F87-F90.
[106] Swerdlow AJ, De Stavola B, MacOnochie N, et al. A population-based study of cancer risk in twins: relation-ships to birth order and sexes of the twin pair. Int J Cancer, 1996, 67: 472-478.
[107] Swerdlow AJ, De Stavola BL, Swanwick MA, et

[107] al. Risks of breast and testicular cancers in young adult twins in England and Wales: evidence on prenatal and genetic aetiology. Lancet, 1997, 350: 1723-1728.

[108] TambyRaja RL, Ratnam SS. Plasma steroid changes in twin pregnancies. Prog Clin Biol Res, 1981, 69A: 189-195.

[109] Tapanainen J, Koivisto M, Vihko R, et al. Enhanced activity of the pituitary-gonadal axis in premature human infants. J Clin Endocrinol Metab, 1981, 52: 235-238.

[110] Thiery M, Dhont M, Vandekerckhove D. Serum HCG and HPL in twin pregnancies. Acta Obstet Gynecol Scand, 1977, 56: 495-497.

[111] Tomatis L. Prenatal exposure to chemical carcinogens and its effect on subsequent generations. Natl Cancer Inst Monogr, 1979, 51: 159-184.

[112] Tot T. DCIS, cytokeratins and the theory of the sick lobe. Virchows Arch, 2005, 447: 1-8.

[113] Tot T. The theory of the sick lobe and the possible conse-quences. Int J Surg Pathol, 2007, 15: 369-375.

[114] Tot T, Tabár L, Dean PB. Practical breast pathology. Thieme, Stuttgart, 2002: pp 116-123.

[115] Trichopoulos D. Hypothesis: does breast cancer origi-nate in utero? Lancet, 1990a, 335: 939-940.

[116] Trichopoulos D. Is breast cancer initiated in utero. Epidemiology, 1990b, 1: 95-96.

[117] Trichopoulos D, Lagiou P, Adami HO. Towards an integrated model for breast cancer etiology: the crucial role of the number of mammary tissue-specifc stem cells. Breast Cancer Res, 2005, 7: 13-17.

[118] Troisi R, Potischman N, Roberts J, et al. Associations of maternal and umbilical cord hormone concentrations with maternal, gestational and neonatal factors (United States). Cancer Causes Control, 2003a, 14: 347-355.

[119] Troisi R, Potischman N, Roberts JM, et al. Correlation of serum hormone concentrations in maternal and umbilical cord samples. Cancer Epidemiol Biomarkers Prev, 2003b, 12: 452-456.

[120] Troisi R, Hatch EE, Titus-Ernstoff L, et al. Cancer risk in women prenatally exposed to diethylstilbestrol. Int J Cancer, 2007, 121: 356-360.

[121] Tulchinsky D, Hobel CJ, Korenman SG. A radioligand assay for plasma unconjugated estriol in normal and abnor-mal pregnancies. Am J Obstet Gynecol, 1971, 111: 311-318.

[122] Vatten LJ, Nilsen TI, Tretli S, et al. Size at birth and risk of breast cancer: prospective population-based study. Int J Cancer, 2005, 114: 461-464.

[123] Vogel PM, Georgiade NG, Fetter BF, et al. The correlation of histologic changes in the human breast with the menstrual cycle. Am J Pathol 104: 23-34.

[124] Wei Q, Matanoski GM, Farmer ER, et al. DNA repair and aging in basal cell carcinoma: a molecular epidemiology study. Proc Natl Acad Sci USA, 1993, 90: 1614-1618.

[125] Weiss HA, Potischman NA, Brinton LA, et al. Prenatal and perinatal risk factors for breast cancer in young women. Epidemiology, 1997, 8: 181-187.

[126] Weiss-Salz I, Harlap S, Friedlander Y, et al. Ethnic ancestry and increased paternal age are risk factors for breast cancer before the age of 40 years. Eur J Cancer Prev, 2007, 16: 549-554.

[127] Wellings SR, Jensen HM, Marcum RG. An atlas of subgross pathology of the human breast with special reference to possible precancerous lesions. J Natl Cancer Inst, 1975, 55: 231-273.

[128] White E, Lee CY, Kristal AR. Evaluation of the increase in breast cancer incidence in relation to mammography use. J Natl Cancer Inst, 1990, 82: 1546-1552.

[129] Xu X, Dailey AB, Peoples-Sheps M, et al. Birth weight as a risk factor for breast cancer: a meta-analysis of 18 epidemiological studies. J Womens Health (Larchmt), 2009, 18: 1169-1178.

[130] Xue F, Michels KB. Intrauterine factors and risk of breast cancer: a systematic review and meta-analysis of current evidence. Lancet Oncol, 2007a, 8: 1088-1100.

[131] Xue F, Michels KB. Diabetes, metabolic syndrome, and breast cancer: a review of the current evidence. Am J Clin Nutr, 2007b, 86: s823-s835.

[132] Xue F, Colditz GA, Willett WC, et al. Parental age at delivery and incidence of breast cancer: a prospective cohort study. Breast Cancer Res Treat, 2006, 104: 331-340.

[133] Yu H, Jin F, Shu XO, et al. Insulin-like growth factors and breast cancer risk in Chinese women. Cancer Epidemiol Biomarkers Prev, 2002, 11: 705-712.

[134] Zapf J, Schmid C, Froesch E. Biological and immuno-logical properties of insulin-like growth factors (IGF) I and II. Clin Endocrinol Metab, 1984, 13: 7-12.

[135] Zeisler H, Jirecek S, Hohlagschwandtner M, et al. Concentrations of estrogens in patients with preeclampsia. Wien Klin Wochenschr, 2002, 114: 458-461.

[136] Zhang Y, Cupples LA, Rosenberg L, et al. Parental ages at birth in relation to a daughter's risk of breast cancer among female participants in the Framingham Study (United States). Cancer Causes Control, 1995, 6: 23-29.

[137] Zhu BT, Conney AH. Functional role of estrogen metabolism in target cells: review and perspectives. Carcinogenesis, 1998, 19: 1-27.

第 4 章 正常及恶性乳腺组织中的基因改变

Chanel E. Smart, Peter T. Simpson,
Ana Cristina Vargas, Sunil R. Lakhani

缩　写

ADH	不典型导管增生
ALDH1	乙醛脱氢酶1
ALH	不典型小叶增生
CAF	肿瘤相关成纤维细胞
CCL	柱状细胞病变
CGH	比较基因组杂交
DCIS	导管原位癌
ECM	细胞外基质
FEA	平坦型上皮非典型增生
FFPE	甲醛固定石蜡包埋
G6PD	葡萄糖-6-磷酸脱氢酶
HR	同源重组
HUT	正常增生
ILC	浸润性小叶癌
IDC	浸润性导管癌
LCIS	小叶原位癌
LOH	杂合性缺失
NS	正常实质
PLC	多形性小叶癌
ROH	杂合性保留
SNP	单核苷酸多态性
TDLU	末端导管小叶单元

S. R. Lakhani
University of Queensland Centre for Clinical Research,
School of Medicine, and Pathology Queensland,
The Royal Brisbane & Women's Hospital, Brisbane,
Queensland, Australia
e-mail: s.lakhani@uq.edu.au

4.1 背　景

乳腺癌是一种高度异质性疾病，形态学上存在很多亚型，临床表现差异很大。通过很长时间的努力，病理学家用分子亚型、病理分期等方式构建了独特的病理系统，它能够记录肿瘤的相关信息，这些信息既反映了肿瘤的异质性，也为预测治疗效果和预后提供了信息。分子亚型、分级和分期提供了预后的信息（Ellis, et al 1992; Elston, Ellis, 1991），激素受体的分析，如HER2的过表达和扩增提供了治疗所需的预后和预测的数据（Oldenhuis, et al, 2008）。然而，这一系统存在局限性。临床工作者深有体会，即便是同一亚型（如小管癌）或同一分期（如腋窝淋巴结阳性），肿瘤细胞的生物学行为都存在很大的不同。理解疾病背后的分子异常，能够赋予我们"一击而中"的能力。

4.2 肿瘤的遗传基础

目前，肿瘤被认为是一种遗传性疾病：由细胞内DNA驱动发生。某些突变从胚胎遗传而来，遍布所有的体细胞，个体因而增加了罹患某种肿瘤的风险。其他某些体细胞的突变可能是由环境造成的，例如化学致癌物、放射线或DNA修复机制的缺陷，后者在肿瘤发生过程中失效。肿瘤演进中单基因/基因组的改变类型和程度十分复杂，推动肿瘤形成不同的表现型。这些改变包括：①大段的染色体的获得和缺失，这会影响数量众多的基因的表达情况；②某些部分的基因片段增加，导致这些基因反复被复制，其中可能含有原癌基因，促进了肿瘤的生长（例如 ERBB2/HER2 的扩增和过表达）；③由于任何纯合子/半合子基因的删除、甲基化、基因变异或转录抑制导致的重组，使肿瘤或转移抑制基因失活（如小叶癌中 E-cadherin 的失活）；④基因融合导致基因组重排（如分泌型乳腺癌中 ETV6-NTRK3 融合基因，Tognon, et al, 2002）。

近20年来，学术界对人类基因组测序和疾病分子机制的研究为揭开疾病背后的基因基础提供了技术。杂合性缺失（loss of heterozygosity, LOH）或候选基因/基因组突变位点分析技术有助于辨别特殊的基因改变。为了获得肿瘤基因组中体细胞突变（DNA拷贝数目的改变）的更多更复杂的特征信息，科研工作者使用比较基因组杂合技术（comparative genomic hybridization, CGH）进行全基因组分析。通常，该技术解析度低，仅能提供有限的全染色体异常的模式分析（Reis Fihlo, et al, 2005），但是，毫无疑问的是，该技术也揭示了不同个体间肿瘤发生的关键事件和分子特征存在差异的重要机制。基因芯片CGH（aCGH）的出现革新了这项技术，解析度可达100bp，能够分辨基因组改变的细节特征并精确定位。而且，为了确认与疾病有关的基因（基因组相关研究）推动了高密度单核苷酸多态性（single nucleotide polymorphism, SNP）检测技术的发展，该技术能够从等位基因的水平检测基因组拷贝数目的改变。当然，伴随基因组测序谱的巨大进步，基因组表达谱的研究也迅猛前进，这些研究使人们进一步了解基因对肿瘤细胞表现型这一新的水平的复杂调控机制。目前，肿瘤基因组分子分析的金标准是高通量基因组和转录组测序。尽管这项技术还不能广泛开展，但是该技术能够在核苷酸的水平辨认基因组的重排和变异，并且无偏移地评价mRNA和microRNA的表达水平（Stratton, et al, 2009）。

这些技术揭示了乳腺癌基因组的复杂性，并且彻底改变了我们对于乳腺疾病生物学的理解。这些研究已经确认了疾病进展中的重要突变，可用于治疗的分子靶标（如ER和HER2），证实了某些早期病变会发展成浸润性癌，以及对疾病的分类（Alizadeh, et al, 2001; Buerger, et al, 1999b; Lakhani, 1997; Nishizaki, et al, 1997; Pollack, et al, 1999; Reis-Filho, et al, 2005; Simpson, et al, 2005b; Perou, et al, 2000; Sorlie, et al, 2001）。

4.3 浸润性乳腺癌的分子分析

浸润性乳腺癌的分子分析发现了常见的基因组改变，如染色体1q、8q、17q和20q处核苷酸的增加，染色体4q、5q、8q、11q、13q和16q处的减少。在1q32、8p12、8q24、11q13、17q12和20q13处多出现高水平的基因组扩增。基因组改变的特点与组织学分级、分子分型密切相关，与组织学类型也有关系。这些分子水平的发现证实，低级别乳腺癌与高级别乳腺癌在分子水平存在不同，导致了不同级别乳腺癌是经不同路径发展而来的假设（Buerger, et al, 1999a、b, 2000; Roylance, et al, 2006; Stratton, et al, 1995）。总的来说，低级别导管癌和小管癌的基因组不稳定性较低，16号染色体的q端丢失，1号染色体q端增加是其特点，其他重复改变少见。高级别乳腺癌的基因组不稳定性较高，基因组改变复杂，17q12、8q24和20q13处的基因序列高度增加（扩增）。LOH和染色体CGH分析技术发现了这些数据，因此研究者认为来自于正常乳腺组织的低级别肿瘤的发生发展与高级别肿瘤不同。低级别肿瘤细胞中16号染色体q端片段的丢失很常见，甚至整个染色体臂；但是高级别肿瘤极少发生16q处序列的丢失，即使出现了基因片段的丢失，其背后的机制也有所不同（有丝分裂重组的LOH）（Roylance, et al, 2002, 2006; Cleton-Jansen, et al, 2004; Natrajan, et al, 2009a）。

但是，也有例外存在，20%的高级别浸润性导管癌（IDC）存在整个16q的缺失。无论形态学还是分子水平，组织学Ⅲ级IDCs的异质性很高。最近，高级别IDC的aCGH分析显示，16q丢失的瘤组织的主要部分为ER阳性。这提示肿瘤组织可能是从低级别/ER+发育为高级别/ER+的乳腺癌（Natrajan, et al, 2009a）。对多形性小叶癌（PLC）的研究也支持这一观点。PLC是典型浸润性小叶癌（ILC）的变异形式（Eusebi, et al, 1992; Middleton, et al, 2000; Weidner, Semple, 1992; Palacios, et al, 2003; Sneige, et al, 2002; Simpson, et al, 2003），生物学行为不良（Orvieto, et al, 2008; Buchanan, et al, 2008）。简言之，多形性小叶原位癌（LCIS）和ILC具有小叶癌典型的松散的形态学特征，缺乏E钙联素的表达；然而，PLC具备高级别肿瘤的特点，且出现极性分化的特征。尽管PLC的分子数据还比较缺乏，但是，它的基因改变与典型的ILC和Ⅲ级浸润性导管癌存在一定程度的交叉。PLC存在16q的丢失，整个基因组与ILC类似。这些数据提示，PLC可能与ILC的进化路径相同。高级别肿瘤中更常见的散发性的基因改变的累积（*HER2*、*p53*、*MYC*）可能进一步加强了其恶性的生物学行为（Simpson, et al, 2008）。

CGH和传统的细胞基因学研究已经发现，在浸润性乳腺癌的不同亚型间存在一定程度的基因变异的改变。尽管这种差别在不同组织学亚型间确实存在，但是，在组织学分级方面，这种关系不是那么明显（Buerger, et al, 1999a; Reis-Filho, Lakhani, 2003）。IDC和ILC间的比较分析已经显示，相对于IDC，ILC整体上基因改变较少。尽管某些染色体异常的频率在不同的组织学类型中有明确的不同，但是，这可能仅仅提示了一个事实，即绝大多数ILC都是低核级别的肿瘤。几种反复错乱的改变，包括16号染色体的q臂消失，在ILC和IDC中都普遍存在。这说明ILC和低级别的IDC可能来自同一条进化路径。

鉴于此，一些作者提出了疑问，如是否应该取消导管和小叶病变之间的界限，"导管"和"小叶"的命名是否合适。乳腺癌的细胞主体来自于末梢导管–小叶单元（TDLU），"导管"和"小叶"术语不是用来反映解剖位置的起源，而是细胞形态和生物学的特点（Simpson, et al, 2003）。因此，必须强调的一点是，尽管在Ⅰ级IDC和ILC中都存在16q的丢失，但是，这一丢失导致的基因改变可能不同。在ILC中，16q丢失最可能影响的抑癌基因是位于16q22.1的*CDH*1（E钙黏素）（Cleton-Jansen, et al, 2004; Palacios, et al, 2003; Simpson, et al, 2003）。16q丢失、基因突变、启动子甲基化或*CDH*1的再丢失在ILC中很常见。E钙黏素是一种关键的细胞间黏附分子，它的减少反映了单个细胞间松散的特点，以及小叶癌的整体生长模式。但是，在组织学Ⅰ级的IDC中，E钙黏素表达的丢失和*CDH*1基因突变非常少见，*CDH*1基因不是此类型乳腺癌的特征改变基因。与Ⅰ级IDC有关的肿瘤抑制基因的研究还在继续（Cleton-Jansen, 2002; Rakha, et al, 2004b; Roylance, et al, 2003）。

4.4 浸润性乳腺癌的分子分类

使用芯片CGH和基因表达分析技术，研究者对乳腺癌的分子表型进行了新的分类。基因组和后续基因表达的改变控制着肿瘤的表现型，这之间存在千丝万缕的联系。

最近，通过使用芯片分析乳腺癌的基因表达，研究者们将乳腺癌分为了5种不同的类型，进一步反映了这种疾病的异质性。这5种类型是：腔面A型、腔面B型、HER2型、基底样型和正常型（Perou, et al, 2000; Sorlie, et al, 2001, 2003），这些分型间主要的差别是ER水平。ER阳性会降低肿瘤的恶性程度，这类肿瘤与正常乳腺上皮有类似的基因表达，表达低分子量的角蛋白，如CK8/18，ER及其他基因。这类腔面型肿瘤进一步被分为A型和B型，后者有更高的增殖指数和更差的预后，分级更高。尽管被分为两群，但是，这类型肿瘤本质上还是存在相互联系的。来自小叶癌的数据显示（腔面A型是典型病变；腔面B型是多形性的变化体），腔面A型肿瘤能够因随机的基因突变，如预后不良的TP53突变和HER2过表达，而进化为腔面B型。

ER阴性的群体异质性更高。正常型的存在很难令人信服，可能是研究中正常细胞的污染所致。原研究中，HER2型和基底样型的预后最差。然而，一些研究显示，基底样肿瘤是一群极度异质性的细胞群体，其预后有好有坏。基底样肿瘤的命名是因为这类肿瘤的基因表达类型非常类似于正常乳腺的基底/肌上皮细胞，包括表达高分子量角蛋白（CK14、5/6和17）、P钙黏蛋白、P63、S100和上皮生长因子受体（EGFR/HER1）。这型肿瘤的形态学特征比较特异，中央多无细胞、有坏死区域、边界受挤压推移、高度多形性、高有丝分裂指数以及鳞状和纺锤形细胞分化（Fulford, et al, 2006）。基底样型乳腺癌多为三阴性（ER、PR和HER2阴性），偶有例外。HER2型组织学分级也较高，HER2及HER2路径上的基因都过表达。然而，临床实践中，一些HER2过表达的肿瘤被分入腔面B型中。芯片分析还将ER阴性乳腺癌亚型进一步分为"分泌型"亚型（Farmer, et al, 2005）、"干扰素"亚型和"紧密连接缺乏"型（Hennessy, et al, 2009）。这些亚型的临床和生物学意义还不清楚。

通过芯片CGH分析后，浸润性癌的基因组结构被分为"单纯型（Simplex）"、"复杂-狂暴型（Complex-Firestorm）"或"复杂-锯齿型（Complex-Sawtooth）"（Hicks, et al, 2006; Bergamaschi, et al, 2006; Natrajan, et al, 2009b），这些类型与因基因表达类型不同而分类的分子类型亦有关联。"单纯型"预后较好，是典型的腔面型癌，常同时出现1q的获得和16q的丢失。相比之下，复杂型预后较差。"狂暴型"的基因扩增区域很复杂，包括11q13、8p12、8q和17q12，多为HER2和腔面B型。"锯齿型"有很多短小的基因序列出现复制和丢失，遍及全部染色体和基因组的主体，但很少出现扩增，多见于"基底样癌"。这些基因拷贝数目的特点可能与这些肿瘤中DNA修复缺陷/不稳定的类型不同有关。

尽管新的分子分型让研究者兴奋不已，但是，我们还是应该牢记，随着我们对乳腺疾病认识的深入，分型会不断改变。例如，由于"腔面型"表达腔面细胞类的角蛋白，"基底型"表达肌上皮角蛋白，因此，新分类法将这两类可能分别来源于腔面上皮细胞和基底/肌上皮细胞或干细胞的乳腺癌分开。然而，对正常细胞与其前体细胞的研究数据显示，基底样癌可能来自腔面祖细胞（Lim, et al, 2009）。为了理解正常细胞系的分化和单个细胞类型的可塑性，我们还有很多的工作要做。在对疾病的组织学进行分类时，我们应该小心谨慎，不应草率下结论。

4.5 浸润前乳腺癌的分子分析

浸润性癌与增生性病变常共同出现，形态学有相似的地方，病理学家因此认为二者之间在生物学上有相关性（如LCIS和ILC，DCIS与IDC）（Reis-Filho, Lakhani, 2003）。新的分子病理学方法深入地研究了这种复杂的相关性，并且，通过观察不典型导管增生（ADH）DCIS病变和不典型小叶增生（ALH）LCIS病变中存在浸润性导管和小叶癌这种现象，研究者们最终总结出了基因型或表现型模式（Buerger, et al, 1999a, b; Lakhani, et al, 1995; Lu, et al, 1998; O'Connell, et al, 1998）。不同分级的浸润性癌存在不同的分子基因特征，这也反映了形态学类似的浸润前病变存在（Buerger, et al, 2000; Reis-Filho, Lakhani, 2003）。

回顾看来，在乳腺癌演进的多步骤模型中，清晰地存在两条主线：一条是温和的、分化良好的DCIS（低级别）演进为Ⅰ级IDC；另一条是分化差（高级别）的DCIS演进为Ⅲ级IDC。在"低级别"主线，这些原位和浸润性肿瘤核级别低，ER和PR多阳性，HER2和基底样标志物阴性，基因较稳定，16q序列存在。在"高级别"主线，病变的细胞核不典型性高，激素受体多阴性，HER2阳性或基底样标志物阳性，基因背景改变较多，如多种基因改变重复且共同出现：8p、11q、13q和14q的丢失；1q、5p、8q和17q的增加；6q22、8q22、11q13、17q12和17q22~24及20q13的扩增。无论是基因特点还是病理特点，典型的LCIS和ILC与"低级别"主线的那些肿瘤非常类似（Lu, et al, 1998; Simpson, et al, 2003）。与分化良好的DCIS/Ⅰ级IDC相比，这些肿瘤的主体成分缺乏E钙黏素的表达，这与*CDH*1基因的序列和（或）表观遗传改变有关（Rakha, et al, 2004a; Roylance, et al, 2003）。另一方面，PLCIS与PLC之间形态学上的共同特点，即既有典型小叶病变又存在Ⅲ级别的癌灶，E钙黏素（16q）丢失且HER2阳性率低（Eusebi, et al, 1992; Palacios, et al, 2003; Sneige, et al, 2002; Reis-Filho, et al, 2005）。这些表现又提示乳腺癌演进的分子通路很复杂。

ADH和ALH在形态学和基因表型上极度类似低级别DCIS和LCIS。除此以外，其他的非必然/癌前病变更难以定性，难以在多步骤的演进路径上定位它们的位置（O'Connell, et al, 1994, 1998; Reis-Filho, Lakhani, 2003）。ADH和低级别DCIS有相同的免疫表型，染色体异常和16q的重复丢失都很少。ALH和LCIS在形态学、免疫组化和基因水平也很类似（Simpson, et al, 2003）。实际上，ALH和LCIS是通过微小的定量而非形态学定性的方法进行区分，这种区分方法很主观。因此，学术界广泛认同这样的观点，即ADH和ALH都不是低级别DCIS和LCIS的必然前期病变。换句话说，我们可以将ADH和ALH视为微小的DCIS或LCIS病变，尽管这种观点未能被广泛接受。

肿瘤内形态学和基因的异质性提示了细胞克隆多样性的存在。这种多样性进一步增加了模型的复杂性，可能是临床上肿瘤性质多变的部分原因。同一个肿瘤内部，多个新生细胞克隆的发育导致基因不稳定性的进一步增加可能是多样性的原因。DCIS中发现了克隆多样性，多达50%的病例研究显示细胞分级存在异质性，9%的低级别DCIS也存在中高级别的区域。这类病例的免疫组化标志物表达水平不定，特别与p53阳性有关（Allred, et al, 2008）。作者指出，在某些病例中，ADH（低级别DCIS的前期病变）也可能是高级别DCIS的前期病变，后续演进为Ⅲ级IDC。低级别疾病与高级别疾病分子数据的不同也提示，相比细胞克隆的互相演进，不同级别细胞克隆独立出现并共存的可能性更大。

多年以来，普通增生（Hyperlasia of Usual Type HUT）一直被认为是ADH和DCIS的前期病变。然而，它在乳腺癌多步骤演进模型中的地位受到了质疑（Aubele, et al, 2000; Jones, et al, 2003; Lakhani, et al, 1996）。HUTs的形态学特点和免疫表型与那些已知的前期病变都有所不同，前者是一大群比例不定的细胞集合，ER、PR阳性的腔面细胞，肌上皮/基底标志物阳性细胞等。在分子水平，几乎没有随机的染色体改变出现（Aubele, et al, 2000; Jones, et al, 2003; Lakhani, et al, 1996）。尽管如此，目前的技术显示，在HUTs中存在极小的部分细胞具备克隆、恶性增生的能力（类似克隆性腺瘤），它们具有演进为ADH或DCIS的潜力。而没有任何证据显示HUTs的主体部分具有上述潜能。当前，绝大多数作者认为，这类型的病变在肿瘤的演进过程中作用不大，它们演进的方向是个"死胡同"。

ADH和低级别DCIS的另一个可能的前期病变是柱状细胞病变（CCL）（Fraser, et al, 1998; Schnitt, Vincent-Salomon, 2003; Simpson, et al, 2005a）。这包含了一系列程度不同的结构和核异常病变，其中异常程度最轻的病变是柱状细胞改变和增生，程度最重时，不典型改变明显，包括"扁平上皮不典型增生（FEA）"和典型的ADH。在整个系列中，CCLs的免疫表型与ADH/低级别DCIS类似（Schnitt, Vincent-Salomon, 2003）。然而，CGH技术显示，增生、结构和细胞的异常程度与基因水平的改变一致，染色体拷贝数目的数量和复杂程度都在逐级递增（Simpson, et al, 2005a）。而且，"低级别"病变的基因改变的特征性事件——16q的丢失，是最常被检测到的重复出现的改变。CCL的分子基因表型与相关的高级别病变之间存在一定程度的重叠（Moinfar, et al, 2000 b; Simpson, et al, 2005a）。有意思的是，在多灶性CCLs存在时，ALH/LCIS很少见。因此，CCLs可能是正常乳腺和ADH之间的演进环节，也是"导管性"和"小叶性"肿瘤形成之间的环节（Abdel-Fatah, et al, 2007, 2008）。分化差的DCIS的前期病变依旧是个谜。从形态学、免疫组织化学和分子研究的结果看，CCL、ADH和低级别DCIS可能都不是正确答案。

尽管乳腺组织的分泌型改变一向被认为是与衰老有关的化生性变化，但是，随着分子研究的深入，这一观点已经遭遇挑战（Jones, et al, 2001; Selim, et al, 2000, 2002）。至少分泌型的部分病变出现了基因改变，包括1p（*MYCL*1）、11q（*INT*2）、13q、16q和17q的LOH/等位基因失衡，以及反复出现的染色体改变，包括1p、2p、10q、16q、17q和22q的丢失，以及1p、2q和13q的获得。与分泌型囊肿相比，这些改变多在分泌型腺病和增生中出现。这些发现多被忽视。这样做是否合理有待探讨。但是，我们认为有确实的分子数据显示，至少是一部分病变可能是高级别DCIS和浸润性癌的前期病变。

4.6 正常乳腺的分子改变

随着许多潜在的前期病变的基因改变被发现，研究者逐渐关注浸润前和浸润性癌邻近的"正常"组织是否也存在基因突变。随着1990年代微切片技术的进步，Deng等（1996）报道称浸润性癌中常见的LOH在邻近癌组织的正常乳腺小叶中也能检测到。由于该研究是采用了石蜡包埋的微切片法，肿瘤细胞通过形变进入小叶中的可能性不能被排除。因此，存在3种可能的解释：①LOH来自于迁移进入正常小叶的邻近的浸润性癌的癌细胞。②LOH确实来自那些形态学正常的细胞。第二种假设暗示那些存在基因突变的貌似"正常"的乳腺组织促进了浸润性癌的发展。③肿瘤可能来自这些"正常"细胞。这些早期病变是如何产生的，这是病变小叶理论的一个主要议题（Tot, 2005）。

病变小叶理论指出，乳腺上皮细胞在其发育过程中出现的改变能够导致整个小叶或乳腺区段对进一步变化（成人时期）更敏感，结果导致了癌症的发生（图4.1A、B）。很可能这种改变是发生于基因水平的突变，最初是在单细胞内，后来传代至后续所有的细胞，这些细胞构成了乳腺的一个小叶。该理论指出正常小叶是单克隆性的，从而也引出了祖细胞或干细胞存在与否的疑问，这些原始细胞能分化为构成小叶的全部上皮细胞。目前已经有数个研究支持这个观点。

Lakhani等（1999）使用细胞克隆技术试图从无肿瘤细胞污染的乳腺样本中寻找LOH，并分别在乳腺的腔面细胞和肌上皮细胞中独立地检测LOH。研究者选择了浸润性乳腺癌中高频率的LOH位点，检测了来自乳腺癌患者的"正常"组织和行乳腺缩小术患者的组织。前者为来自石蜡包埋组织的导管小叶单元，后者是离体培养的新鲜组织的"正常"腔面和肌上皮细胞。不同类型上皮间的区分能力是非常重要的，它能确认改变是否发生在祖细胞或干细胞。研究发现，10例乳腺癌标本中有5例的正常组织中存在LOH，3个乳腺缩小术的标本中有1例存在LOH。无论肿瘤附近还是远处的正常细胞内都检测到了LOH。

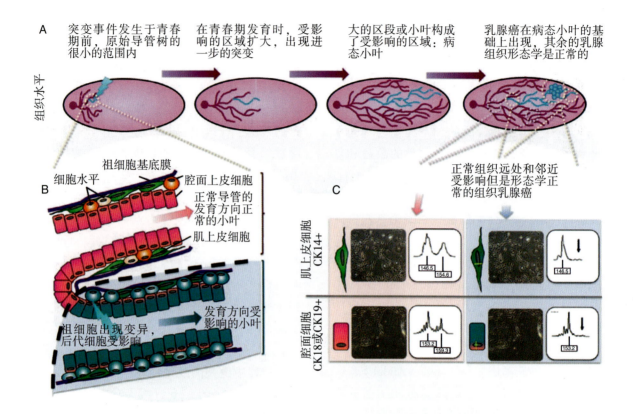

图4.1 基因改变影响病态小叶的可能机制

A. 简单的示意图显示发育中的乳腺内的管状上皮的基因改变，并将其传递给后代细胞形成"病态小叶"。正常的管状上皮为红色，病态的上皮为蓝色。B. 示意图描述了正常与病态小叶交界处的可能的细胞构成。当乳腺干细胞或祖细胞发生突变后，这种改变可以在所有后代细胞中发现，包括腔面细胞和肌上皮细胞以及其他祖细胞。细胞类型、功能和受影响区域的分子特征都会改变（蓝色），尽管用传统的组织化学方法可能无法检测出这些改变。C. 因此，成体乳腺是由正常小叶和病态小叶构成，后者的突变基因使细胞更易感。Clarke等的研究支持这一模型。来自BRCA1/2携带者的新鲜组织中培养的细胞克隆显示，腔面细胞是CK18/19阳性，肌上皮细胞是CK14阳性。尽管大多数克隆的DNA保留了杂合性（ROH），但还是有少数的克隆，包括腔面细胞和肌上皮细胞的BRCA1/2位点丢失了杂合性（LOH）。这些形态学上正常的细胞与残存的肿瘤细胞存在一样的突变，说明这种突变促进了肿瘤的产生。实际上，LOH（尤其是抑癌基因，如BRCA）的出现被认为是肿瘤形成的第一步。而且，腔面细胞和肌上皮细胞都存在相同的基因改变，说明最初的改变应该在祖细胞

3个乳腺缩小术标本培养了93株细胞克隆，其中1株显示出染色体13q上的等位基因的丢失。1例患者的标本中，所有的腔面和肌上皮细胞中都显示出同样的染色体13q的等位基因丢失。这些数据证实，LOH独立地存在于正常组织、腔面类型细胞和肌上皮类型细胞中。这说明，改变发生于细胞分化前的祖细胞或干细胞。微切片技术显示改变发生于全部类型的细胞中，这说明这种细胞克隆程度的改变可能主要发生于干细胞水平。

在人类样本中辨认克隆斑（clonal patch）很难，但是很重要。非常多的研究使用了X染色体连锁的失活法，结论都认为乳腺病变本质上存在克隆化的特点。一些专家没有意识到，如果没有克隆斑大小的概念，那么这些数据是没有意义的。如果克隆斑足够大，那么组织可能来自于多个细胞，并且在X连锁的检测方法下呈现单细胞克隆的特征。为了检

测出正常组织的克隆化结构，必须采用某种细胞标志物来确认细胞的胚系传代来源。使用嵌合体（mosaic）的动物实验可以达到这个目的。

因为X染色体失活，存在X染色体连锁多态性（杂合）的女性在mRNA和蛋白水平都是嵌合体。早期的研究使用了X连锁基因，例如葡萄糖-6-磷酸脱氢酶（G6PD）（Fialkow 1976）或不考虑斑块的尺寸时，使用限制性片段长度多态性法（Vogelstein, et al, 1985）。在雌性哺乳动物，胚胎时期X染色体失活（人类女性是胚胎第16天）。通过CpG岛的甲基化，两条X染色体的某一条的绝大多数基因被随机失活（Lyon, 1972）。甲基化非常稳定，会遗传给所有后代细胞。据报道，在肿瘤演进的过程中，X染色体失活也很稳定（Jones, 1996）。由于X染色体失活发生于胚胎形成的早期阶段，尽管后来随着发育有少数细胞不可避免地混杂进来，但是，在成年哺乳动物中从单个X染色体失活的胚胎细胞而来的后代细胞多聚集在一起。在上皮中，这些具有相同的X失活模式的细胞群就被称为细胞斑（patch）。斑块是由1或几个具有相同X染色体失活模式的细胞的后代细胞构成。因此，某个斑块内的细胞表现型相同，但来源可能是单克隆或多克隆。Novelli等（2003）收集了撒丁岛女性的切除标本，这些女性的G6PD存在地中海突变（563 C→T），基因型是杂合型。所有女性的G6PD酶活性都存在降低，突变情况经PCR（聚合酶链反应）证实。通过免疫组织化学技术，研究者证实乳腺中的细胞克隆斑的范围很广泛，包含整个导管和小叶单元。研究结果进一步支持了从LOH数据产生的假设。

Lakhani等（1999）报道了1个病例，患者的BRCA1存在胚系来源的截短，33个正常的克隆中有3个存在17q的LOH，其中一个克隆丢失了野生型的等位基因，提示了基因失活的存在。并且，11p和13q也存在LOH，这说明同源重组（homologous recombination, HR）丢失后，基因组的不稳定性进一步加重。后续对胚系BRCA1/2突变的分析是上述研究的延续。Clarke等（2006）研究了992株正常细胞克隆的BRCA1/2位点，这些细胞来自4例BRCA1/2突变携带者的正常组织。克隆中的LOH率很低（1.01%），但是4例标本中都有，无论是否有肿瘤存在。而且，在全部的腔面细胞克隆和肌上皮细胞克隆中，LOH都可以检测到。这说明不仅全部细胞都携带了这种基因突变（图4.1C），而且由于突变完全相同，说明这些细胞都来自同一种祖细胞。考虑到这些细胞体外培养的过程，这些细胞克隆也可能都来自同一个定向祖细胞。定位研究发现，某些病例的基因改变成簇状节段性地分布。该研究证实，基因不稳定的范围可存在于肿瘤周围，远大于TDLU以外。尽管后续再无类似研究进一步证实，但是，从表面看来，该研究提示外科手术时范围一定要足够以避免局部复发。同时，它也提出了疑问，即是否这就是肿瘤"完全切除"后部分病例局部复发的原因。

其他两个研究进一步发现，BRCA突变携带者的正常乳腺组织已经出现了改变，与肿瘤的早期改变类似。Max Wicha的课题组不仅观察到BRCA1突变携带者的形态学正常的乳腺组织存在BRCA1 LOH（Liu, et al, 2008），他们还发现ALDH1可以用来标记那些出现了基因改变的乳腺小叶组织。前者是一种潜在的干细胞标志物。尽管健康人体内ALDH1阳性细胞极其少见，但是，BRCA1突变携带者体内的ALDH1阳性细胞数较多，似乎构成了整个小叶组织。这个发现具有重要的意义，因为它提供了重要的证据，即BRCA1突变者的乳腺组织从基因到分子上都是不同的，尽管形态学是正常的。从这个角度看，图4.1a中用彩色线勾画出的病态小叶的范围也可以代表ALDH1的活性范围，改变发生的越早，范围就越大。不但如此，由于ALDH1是一种潜在的干细胞标志物，突变者乳腺中高水平ALDH1的表达提示初始的基因改变可能发生于乳腺干细胞，后者尽管分裂形成了腺泡，但是仍然存在某种分化缺陷，持续表达这种标志物。另一项研究在 BRCA1 突变携带者的乳腺全切除标本中发现了一群异常的腔面祖细胞，这进一步证实了上述假设，尽管研究者没有进行基因差异方面的检测（Lim, et al, 2009）。

4.7 病态的间质组织

Moinfar等（2000a）检查了乳腺癌患者的乳腺间质的LOH。研究者在石蜡标本中应用11个DNA标志物进行检测，结果发现在11%~57%的病例中形态学正常的间质组织存在LOH。对上皮和间质细胞的LOH进行比较发现，73%的病例在两种组织间至少有1个完全相同的LOH改变。这个有趣的结果提示上皮和间质细胞可能存在共同的祖细胞；然而，该研究结果还需进一步验证，其他研究也存在不同结论。Kurose等（2001）确认了上皮细胞的基因改变在先，间质细胞的LOH改变在后。

绝大多数cDNA芯片研究都关注乳腺上皮的恶性转化。最近的一些研究使用基因表达图谱来研究乳腺癌演进过程中乳腺实质的角色。一共14例患者，Ma等（2003）对DCIS、IDC、正常上皮、IDC间质（IDC-S）、DCIS间质（DCIS-S）和正常间质（NS）的基因表达进行了研究，结果发现在肿瘤演进的过程中间质组织也出现了基因改变，这说明肿瘤间质可能也与恶性上皮组织共同演进，甚至早于恶性转化发生之前。这些改变的基因主要涉及细胞外基质（extra cellular matrix, ECM）和重塑ECM所需的金属基质蛋白酶（matrix metalloproteases, MMP）。细胞质的核糖体蛋白下降了，但是线粒体的核糖体蛋白的基因表达上升。IDC-S和NS间的差异基因包括WNT受体信号通路的拮抗蛋白，该通路受TGFb家族成员调控。间质内与增殖相关的基因表达上调，如ECM、MMP和细胞周期相关基因。特别的是，与DCIS-S相比，ICD-S的间质内MMP11、MMP2、MMP14和MMP13的表达量明显升高，说明MMPs在原位癌向浸润性癌的转化过程中发挥作用（Fleming, et al, 2008; Ma, et al, 2009）。

Allinen等（2004）开发出了一种能从乳腺组织中纯化细胞的方法。该方法使用了细胞表面标志物与磁珠。BerEP4分选上皮细胞，CD45分选白细胞，P1H12分选上皮细胞，CD10用于后续分离肌上皮和肌成纤维细胞。去除这些组分后的未分离的细胞即被认为是富含成纤维细胞的实质部分。但是，很难进一步将肌成纤维细胞和肌上皮细胞分开。经过aCGH分析，DCIS和IDC来源的肌上皮细胞/肌成纤维细胞间并无基因差异，主要的基因差异还是肿瘤的上皮细胞之间。邻近肿瘤的正常组织并没有表现出基因改变。SNP检测和LOH检测也证实，在来自DCIS/IDC的纯化的间质细胞中并无LOH的存在。因此，与Lakhani等和Clarke等的研究结果不同，上述研究仅在腔面上皮细胞内检测到了基因的改变（Allinen, et al, 2004）。

对肿瘤有关的成纤维细胞/肌成纤维细胞的基因组改变的研究结果并不一致。Qiu等（2008）使用SNP检测法，对肿瘤相关的成纤维细胞（CAFs）进行了研究。这些细胞来自人类卵巢癌和乳腺癌的冰冻切片以及体外培养组织。来自切片的10个CAFs中没有拷贝数的改变，也没有染色体LOH的改变。但是，体外培养的样本中，有1个出现了7号和10号染色体的增加。另一个有意思的现象是，当将并未检测出改变的CAF和正常乳腺间质成纤维细胞分别注射入异种成瘤的动物体内后，前一种动物体内的肿瘤生长非常迅速。

尽管基因组未出现改变，但是，表观遗传学改变存在。Qiu等（2008）的研究同时发现，与正常的成纤维细胞相比，来自肿瘤的CAFs的甲基化和基因表达方式都不同。这说明间质基因未改变，但是培养的CAF存在不同的表现型（Qiu, et al, 2008）。随后，通过基因组甲基化检测、亚硫酸钠测序和羧基端甲基化免疫组化检测，研究者证实肌成纤维细胞的整体甲基化水平下降。胃癌的转基因小鼠模型证实去甲基化是肿瘤演进的早期事件；然而，确切的原因还未知(Jiang，et al，2008)。

因此整体而言，正常的组织存在分子改变，上皮细胞内存在基因突变是不争的结论；但是，间质细胞是否存在突变，没有突变时是否存在基因表达改变，这些疑问还需要研究进一步澄清。研究者们都确信，正常组织的改变在乳腺癌的演进中发挥了重要作用。

4.8 假　设

总结之前的研究结果，肿瘤演进的第一步可能起源于干/祖细胞。由于大多数突变都是在细胞分裂DNA复制时发生，因此，这些祖细胞群的基因突变也很有可能是在细胞分裂时发生，例如青春期时细胞分裂成为成熟乳腺细胞时。可以想象，干/祖细胞的基因改变会形成规模很大的携带突变的克隆斑（细胞群）。这些突变使得组织更易进一步改变，是肿瘤形成的第一步。尽管这个理论假设未能解释LCIS时的多灶性病变，但是，的确能够解释某些类型的乳腺病变的区段性分布的特点，如DCIS。我们推测，多灶性的情况可能是胚系突变导致的易感性与间质导致的易感性混杂存在，从而形成了临床中的风险和疾病表现。随着当前间质组织中分子改变的数据的积累，以及对间质上皮交互作用认识的深入，研究者们逐渐认识到，"病态"小叶中的间质和上皮成份可能都存在异常。

4.9 结论：与临床实践的关系

这个问题和"假设是否正确"一样难以回答。研究者们会告诉医生：复发或许是一种新的肿瘤，来源于已然不稳定的克隆斑（细胞群），由于医生不了解这些细胞的范围，因此上次手术后被残留下来。当前的技术条件不容许做解剖精度如此高的手术。或许在未来，出现了能够体内标识异常细胞的技术，采用导管内或导管外的方式切除导管树就变得可行。当然，这并未将重要角色的间质考虑在内，实际上的治疗会比我们想象的更复杂。

未来的10年非常关键，新的技术和传统病理学的结合能够揭示乳腺癌演进的生物学过程，并为我们如何治疗乳腺癌提供帮助。

参考文献

[1] Abdel-Fatah TM, Powe DG, Hodi Z, et al. High frequency of coexistence of columnar cell lesions, lobular neoplasia, and low grade ductal carcinoma in situ with invasive tubular carcinoma and invasive lobular carcinoma. Am J Surg Pathol, 2007, 31：417-426.

[2] Abdel-Fatah TM, Powe DG, Hodi Z, et al. Morphologic and molecular evolutionary pathways of low nuclear grade invasive breast cancers and their putative precursor lesions：further evidence to support the concept of low nuclear grade breast neoplasia family. Am J Surg Pathol, 2008, 32：513-523.

[3] Alizadeh AA, Ross DT, Perou CM, et al. Towards a novel classifcation of human malignancies based on gene expression patterns. J Pathol, 2001, 195：41-52.

[4] Allinen M, Beroukhim R, Cai L, et al. Molecular characterization of the tumor microenvironment in breast cancer. Cancer Cell, 2004, 6：17-32.

[5] Allred DC, Wu Y, Mao S, et al. Ductal carcinoma in situ and the emergence of diversity during breast cancer evolution. Clin Cancer Res, 2008, 14：370-378.

[6] Aubele MM, Cummings MC, Mattis AE, et al. Accumulation of chromosomal imbalances from intraductal proliferative lesions to adjacent in situ and invasive ductal breast cancer. Diagn Mol

Pathol, 2000, 9: 14-19.

[7] Bergamaschi A, Kim YH, Wang P, et al. Distinct patterns of DNA copy number alteration are associated with different clinicopathological features and gene-expression subtypes of breast cancer. Genes Chromosomes Cancer, 2006, 45: 1033-1040.

[8] Buchanan CL, Flynn LW, Murray MP, et al. Is pleomorphic lobular carcinoma really a distinct clinical entity. J Surg Oncol, 2008, 98: 314-317.

[9] Buerger H, Otterbach F, Simon R, et al. Comparative genomic hybridization of ductal carcinoma in situ of the breast-evidence of multiple genetic pathways. J Pathol, 1999a, 187: 396-402.

[10] Buerger H, Otterbach F, Simon R, et al. Different genetic pathways in the evolution of invasive breast cancer are associated with distinct morphological subtypes. J Pathol, 1999b, 189: 521-526.

[11] Buerger H, Simon R, Schafer KL, et al. Genetic relation of lobular carcinoma in situ, ductal carcinoma in situ, and associated invasive carcinoma of the breast. Mol Pathol, 2000, 53: 118-121.

[12] Clarke CL, Sandle J, Jones AA, et al. Mapping loss of heterozygosity in normal human breast cells from BRCA1/2 carriers. Br J Cancer, 2006, 95: 515-519.

[13] Cleton-Jansen AM. E-cadherin and loss of heterozygosity at chromosome 16 in breast carcinogenesis: different genetic pathways in ductal and lobular breast cancer. Breast Cancer Res, 2002, 4: 5-8.

[14] Cleton-Jansen AM, Buerger H, Haar N, et al. Different mechanisms of chromosome 16 loss of heterozy-gosity in well-versus poorly differentiated ductal breast cancer. Genes Chromosomes Cancer, 2004, 41: 109-116.

[15] Deng G, Lu Y, Zlotnikov G, et al. Loss of heterozygosity in normal tissue adjacent to breast carcinomas. Science, 1996, 274: 2057-2059.

[16] Ellis IO, Galea M, Broughton N, et al. Pathological prognostic factors in breast cancer. II. Histological type. Relationship with survival in a large study with long-term follow-up. Histopathology, 1992, 20: 479-489.

[17] Elston CW, Ellis IO. Pathological prognostic factors in breast cancer. I. The value of histological grade in breast cancer: experience from a large study with long-term follow-up. Histopathology, 1991, 19: 403-410.

[18] Eusebi V, Magalhaes F, Azzopardi JG. Pleomorphic lobular carcinoma of the breast: an aggressive tumor showing apocrine differentiation. Hum Pathol, 1992, 23: 655-662.

[19] Farmer H, McCabe N, Lord CJ, et al. Targeting the DNA repair defect in BRCA mutant cells as a therapeutic strategy. Nature, 2005, 434: 917-921.

[20] Fialkow PJ. Clonal origin of human tumors. Biochim Biophys Acta, 1976, 458: 283-321.

[21] Fleming JM, Long EL, Ginsburg E, et al. Interlobular and intralobular mammary stroma: genotype may not refect phenotype. BMC Cell Biol, 2008, 9: 46.

[22] Fraser JL, Raza S, Chorny K, et al. Columnar alteration with prominent apical snouts and secretions: a spectrum of changes frequently present in breast biopsies performed for microcalcifcations. Am J Surg Pathol, 1998, 22: 1521-1527.

[23] Fulford LG, Easton DF, Reis-Filho JS, et al. Specifc morphological features predictive for the basal phenotype in grade 3 invasive ductal carcinoma of breast. Histopathology Jul, 2006, 49 (1): 22-34.

[24] Hennessy BT, Gonzalez-Angulo AM, Stemke-Hale K, et al. Characterization of a naturally occurring breast cancer subset enriched in epithelial-to-mesenchymal transition and stem cell characteristics. Cancer Res, 2009, 69: 4116-4124.

[25] Hicks J, Krasnitz A, Lakshmi B, et al. Novel patterns of genome rearrangement and their association with survival in breast cancer. Genome Res, 2006, 16: 1465-1479.

[26] Jiang Y, Tong D, Lou G, et al. Expression of RUNX3 gene, methylation status and clinicopathological signifcance in breast cancer and breast cancer cell lines. Pathobiology, 2008, 75: 244-251.

[27] Jones PA. DNA methylation errors and cancer. Cancer Res, 1996, 56: 2463-2467.

[28] Jones C, Damiani S, Wells D, et al. Molecular cytogenetic comparison of apocrine hyper-plasia and apocrine carcinoma of the breast. Am J Pathol, 2001, 158: 207-214.

[29] Jones C, Merrett S, Thomas VA, et al. Comparative genomic hybridization analysis of bilateral hyperplasia of usual type of the breast. J Pathol, 2003, 199: 152-156.

[30] Kurose K, Hoshaw-Woodard S, Adeyinka A, et al. Genetic model of multi-step breast carcinogenesis involving the epithelium and stroma: clues to tumour-microenvironment interactions. Hum Mol Genet, 2001, 10: 1907-1913.

[31] Lakhani SR. Is there a benign to malignant progression. Endocr Relat Cancer, 1997, 4: 93-104.

[32] Lakhani SR, Collins N, Stratton MR, et al. Atypical ductal hyperplasia of the breast: clonal proliferation with loss of heterozygosity on chromosomes 16q and 17p. J Clin Pathol, 1995, 48: 611-615.

[33] Lakhani SR, Slack DN, Hamoudi RA, et al. Detection of allelic imbalance indicates that a proportion of mammary hyperplasia of usual type are clonal, neoplastic proliferations. Lab Invest, 1996, 74: 129-135.

[34] Lakhani SR, Chaggar R, Davies S, et al. Genetic alterations in 'nor-mal' luminal and myoepithelial cells of the breast. J Pathol, 1999, 189: 496-503.

[35] Lim E, Vaillant F, Wu D, et al. Aberrant luminal progenitors as the candidate target population for basal tumor development in BRCA1 mutation carriers. Nat Med, 2009, 15: 907-913.

[36] Liu S, Ginestier C, Charafe-Jauffret E, et al. BRCA1 regulates human mammary stem/progenitor cell fate. Proc Natl Acad Sci USA, 2008, 105: 1680-1685.

[37] Lu YJ, Osin P, Lakhani SR, et al. Comparative genomic hybridization analysis of lobular carcinoma in situ and atypical lobular hyperplasia and potential roles for gains and losses of genetic material in breast neoplasia. Cancer Res, 1998, 58: 4721-4727.

[38] Lyon MF. X-chromosome inactivation and developmental patterns in mammals. Biol Rev Camb Philos Soc, 1972, 47: 1-35.

[39] Ma XJ, Salunga R, Tuggle JT, et al. Gene expression profiles of human breast cancer progression. Proc Natl Acad Sci USA, 2003, 100: 5974-5979.

[40] Ma XJ, Dahiya S, Richardson E, et al. Gene expression profiling of the tumor microenvironment during breast cancer progression. Breast Cancer Res, 2009, 11: R7

[41] Middleton LP, Palacios DM, Bryant BR, et al. Pleomorphic lobular carcinoma: mor-phology, immunohistochemistry, and molecular analysis. Am J Surg Pathol, 2000, 24: 1650-1656.

[42] Moinfar F, Man YG, Arnould L, et al. Concurrent and independent genetic alterations in the stromal and epithelial cells of mammary carcinoma: implications for tumorigenesis. Cancer Res, 2000a, 60: 2562-2566.

[43] Moinfar F, Man YG, Bratthauer GL, et al. Genetic abnormalities in mammary ductal intraepi-thelial neoplasia-fat type ("clinging ductal carcinoma in situ"): a simulator of normal mammary epithelium. Cancer, 2000b, 88: 2072-2081.

[44] Natrajan R, Lambros MB, Geyer FC, et al. Loss of 16q in high grade breast cancer is associated with estrogen receptor status: evidence for progression in tumors with a luminal phenotype. Genes Chromosomes Cancer, 2009a, 48: 351-365.

[45] Natrajan R, Lambros MB, Rodríguez-Pinilla SM, et al. Tiling path genomic profiling of grade 3 invasive ductal breast cancers. Clin Cancer Res, 2009b, 15: 2711-2722.

[46] Nishizaki T, Chew K, Chu L, et al. Genetic alterations in lobular breast cancer by comparative genomic hybridization. Int J Cancer, 1997, 74: 513-517.

[47] Novelli M, Cossu A, Oukrif D, et al. X-inactivation patch size in human female tissue confounds the assessment of tumor clonality. Proc Natl Acad Sci USA, 2003, 100: 3311-3314.

[48] O'Connell P, Pekkel V, Fuqua S, et al. Molecular

genetic studies of early breast cancer evolution. Breast Cancer Res Treat, 1994, 32: 5-12.

[49] O'Connell P, Pekkel V, Fuqua SA, et al. Analysis of loss of heterozygosity in 399 premalignant breast lesions at 15 genetic loci. J Natl Cancer Inst, 1998, 90: 697-703.

[50] Oldenhuis CN, Oosting SF, Gietema JA, et al. Prognostic versus predictive value of biomarkers in oncol-ogy. Eur J Cancer, 2008, 44: 946-953.

[51] Orvieto E, Maiorano E, Bottiglieri L, et al. Clinicopathologic characteristics of invasive lobular carcinoma of the breast: results of an analysis of 530 cases from a single institution. Cancer, 2008, 113: 1511-1520.

[52] Palacios J, Sarrio D, Garcia-Macias MC, et al. Frequent E-cadherin gene inactivation by loss of heterozygosity in pleomorphic lobular carcinoma of the breast. Mod Pathol, 2003, 16: 674-678.

[53] Perou CM, Sorlie T, Eisen MB, et al. Molecular portraits of human breast tumours. Nature, 2000, 406: 747-752.

[54] Pollack JR, Perou CM, Alizadeh AA, et al. Genome-wide analysis of DNA copy-number changes using cDNA microarrays. Nat Genet, 1999, 23: 41-46.

[55] Qiu W, Hu M, Sridhar A, et al. No evidence of clonal somatic genetic alterations in cancer-associated fibroblasts from human breast and ovarian carcinomas. Nat Genet, 2008, 40: 650-655.

[56] Rakha EA, Pinder SE, Paish CE, et al. Expression of the transcription factor CTCF in invasive breast cancer: a candidate gene located at 16q22.1. Br J Cancer, 2004a, 91: 1591-1596.

[57] Rakha EA, Pinder SE, Paish EC, et al. Expression of E2F-4 in invasive breast carcinomas is associated with poor prognosis. J Pathol, 2004b, 203: 754-761.

[58] Reis-Filho JS, Lakhani SR. The diagnosis and management of preinvasive breast disease: genetic alterations in preinvasive lesions. Breast Cancer Res, 2003, 5: 313-319.

[59] Reis-Filho JS, Simpson PT, Jones C, et al. Pleomorphic lobular carcinoma of the breast: role of comprehensive molecular pathology in characterization of an entity. J Pathol, 2005, 207 (1): 1-13.

[60] Reis-Filho JS, Simpson PT, Gale T, et al. The molecular genetics of breast cancer: the contribution of comparative genomic hybridization. Pathol Res Pract, 2005, 201: 713-725.

[61] Roylance R, Gorman P, Hanby A, et al. Allelic imbalance analysis of chromosome 16q shows that grade I and grade III invasive ductal breast cancers follow different genetic pathways. J Pathol, 2002, 196 (1): 32-36.

[62] Roylance R, Droufakou S, Gorman P, et al. The role of E-cadherin in low-grade ductal breast tumourigenesis. J Pathol, 2003, 200: 53-58.

[63] Roylance R, Gorman P, Papior T, et al. A comprehensive study of chromosome 16q in invasive ductal and lobular breast carcinoma using array CGH. Oncogene, 2006, 25: 6544-6553.

[64] Schnitt SJ, Vincent-Salomon A. Columnar cell lesions of the breast. Adv Anat Pathol, 2003, 10: 113-124.

[65] Selim AG, El-Ayat G, Wells CA. C-erbB2 oncoprotein expression, gene amplifcation, and chromosome 17 aneusomy in apocrine adenosis of the breast. J Pathol, 2000, 191: 138-142.

[66] Selim AG, El-Ayat G, Wells CA. Expression of cerbB2, p53, Bcl-2, Bax, c-myc and Ki-67 in apocrine metaplasia and apocrine change within sclerosing adenosis of the breast. Virchows Arch, 2002, 441: 449-455.

[67] Simpson PT, Gale T, Fulford LG, et al. The diagnosis and management of pre-invasive breast disease: pathology of atypical lobular hyperplasia and lobular carcinoma in situ. Breast Cancer Res, 2003, 5: 258-262.

[68] Simpson PT, Gale T, Reis-Filho JS, et al. Columnar cell lesions of the breast: the missing link in breast cancer progression. A morphological and molecular analysis. Am J Surg Pathol, 2005a, 29: 734-746.

[69] Simpson PT, Reis-Filho JS, Gale T, et al. Molecular evolution of breast cancer. J Pathol, 2005b, 205: 248-254.

[70] Simpson P, Reis-Filho J, Lambros M, et al. Molecular profling pleomorphic lobular carcinomas of the breast: evidence for a com-mon molecular genetic pathway with classic lobular carcinomas. J Pathol, 2008, 215: 231-244.

[71] Sneige N, Wang J, Baker BA, et al. Clinical, histopathologic, and biologic features of pleomorphic lobular (ductal-lobular) carcinoma in situ of the breast: a report of 24 cases. Mod Pathol, 2002, 15: 1044-1050.

[72] Sorlie T, Perou CM, Tibshirani R, et al. Gene expression patterns of breast carcinomas distinguish tumor subclasses with clinical implications. Proc Natl Acad Sci USA, 2001, 98: 10869-10874.

[73] Sorlie T, Tibshirani R, Parker J, et al. Repeated observation of breast tumor subtypes in independent gene expression data sets. Proc Natl Acad Sci USA, 2003, 100: 8418-8423.

[74] Stratton MR, Collins N, Lakhani SR, et al. Loss of heterozygosity in ductal carcinoma in situ of the breast. J Pathol, 1995, 175: 195-201.

[75] Stratton MR, Campbell PJ, Futreal PA. The cancer genome. Nature, 2009, 458: 719-724.

[76] Tognon C, Knezevich SR, Huntsman D, et al. Expression of the ETV6-NTRK3 gene fusion as a primary event in human secretory breast carcinoma. Cancer Cell, 2002, 2: 367-376.

[77] Tot T. DCIS, cytokeratins, and the theory of the sick lobe. Virchows Arch, 2005, 447: 1-8.

[78] Vogelstein B, Fearon ER, Hamilton SR, et al. Use of restriction fragment length polymorphisms to determine the clonal origin of human tumors. Science, 1985, 227: 642-645.

[79] Weidner N, Semple JP. Pleomorphic variant of invasive lobular carcinoma of the breast. Hum Pathol, 1992, 23: 1167-1171.

第5章 乳管灌洗法的作用——一个发人深省的故事

Susan M.Love, Dixie J.Mills

5.1 背 景

近100年前,英国医生及作家杰弗里·凯恩斯先生认为"乳腺是一个腺体,在人的一生中不停地分泌一些物质,哺乳期与非哺乳期乳腺的区别主要在于以下两个方面,一是分泌的程度不同,二是分泌物的化学成分不同"(Keynes,1923)。近几年来,尽管人们对乳腺癌病理组织学的认识已经有了显著进展,但是,在非哺乳期或静息期乳房的腔内细胞和乳管系统的分泌物仍很少受到关注。大多数病理学家认为,这些细胞和分泌物逐渐退变成脱落的上皮和蛋白质样物质,并且没有生物学活性(Petrakis,1986)。然而,仔细地观察这种分泌物并确定其生理及临床意义是非常有价值的。

5.2 乳头抽吸液 (NAF)

早在1958年,Papanicolaou就有应用吸奶器抽吸乳头从乳管中获得少量乳头抽吸液(NAF)的描述(Papanicolaou, et al,1958)。人们希望这些抽吸液可以像宫颈涂片对宫颈癌的预测一样用来检测早期乳腺癌。但是,由于这些抽吸液几乎没有细胞存在,且很少有阳性结果,因此,该技术并没有得到广泛应用。

在1970年代,许多研究人员重新评估和恢复了Papanicolaou的研究方法(Buehring,1979; Sartorius,1973; Sartorius, et al,1977)。他们通过应用一个使用短塑料管连接到10mL注射器上的吸盘,从更多的女性乳头中得到抽吸液。他们还发现这种方法可以清除任何封闭孔洞的角质栓,从而达到清洗乳头的作用。这种吸引器可以产生更强的负压,经过多次尝试,研究人员从近70%的女性患者乳房中抽取了乳头抽吸液。乳头抽吸液容易从有湿型耵聍的绝经前白种妇女中获得,亚裔美国人和绝经后妇女是最不容易获得乳头抽吸液的人群。经研究发现,NAF中含有脂质、胆固醇、激素和其他一些不同种类的物质,如巴比妥类、咖啡因、尼古丁和农药(Petrakis,1986)。NAF的细胞病理学检查显示其含有导管上皮细胞、分泌细胞、泡沫细胞即巨噬细胞(King, et al,1975)。目前的研究主要集中在NAF中的上皮细胞,因为通过观察其由正常上皮细胞逐渐通过增生、不典型增生、原位癌到浸润癌的演变,我们可以更好地理解乳腺癌的病理生理。

Wrensch和Petraskis认为,在NAF中发现上皮细胞与患乳腺癌是有关联的,这种风险在30岁后增加21%。此外,与没有抽出液体的女性相比,在NAF中发现异形细胞的女性患乳腺癌的风险是她们的2.8倍(Wrensch, et al,2001)。然而,NAF中的异形细胞并非一定是

S. M. Love
Dr. Susan Love Research Foundation, Santa Monica, CA, USA
e-mail: susan.love@dslrf.org

乳腺癌的前奏，因为只有11%的女性发展成乳腺癌。3个大型临床研究经过20年的随访观察证实，存在乳头溢液尤其是其内发现异形细胞的女性患乳腺癌的风险更高（Wrensch, et al, 2001; Buehring, et al, 2006;Baltzell, et al, 2008）（表5.1）。然而，NAF作为筛选乳腺癌的一个危险因素是有条件限制的，包括其技术限制及存在相当数量的没有抽出液体的女性，更重要的是，在NAF中上皮细胞的数量相当有限，需要受过严格训练的病理学家来读取样本。

5.3 导管灌洗（DL）

乌拉圭的一名叫Leborgne的医生在60多年前首次提出这种研究乳管及乳头溢液的方法（Leborgne，1946）。他描述的这种方法是：用一根细管经过乳头插入乳管中，进而通过细管注入生理盐水，然后拔出细管，按摩乳房，进而收集流出的液体。这种程序被称为"乳管灌洗"。随着放射影像技术的提高，乳腺增强X线检查被应用于乳头溢液的术前评估（Love, Barsky, 1996）。尽管乳腺导管树在X线下清晰地显影，但获得图像清晰的X线片的难度以及对比剂的副作用均使其广泛应用受到了限制（图5.1）。然而，随着对宫颈细胞学检查意义的认可，人们对乳管灌洗又产生了新的兴趣。Otto Sartorius及其同事把乳管对比造影和造影后灌洗液检查结合到一起，通过这一技术获得了更多的阳性结果（Sartorius, et al, 1977）。直到Love发明了一种独特的微导管，乳管灌洗才得到了较广泛的应用。这种微导管与双腔导管相通，并能保持导管的通畅性（Love, Barsky, 1996）（图5.2）。基于对导管原位癌和浸润性导管癌局限于一个导管系统的观察结果，DL和微导管（Cytyc catheter）逐渐发展成为观察某一特定导管的方法并被商业化（Holland, et al, 1985;Mai, et al, 2000）。

有证据表明，DL的过程可以将液体（染料或生理盐水）输送到乳腺末端导管小叶单

表5.1 关于NAF与癌症相对危险度的主要前瞻性研究

研究中心	样本数	随访（年）	无乳管液	有乳管液	细胞	异形细胞
Wrensch, et al, 2001	3 627	21	1.0 (3.7%)	1.2 (7.5%)	1.3 (6.6%)	2.1 (11%)
Buehring, et al, 2006	972/1 744	25	1.0		2.27	
Baltzell, et al, 2008	946/1 706	20	1.0	1.4	1.7	2.0

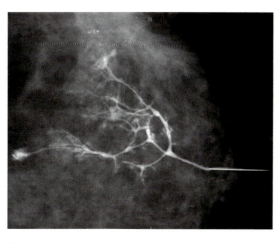

图5.1 使用染料（对比剂）后，乳腺X线片显示深入小叶的导管系统

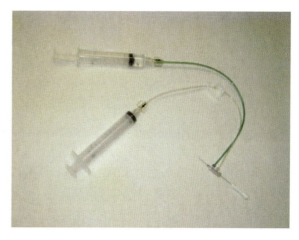

图5.2 DL用微导管

位，同样也可以收集到此处的细胞，包括利用染料显示乳腺灌洗液流通路径在内的多项研究已经证实了乳腺导管系统内小叶-腺泡部分渗透现象的存在（Love，Barsky，1996；Brogi，2003；Khan，2004）。此外，从一位病理确诊的小叶原位癌患者的乳管灌洗液中收集到具有小叶原位癌细胞学特征的脱落细胞（Brogi，et al，2003）。此外，灌洗试验的参加者报告称胸壁和躯干中心区域感受到比室温低的灌洗液循环流动（King，Love，2005）。总之，这些数据表明，通过乳管灌洗我们可以收集到乳腺导管末端脱落的上皮细胞。纳入507例高风险女性样本的第一个多中心研究结果表明，乳管灌洗可获得大量的导管上皮细胞，而且灌洗过程安全，耐受性良好，是一种相比乳头抽吸法获得乳腺异形细胞的敏感性更高的方法（Dooley，et al，2001）。

5.3.1 乳头浅表解剖

事实上，任何一个仔细观察过哺乳期妇女的人都能够明显发现，乳汁像散水壶一样溢出而不是像喷管一样从乳头表面喷出。乳头小孔不允许任何物质反流回乳房，因此被认为是单向导管。通过仔细观察发现，乳头表面存在很多裂隙，乳腺导管的开口并不总是显而易见的。事实上，这些小孔的数量是有争议的。Astley Cooper（Cooper，1845）对死于分娩败血症的患者进行尸体解剖时，通过乳头注入石蜡进行研究。他认为大多数情况下可存在7~10个乳管，最多不超过12个乳管。Love和Barsky（2004）通过对200名哺乳期女性进行观察，认为平均5~9个导管开孔于乳头。他们的以下观点似乎一致，即在乳头的中央组有4~5个导管开口，在乳头的外周同样有4~5个开口。Teboul和Halliwell（1995）报道称对超过6 000名妇女的超声检查结果提示，在乳头中有5~8个乳汁流出道。Ramsay等（2005）研究了21名哺乳期妇女的乳头超声图像，结果发现乳头中有6~12个主导管。而人们引用较多的是对乳头的病理切片中的管腔进行计数，发现乳头中有15~20个管腔（Rusby，et al，2007）。关于乳头精确解剖的研究仍在继续，例如这些乳腺导管是退化的还是直接连通的？导管是否汇合后开口于乳头表面？此外，由于对乳头的横断面切片研究并没有追根到乳腺实质，其代表的意义并不清楚。每个乳腺小叶是单独的还是互有联系，本书其他部分另有涉及。

5.3.2 乳管灌洗技术

因为确定乳管孔是非常困难的，所以乳管灌洗最初仅应用于那些经过乳管抽吸装置可以吸出液体的女性身上（Dooley，et al，2001）。首先，使用温和的研磨乳液将乳头去角质化，由患者自己或医生轻轻按摩乳房至少1min；其次将配有10~20mL注射器的吸杯放置在乳头上，加少量的吸力（7~15mL）。如果没有液体流出，则用手在乳头基底部输乳窦区进行挤压。经过反复按摩乳房和抽吸，直到液体抽出或由研究者确认确实没有液体产生。

第一个关于乳管灌洗的大型研究报道（Dooley，et al，2001）称，多数情况下采用乳头局部浸润或表面麻醉（局麻乳膏：2.5%利多卡因和2.5%普鲁卡因；Astra USA）。大约28%的研究对象在全身麻醉或镇静下进行，这就需要在手术室进行操作。

应用30号针头抽取1%利多卡因于乳晕皮下注射或乳头阻滞麻醉的尝试因受试者产生不适感而被放弃。当乳头抽吸后有多个管道排出液体后，可以立即尝试进行乳管灌洗。一般采用仰卧位，乳头周围皮肤用70%的酒精消毒。乳头麻醉后，应用微扩张器轻轻扩张乳管孔，并在扩张器的尖端涂2%的利多卡因胶浆，以方便插管。为了防止不同导管系统间细胞交叉污染，一个插管对应一个微导管。在插入之前，微导管要用1%利多卡因或生理盐水注满，防止进入空气。将导管插入最大深度1.5cm处，注入2mL生理盐水、羧甲淀粉或乳酸钠林格液，然后挤压或按摩乳房，以促进导管液体的回收。将整个灌洗过程（注入生理盐水、挤压或按摩乳房以及流出物的收集）重复多次，每个导管灌注总量10~20mL的生理盐水，回收5~10mL。将收集到的液体放入离心机，以2 500r/min离心10min，将沉淀的细胞悬浮于20mL的专用溶液（Preservcyt, Hologic, MA）中进行细胞学检查，将上清液冷冻，以备进行其他生物标志物的研究。

5.3.3 改进

最近，Tondre等人（2008）直接应用30号针管经乳头注射以碳酸氢钠缓冲的1%利多卡因（图5.3）。根据受试者的不适程度以及整个灌洗程序的长短，可适当增加利多卡因或布比卡因的量。该技术的疼痛评分不高。这样可以使乳头充血膨胀，导管孔可更加容易显现。扩张器及加强器可以用来判断非排出管道。将乳头轻拉提起，可以将扩张器更容易插入乳管中，使用放大镜也可以起到积极作用。经过几次实践，在短时间内很容易就能找到6~8个非排出乳管（Love, et al, 2009）。

一些研究者（Visvanathan, et al, 2007; Loud, et al, 2009）经随访后报道，该过程耐受性较差并且具有较高的损耗率（25%）。乳管灌洗可作为BRCA1和BRCA2基因突变携带者或具有其他高风险因素的女性的健康筛查方式。事实上，患者精神越紧张，乳管灌洗造成的身体不适就比想象的越明显（Loud, et al, 2009）。有关报道（Tondre, et al, 2008）称经过6个月的随访，其回访率在健康志愿者身上可高达90%，在高风险女性身上高达95%（Twelves, Gui, 2008）。当然，这与受试者的参与及理解以及临床医生对乳管灌洗投入的热情是分不开的。对有些人来讲，乳管灌洗较乳腺钼靶检查更容易接受，其他人则相反，因此其作为常规乳腺筛查的工具再度受到质疑。

我们可以结合乳管灌洗与超声技术来识别乳腺导管是管状结构还是穿孔。在乳管镜检查之后它可以再次识别和确认乳腺导管是管状结构而不是穿孔（Tondre, et al, 2008）（图5.4、图5.5）。Danforth等提出了一个可行性研究，即在乳管灌洗之后，应用乳管内镜连接一个刷子、线圈或抽吸装置，对11个受试者的乳腺进行取样（Danforth, et al, 2006）。后来的取样研究可以在对乳管损伤较小的前提下，获得更多的细胞或样品数量。这项研究是在静脉镇静下完成的。

5.4 研究和经验教训

乳管灌洗成功的报告引发了多个研究中心对该方法应用于患癌风险评估价值的研究。大多数中心及研究对象主要来源于乳腺癌高危人群。关于乳管灌洗的管理及建议早在2003年就已经被刊登了（Danforth, et al, 2006）。冲洗液细胞学检查若为良性，则需要1~3年复查一次；若为轻度不典型增生，则需要在1年内复查一次或考虑预防性治疗（图5.6）；若为重度不典型增生或恶性，则需要进一步检查以确认结果，如乳腺磁共振成像，乳管镜或乳腺导管造影摄片。如果确认病变或乳管灌洗的结果需要进行预防性治疗时，组织活检可能是必要的。并不推荐仅基于乳管灌洗结果而开展手术治疗。然而，由于乳

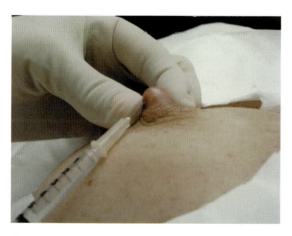

图5.3 使用30号针头进行乳头阻滞麻醉，注意针头方向和注射点

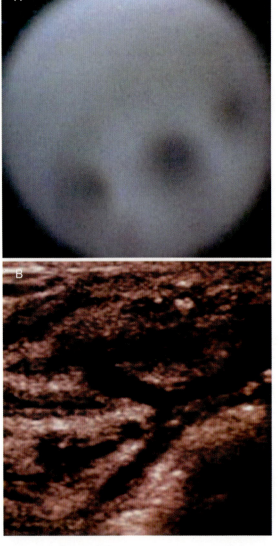

图5.4 导管镜下导管的3个分支（A）以及灌洗时超声显示管道的扩张（B）

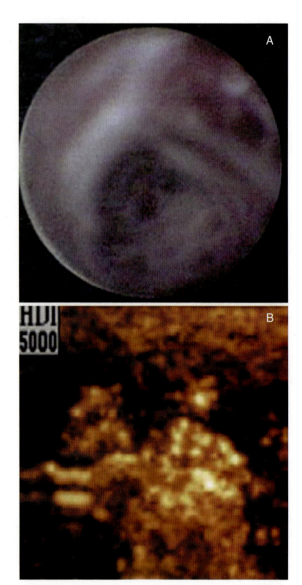

图5.5 穿孔在镜下表现出不规则和高亮的特征（A），超声下显示出信号集中增强（B）

管灌洗结果判定所依据的假说并不完全准确，人们对乳管灌洗的研究正由最初的狂热逐渐衰减。

5.4.1 溢液导管的重要性

最初的假设是那些分泌最活跃且最容易受影响的、被称为前哨导管的那部分导管代表着整个乳腺的情况（Dooley, et al, 2001）。事实上，如果乳头抽吸液代表整个乳房的某部分有缺陷的话，那么人们期望得到的结果是任何患有乳腺癌的部分导管中抽出的液体都有不典型增生的细胞。Khan等（2004）和Brogi等（2003）的研究发现并非如此。另一种假设是溢液的乳管最有可能储藏不典型细胞和恶性细胞，因此乳管抽吸液（NAF）和乳管灌洗（DL）的结果在一定程度上是相似的。根据上述对乳管抽吸液的研究，有人提出这样的假设：产生乳头抽吸液的那部分导管极有可能是异常的。然而，最近一些研究证明，不分泌液体的导管与分泌液体的导管内同样有可能含有不典型细胞（Kurian, et al,

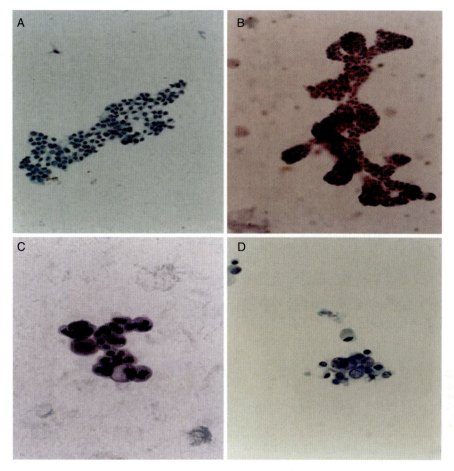

图5.6　DL的细胞病理学。A. 良性。B. 轻度异型。C. 明显异型。D. 恶性

2005; Bhandare, et al, 2005; Maddux, et al, 2004），这些研究显示，不典型细胞在分泌性和非分泌性导管的发生率是一致的。Khan等（2005）的研究证明，大多数存在原位癌的导管并不产生乳管抽吸液。这些研究结果并不令人惊讶，因为在原位癌或浸润癌中，只有5%表现为血水性或浆液性溢液（Cabioglu, et al, 2003）。

5.4.2 细胞学不典型增生表现的意义及临床应用

Dupont和Page在1985年证实，从乳房组织活检中查出的不典型增生导管是一种乳腺癌的高风险因素（Dupont, Page, 1985）。在乳管抽吸液中查出细胞异型也被 Wrensch、Buehring和Baltzell等的研究证明是一种高风险因素，虽然风险性较组织学检查低（Wrensch, et al, 2001; Buehring, et al, 2006; Baltzell, et al, 2008）。但乳管灌洗液中发现异型的患病风险仍只是推测。将乳管灌洗液标本中的异形细胞作为罹患乳腺癌的风险因素，目前仍缺乏大规模样本的调查及前瞻性数据分析。一项多中心研究——导管上皮细胞的系列评价试验（SEDE）被提前结束，该试验的目的是解决关于乳管灌洗的很多问题及其风险性评估（Linder, 2004）。乳管灌洗液标本主要来自高风险妇女，以6个月为间隔进行抽取，标本的细胞形态学已经得到研究，其离心后的上清液也被冷冻，可在将来进行生物标记物的研究。这些患者的随访和标本检查仍在进行中。

最初，在乳管灌洗液标本中，细胞学的异型性研究被认为对临床试验研究有益。然而，随着时间的推移，乳管灌洗中异形细胞的重复性并没有被认可，因此，其在风险评估中的有效性受到了质疑。一项Johnson-Maddox研究发现：在乳管灌洗液中初次发现异形细胞者，经再次取样，仅有不到一半的女性再次发现异形细胞（Johnson-Maddox, et al, 2005）。Patil（Pail, et al, 2008）在研究中提出：在被确诊为良性增生的患者中，58%的患者在6个月之后的随访中，细胞学检查变为良性，有20%良性改变的女性在6个月之后变为轻度不典型增生。由Hartman等（2004）进行的一项样本量较小的研究显示：只有1/4的轻度不典型增生女性重复多次进行的乳管灌洗结果保持前后一致。Visvanathan等（2007）对乳管抽吸液与乳管灌洗液的可靠性进行对比评估，他们对14名女性的24个导管间隔6个月灌洗检查了2次。在这些导管中，前后2次灌洗出来的细胞数量是不一致的，相比较仅仅细胞学程度比较一致。我们对100个风险因素不确定的普通女性进行研究后发现：在对3个导管进行间隔6个月的灌洗后，只有1/17的导管灌洗前后不典型增生的结论保持一致。该检查在各种风险水平的女性中可重复性均较低。

从这些研究中可以得出这样的结论：导管上皮细胞需要6个月以上的时间才能完全再生——它与脱落细胞中出现异型性细胞代表细胞增殖的过程的理念相左。Euhus等（2007）最近对取自150名女性的514个导管液样本进行细胞异型性及DNA甲基化程度评估，发现细胞异型性及甲基化是两个独立的危险因素。这些观察不得不使我们产生怀疑，是不是所有的细胞异型性都代表着癌前病变前期的增殖状态，还是代表着可能导致癌症产生的其他病理过程，例如慢性炎症持续存在引起的低分化状态。因此，我们建议，对于乳管灌洗查出轻度不典型增生的结果解读可参照ASCUS宫颈涂片检查结果，但其仍存在不确定因素。

5.4.3 细胞学和其他生物标志物作为肿瘤筛查和化学预防的指标

尽管细胞学异型的重复性受到质疑，但是，很少有成熟的试图证明细胞学异型性确实是乳腺癌的风险因素的细胞灌洗研究。仅有1项纳入116例高风险妇女，随访1~4年的研究，其结果显示：尽管25例女性乳管灌洗液中发现异形细胞，但在进一步的病理学检查中，她们没有1人被发现存在不典型增生或发展成为乳腺癌。试验中2例女性确实发展成为乳腺癌，但其乳管灌洗液显示为良性且并没有发现异形细胞。因此，研究组不再将乳管灌洗作为筛查高危患者的检查方法（Carruthers, et al 2007）。

在过去的10年中，随着生物标志物领域新发现的不断增加，许多研究人员探索将乳管抽吸和乳管灌洗作为某种手段，寻找乳腺肿瘤标记物以了解患病风险、患病情况、对治疗的反应和（或）复发情况的方法（Dua,et al,2006）。经细胞学、基因突变以及蛋白质谱分析技术进行分析，各项结果存在较大变异，且可重复性差，其原因可能是由于缺乏精确的测量技术和试剂。一些研究者对乳管灌洗液进行配对研究，他们对细胞学和生物标志物进行了探讨和比较（表5.2）。结果再次说明，细胞学检查敏感度较低，尽管一些生物标记物尤其是FISH有较高的敏感性和特异性。其他的生物标记物，如DNA甲基化在乳管灌洗液标本中也被检测。Euhus发现细胞异型性和甲基化是相互独立的危险因素，并与Gail模型的风险度有关(Euhus, et al, 2007)。Fackler等（2006）报道，当在乳管灌洗液样品中检测沉默的肿瘤抑制基因时，定量多重甲基化特异性聚合酶链反应（PCR）识别癌症的敏感性是单纯应用细胞形态学检测的2倍。

人们在乳管抽吸液及灌洗液中研究生殖激素的水平，并且发现，雌激素在乳腺排出的液体中的浓度明显高于血清中的浓度，并且该浓度与月经周期或绝经等因素无关(Petrakis, et al, 1993; Chatterton, 2005)。激素作为一

表5.2 乳管灌洗的细胞学检查和生物标记物的配对研究

液体	细胞学检查		生物标记物			参考文献
	敏感度（%）	特异度（%）	检测方法	敏感度（%）	特异度（%）	
灌洗	33	89	FISH	100	100	Yamamoto, et al.（2003）
灌洗	47	79	FISH	71	89	King, et al.（2003）
灌洗	31	100	SELDI-TOF MS	75	NA	Mendrinos, et al.（2005）

细胞学和生物标志物的配对研究中，乳房的液体从拟行乳房组织切除活检或乳房切除术的女性中术前收集而来。未做特别说明时，灵敏度反映的是浸润性和（或）导管原位癌（DCIS）的检测。FISH：荧光原位杂交；NA：不适合；SELDI-TOF MS：表面增强激光解吸和电离时间飞行质谱分析

种判断风险或治疗后反应的生物标记物尚未被认可。

Khan等（2009）在高风险女性提供的乳管灌洗液中寻找肿瘤标记物，这些女性的共同特点是给予他莫昔芬治疗。在研究期间，他们发现细胞学检查并不适合被用作他莫昔芬治疗反应的标记物。他们还发现，乳管灌洗作为获取乳腺上皮细胞样本的方法是极其昂贵的，乳管灌洗的损耗率可达53%，并且整个过程需要大量时间来完成，消耗很多耗材，花费很多精力对每个妇女的每个导管的灌洗液进行分析。因其结果的不确定性，所以随着应用时间的延长，在高风险女性中应用乳管灌洗获取生物标记物样本的方法遭到了质疑。

然而，在寻找可靠的患癌生物标记物，或是证明肿瘤化学预防有效性的标记物，以及如何获得最好的获取样本等方面的研究仍在继续。因乳管灌洗在危险度分层上的位置并不明确，目前研究的结果似乎并不支持其在这一领域的应用（Fabian，2007）。然而，在科研领域，如细胞的收集（上皮细胞或组织细胞）和其他标记物的寻找，如上清液中内源性激素、蛋白质或外源性致癌物质等，乳管灌洗仍有一席之地。

5.4.4 所有导管都是相同或独一无二的

乳腺应视为一个器官，分为左右两个部分。最近的教科书上写道，乳腺导管呈放射状地将乳腺平均分为若干等份。这与Cooper（Cooper，1845）和Going（Going，Moffat，2004）进行的解剖学研究不一致，他们认为乳腺小叶的大小是不一致的，6大导管系统占整个乳房体积的75%。

有一个问题在许多研究中均未涉及，即在导管间及在不同女性之间，分析同一组内的细胞学、激素以及其他标志物的系数。我们已经发现，同一乳腺内的不同导管的差异性与不同乳腺间的导管的差异性一样大（Tondre, et al, 2006）。目前，更多的数据正在分析中。此外，每个导管独一无二的假说得到了支持。然而，如果每个导管都是不同的，且乳腺癌是一种腺叶疾病（Tot，2005），那么，在没有乳腺和乳头的标准解剖图谱的情况下，获取上皮细胞样本是十分困难的。这需要影像学或其他方法的介入，来准确引导和辨识那些不正常的导管。

5.4.5 患者的选择

起初，那些流行病学上具有乳腺癌风险的女性被认为是乳管灌洗的最佳人选，例如，Gail模型中那些患有对侧乳腺癌或携带如*BRCA*1或*BRCA*2基因突变具有遗传风险的女性。乳管灌洗并没有成为乳腺癌的筛查方法，但是，确实是一种更精确量化罹患乳腺癌风险的方法。人们希望女性可以通过自己的乳管灌洗液结果来选择一种降低患癌风险的药物或采取其他策略。人们还希望乳管灌洗可以作为一种获取乳腺上皮组织样本的方法，来测量

特定的生物标记物以帮助判断新的预防干预措施是否有效（Fabian，2007）。

尽管最初只有高风险的女性，尤其是那些有乳头溢液的女性是乳管灌洗的候选人，但是，随着我们对乳腺基础解剖学和生理学的深入理解，以及未来新的无创的导管成像和导管内治疗方法的出现，乳管灌洗的价值会越来越明确。

5.5 未来展望

由于对细胞学异型性价值的研究并不令人满意，这迫使我们必须寻求乳管灌洗在其他方面的应用。目前，Susan博士爱心研究基金会（DSLRF）正在研究腺管内巨噬细胞和细胞因子的水平，以期待发现一种更有前景的危险因素。由于目前乳腺肿瘤领域正在研究肿瘤的微环境，我们也正在更多地关注导管的微环境。最初，我们在研究导管流出液中生殖激素的结果显示：每个导管都有自己的系统，与其他导管几乎没有联系。

我们重新审视了非哺乳期或静息期乳房的生理状态和分泌活动。Bonser等（1961）发现，成熟的非哺乳期乳房的分泌活动主要在乳腺腺泡、微导管、小导管中进行。他们在兔子的乳腺导管中注射墨汁的混悬液，发现注射的材料从管腔流出，最终进入淋巴系统。此研究可以证明乳腺的分泌活动和重吸收是不断进行的。在过去的50年中，几乎没有针对静息期乳房的生理功能的研究报道。我们基金会正在研究静息期乳房的膜转运机制。我们应用的药物包括：咖啡因、西咪替丁、阿司匹林和甘露醇。这些物质注入经产妇或未产妇的乳房中，经过12h的吸收后，应用乳管灌洗技术获取灌洗液，然后与哺乳期女性乳汁中的水平进行比较。

初步结果显示是有意义的并且存在明显差异（Mills, et al，2009）。在哺乳期妇女，咖啡因能够在1h内迅速扩散到乳汁中，并且反映了血清中的水平。在静息期乳房，咖啡因注射6h后才达到高峰。西咪替丁可以在哺乳期乳汁中检测到，但是静息期乳房灌洗液中并未检测到。由于西咪替丁的转运方式是主动转运，这种模式与仅仅在哺乳时期表达的主动转运蛋白有关。在乳管抽吸液和灌洗液中药物的浓度和时间进程似乎表明，这是由于生理学上的差异产生而非稀释的结果。经产妇和非产妇在咖啡因的浓度和吸收摄取上存在显著差异。最后，乳腺导管中注射甘露醇实验的初步分析正在进行，这将帮助我们更好地理解药物的双向转运以及筛选可以在志愿者身上应用的其他安全药物。

乳管灌洗的经验及在未溢液的乳管中插管的技术为开辟乳腺导管内治疗提供了可能性。以前认为无溢液的乳管是无法经过乳头穿透进入乳腺的，但是，现在我们已经成功地于无溢液的乳管中注入了生理盐水、乳酸钠林格液及甘露醇，并且无后遗症发生。在动物模型中成功进行了导管内治疗的内容，将在本书中的其他章节进行讨论。2项在拟行乳腺切除术的妇女中研究安全性的试验正在进行。DSLRF监督实施的第一个临床试验是在农村地区的原位癌患者身上应用脂质体阿霉素（PLD）进行导管内治疗。这项研究主要是测试这种导管原位癌术前应用的新辅助方法的安全性和可行性。到目前为止，我们已经在9例患者身上证明了我们可以正确识别受累的导管，可以安全注入20mg PLD来观察组织学变化。一旦30例女性患者的获益分析计算完成，我们就将对标记物、磁共振变化以及病理学展开评估（Mahoney，2009）。

虽然对乳管灌洗作为乳腺癌风险评估的研究热情并没有坚持下去，但是，它的应用使得人们重新对静息期乳房的解剖结构及生理功能进行审视。自1999年以来，DSLRF每2年举办一场关于乳腺癌导管内治疗的国际会议。研讨会上的精彩片段、论文摘要及创新基金资助名单将刊登到网上（www.dslrf.org）或印刷到出版物上面《第六届国际论坛研讨会——乳腺癌导管内治疗的方法（2009）》。第六届研讨会于2009年举行，出席会议的有120多位临床医生、研究人员及对该领域有极高兴趣的拥护者。如果乳腺癌的治疗和预防向更合乎逻辑、更无创的方式进化发展，那么，有关导管内入路的导管/小叶系统的基础知识就非常关键。

尽管新颖的乳管灌洗技术及微导管工具可能使一些临床工作者跳过基础知识阶段，但是本文并非徒劳，在这个警示故事中，我们已经介绍了许多经验教训。显然，Keynes引用的关于乳腺分泌活动的程度和组成的细节仍然不甚明晰，亟待进一步探索研究。

参考文献

[1] Rochman S, Mills D, Kim J, et al. Love S State of the Science and the Intraductal Approach for Breast Cancer: Proceedings Summary of the Sixth International Symposium on the Intraductal Approach to Breast Cancer Santa Monica California. BMC Proc 3, 2009, (Suppl 5): 11.

[2] Baltzell KA, Moghadassi M, Rice T, et al. Epithelial cells in nipple aspirate fuid and subsequent breast cancer risk: a historic prospective study. BMC Cancer, 2008, 19: 8-75.

[3] Bhandare D, Nayar R, Bryk M, et al. Endocrine biomarkers in ductal lavage samples from women at high risk for breast cancer. Cancer Epidemiol Biomarkers Prev, 2005, 14: 2620-2627.

[4] Bonser GM, Dossett SA, Jull SW. Human and experimental breast cancer. CC Thomas, Springfeld, 1961.

[5] Brogi E, Robson M, Panageas KS, et al. Ductal lavage in patients undergoing mastectomy for mammary carcinoma: a correlative study. Cancer, 2003, 98: 2170-2176.

[6] Buehring GC. Screening for breast atypias using exfoliative cytology. Cancer, 1979, 43: 1788-1799.

[7] Buehring GC, Letscher A, McGirr KM, et al. Presence of epithelial cells in nipple aspirate fuid is associated with subsequent breast cancer: a 25-year prospective study. Breast Cancer Res Treat, 2006, 98: 63-70.

[8] Cabioglu N, Hunt KK, Singletary SE, et al. Surgical decision making and factors determining a diagnosis of breast carcinoma in women presenting with nipple discharge. J Am Coll Surg, 2003, 196: 354-364.

[9] Carruthers CD, Chapleskie LA, Flynn MB, et al. The use of ductal lavage as a screening tool in women at high risk for developing breast carcinoma. Am J Surg, 2007, 194: 463-466.

[10] Chatterton RT Jr. Characteristics of salivary profles of oestradiol and progesterone in premenopausal women. J Endocrinol, 2005, 186: 77-84.

[11] Cooper A. The anatomy and diseases of the breast. Philadelphia: Lea and Blanchard, 1845.

[12] Danforth DN Jr, Abati A, Filie A, et al. Combined breast ductal lavage and ductal endoscopy for the evaluation of the high-risk breast: a feasibility study. J Surg Oncol, 2006, 94: 555-564.

[13] Dooley WC, Ljung BM, Veronesi U, et al. Ductal lavage for detection of cellular atypia in women at high risk for breast cancer. J Natl Cancer Inst, 2001, 93: 1624-1632.

[14] Dua RS, Isacke CM, Gui GP. The intraductal approach to breast cancer biomarker discovery. J Clin Oncol, 2006, 24: 1209-1216.

[15] Dupont WD, Page DL. Risk factors for breast cancer in women with proliferative breast disease. N Engl J Med, 1985, 312: 146-151.

[16] Euhus DM, Bu D, Ashfaq R, et al. Atypia and DNA methylation in nipple duct lavage in relation to predicted breast cancer risk. Cancer Epidemiol Biomarkers Prev, 2007, 6: 1812-1821.

[17] Fabian CJ. Is there a future for ductal lavage. Clin Cancer Res, 2007, 13: 4655-4656.

[18] Fackler MJ, Malone K, Zhang Z, et al. Quantitative multiplex methylation-specifc PCR analysis doubles detection of tumor cells in breast ductal fuid. Clin Cancer Res, 2006, 12: 3306-3310.

[19] Going JJ, Moffat DF. Escaping from Flatland: clinical and biological aspects of human mammary duct anatomy in three dimensions. J Pathol, 2004, 203: 538-544.

[20] Hartman A, Daniel BL, Kurian AW, et al. Breast magnetic resonance image screening and ductal lavage in women at high genetic risk for breast carcinoma. Cancer, 2004, 100: 479-489.

[21] Holland R, Veling SH, Mravunac M, et al. Histologic multifocality of Tis, T1-2 breast carcinomas. Implications for clinical trials of breast-conserving surgery. Cancer, 1985, 56: 979-990.

[22] Johnson-Maddux A, Ashfaq R, Cler L, et al. Reproducibility of cytologic atypia in repeat nipple duct lavage. Cancer, 2005, 103: 1129-1136.

[23] Keynes G. Chronic mastitis. Br J Surg, 1923, 11: 89-121.

[24] Khan SA, Wiley EL, Rodriguez N, et al. Ductal lavage fndings in women with known breast cancer undergoing mastectomy. J Natl Cancer Inst, 2004, 96: 1510-1517.

[25] Khan SA, Wolfman JA, Segal L, et al. Ductal lavage fndings in women with mammographic microcalcifcations undergoing biopsy. Ann Surg Oncol, 2005, 12: 689-696.

[26] Khan SA, Lankes HA, Patil DB, et al. Ductal lavage is an ineffcient method of biomarker measurement in high-risk women. Cancer Prev Res (Phila Pa), 2009, 2: 265-273.

[27] King BL, Love SM. The intraductal approach to the breast: raison d'être. Breast Cancer Res, 2005, 7: 198-204.

[28] King EB, Barrett D, King M-C, et al. Cellular composition of the nipple aspirate specimen of breast fuid. The benign cells. Am J Clin Pathol, 1975, 64: 728-738.

[29] King BL, Tsai SC, Gryga ME, et al. Detection of chromosomal instability in paired breast surgery and ductal lavage specimens by interphase fuorescence in situ hybridization. Clin Cancer Res, 2003, 9: 1509-1516.

[30] Kurian AW, Mills MA, Jaffee M, et al. Ductal lavage of fuid-yielding and non-fuid-yielding ducts in BRCA1 and BRCA2 mutation carriers and other women at high inherited breast cancer risk. Cancer Epidemiol Biomarkers Prev, 2005, 14: 1082-1089.

[31] Leborgne R. Intraductal biopsy of certain pathologic processes of the breast. Surgery, 1946, 19: 47-54.

[32] Linder J. Editorial: ductal lavage of the breast. Diagn Cytopathol, 2004, 30: 140-142.

[33] Loud JT, Thiébaut AC, Abati AD, et al. Ductal lavage in women from BRCA1/2 families: Is there a future for ductal lavage in women at increased genetic risk of breast cancer. Cancer Epidemiol Biomarkers Prev, 2009, 18: 1243-1251.

[34] Love SM, Barsky SH. Breast-duct endoscopy to study stages of cancerous breast disease. Lancet, 1996, 348: 997-999.

[35] Love SM, Barsky SH. Anatomy of the nipple and breast ducts revisited. Cancer, 2004, 101: 1947-1957.

[36] Love SM, Zhang B, Zhang W, et al. Local drug delivery to the breast: a phase 1 study of breast cytotoxic agent administration prior to mastectomy. BMC Proc, 2009, 3 (Suppl 5): S29.

[37] Maddux AJ, Ashfaq R, Naftalis E, et al. Patient and duct selection for nipple duct lavage. Am J Surg, 2004, 188: 390-394.

[38] Mahoney ME. Intraductal therapy of DCIS with lipo-somal doxorubicin: a preoperative trial in rural California. Sixth international symposium on the intraductal approach to breast cancer. BMC Proc, 2009, 3 (Suppl 5): S26.

[39] Mai KT, Yazdi HM, Burns BF, et al. Pattern of distribution of intraductal and infltrating ductal carcinoma: a three-dimensional study using serial coronal giant sections of the breast. Hum Pathol, 2000, 31: 464-474.

[40] Mendrinos S, Nolen JD, Styblo T, et al. Cytologic fndings and protein expression profles associated with ductal carcinoma of the breast in ductal lavage specimens using surface-enhanced laser des-orption and ionization-time of fight mass spectrometry. Cancer, 2005, 105: 178-183.

[41] Mills D, Chia D, Casano A, et al. Preliminary exploration into the physiology of the resting breast. BMC Proc, 2009, 3 (Suppl 5): S26.

[42] Papanicolaou GN, Holmquist DG, Bader GM, et al. Exfoliative cytology of the human mammary gland

and its value in the diagnosis of cancer and other diseases of the breast. Cancer, 1958, 11: 377-409.

[43] Patil DB, Lankes HA, Najar R, et al. Reproducibility of ductal lavage cytology and cellularity over a six month interval in high risk women. Breast Cancer Res Treat, 2008, 112: 327-333.

[44] Petrakis NL. Physiologic, biochemical and cytologic aspects of nipple aspirate fuid. Breast Cancer Res Treat, 1986, 8: 7-19.

[45] Petrakis NL, Lowenstein JN, Wiencke JK, et al. Gross cystic disease fuid protein in nipple aspirates of breast fuid of Asian and non-Asian women. Cancer Epidemiol Biomarkers Prev, 1993, 2: 573-579.

[46] Ramsay DT, Mitoulas LR, Kent JC, et al. The use of ultrasound to characterize milk ejection in women using an electric breast pump. J Hum Lact, 2005, 21: 421-428.

[47] Rusby JE, Brachtel EF, Michaelson JS, et al. Breast duct anatomy in the human nipple: three-dimensional patterns and clinical implications. Breast Cancer Res Treat, 2007, 106: 171-179.

[48] Sartorius OW. Breast fuid cells help in early cancer detection. (Medical News). JAMA, 1973, 224: 823, 826-827.

[49] Sartorius OW, Smith HS, Morris P, et al. Cytologic evaluation of breast fuid in the detection of breast disease. J Natl Cancer Inst, 1977, 59: 1073-1080.

[50] Teboul M, Halliwell M. Atlas of ultrasound and ductal echography of the breast: the introduction of anatomic intel-ligence into breast imaging. Blackwell Science, Oxford, 1995.

[51] Tondre J, Nejad M, Brennan M, et al. Preliminary analysis of hormones and cells in lavage fuid. Distinct ducts in healthy women//AACR 2006 international conference on frontiers in cancer prevention research, 2006.

[52] Tondre J, Nejad M, Casano A, et al. Technical enhancements to breast ductal lavage. Ann Surg Oncol, 2008, 15: 2734-2738.

[53] Tot T. DCIS, cytokeratins, and the theory of the sick lobe. Virchows Arch, 2005, 447: 1-8.

[54] Twelves D, Gui G. The feasibility of nipple aspiration and ductal lavage as a screening tool in healthy women with increased breast cancer risk. Eur J Surg Oncol, 2008, 34: 1156-1157.

[55] Visvanathan K, Santor D, Ali SZ, et al. The reliability of nipple aspirate and ductal lavage in women at increased risk for breast cancer: a potential tool for breast cancer risk assessment and biomarker evaluation. Cancer Epidemiol Biomarkers Prev, 2007, 16: 950-955.

[56] Wrensch MR, Petrakis NL, Miike R, et al. Breast cancer risk in women with abnormal cytology in nipple aspirates of breast fuid. J Natl Cancer Inst, 2001, 93: 1791-1798.

[57] Yamamoto D, Senzaki H, Nakagawa H, et al. Detection of chromosomal aneusomy by fuorescence in situ hybridization for patients with nipple discharge. Cancer, 2003, 97: 690-694.

第6章 早期乳腺癌的分布模式

Maria P. Foschini, Vincenzo Eusebi

6.1 简 介

近年来，随着大切片技术（macro section）的使用（Foschini, et al, 2006, 2007; Tot, 2003, 2005, 2007a），乳腺标本的病理工作流程改变巨大。Cheatle（1921）、Ingleby和Holly（1939）首次将大切片技术应用于人类组织，从而能够观察肿瘤病灶与周围组织的关系。随后，该技术得到了进一步改进（Wellings, Jensen, 1973; Sarnelli, Squartini, 1986; Faverly, et al, 1992; Foschini, et al, 2002），基于大切片技术的研究也证实了乳腺X线摄影与病理学存在重要的联系，主要是关注肿瘤范围（Egan, Mosteller, 1977; Faverly, et al, 1994; Gallager, Martin, 1969）。

在评估切缘及测量肿瘤的真实大小方面，大切片技术也有用武之地（Foschini, et al, 2002）。因此，Jackson等（1994）比较了两组乳腺癌术后的标本，其中一组采用大切片技术，另外一组采用传统技术。他发现，大切片组的所有标本都能够很好地评估肿瘤的大小，然而，在传统的小切片组，仅有63%的标本可以正确评估肿瘤的尺寸。大切片技术的另外一个优势是评估肿瘤的程度，评估原位癌和浸润癌是单灶还是多灶性病变（多灶和多中心）

M. P. Foschini
Department of Hematology and Oncology,
Section of Pathology "M. Malpighi"
University of Bologna at Bellaria Hospital, Bologna, Italy
e-mail: mariapia.foschini@ausl.bologna.it

（Foschini, et al, 2006, 2007; Tot, 2005）。

6.2 癌细胞的地砖式（mural）播散

在大切片技术的背景下，Wellings和Jensen（1973）提出导管原位癌（DCIS）起源于终末导管单元（TDLU）。此观点统治学术界数十年，近年来才受到挑战（Tot, 2005）。

由于Going和Moffat（2004）、Mai等（2000）和Ohatake等（1995）的原创性研究，现在我们知道乳腺是由11~48个微解剖上独立的小叶构成。从三维结构上看，乳腺小叶可以被看成是尖朝向乳头，底朝向深筋膜的锥体。某些小叶（优势小叶）比例极大，甚至超过一个象限，并且其管道系统插入临近的小叶中，几乎不能被完整分离。放射科医生将造影剂注入乳管后，发现其分布超过1个象限的范围，从影像上观察到了这一现象。Ohtake等（1995）提出，在不同的小叶间或许存在解剖上的交通汇合管。但是，放射科医生尚未发现造影剂能够反向进入其他的小叶系统，因此，该观点尚未得到证实。

交通汇合管的存在与否具有重要意义，因为，它暗示了癌细胞可以从一个小叶播散至另一个小叶，无需入侵实质。我们在佩吉特病（Paget病）的病理改变过程中发现了与此有关的一些现象。去分化的癌细胞能够沿着导管向上皮方向爬行，最终形成了佩吉特病（Marucci, et al,2002）。某些树突状的 *HER*-2阳性的细胞表现的更为明显（图6.1），这种表型是具有移动能力的细胞非常重要的特征（Marucci, et al,2002; Tavassoli, Eusebi, 2009）。导管内播散的另一个特点被称作变形骨炎式（Pagetoid）播散，常在小叶原位癌（LCIS）中出现。Fechner（1973）曾描述了这种"地砖式"的导管播散方式。这种病理形态也见于未分化型的导管癌（图6.2A、B），以及神经内分泌性DCIS（Tsang, Chan, 1996）。然而，这种癌细胞沿导管播散的观点尚未统一（Tot, 2005），而且，确实也很难判断导管中是否存在远离DCIS病灶的孤立的癌细胞。同时，这种现象甚至很难用区域性癌变的理论进行解释（Slaughter, et al,1953; Braaknuis, et al,2004）。

根据DCIS的组织学结构，传统上分类为薄膜状、微乳头状、乳头状、筛状和毛刺状癌（Rosen, Oberman, 1993）。由于50%的病例都为混合形态（Patchefsky, et al,1989），因此，DCIS的这种分类并无实际意义，而且，还毫无预测和预后的信息。Holland等（1994）开创性地提出了新的观点，他废除了DCIS的结构分类法，而根据癌灶的细胞分化程度，对导管内癌进行了分类。该分类法将DCIS分为3类，高分化DCIS表现为细胞核单一，且细胞沿腔面排列；低分化DCIS表现为细胞核多样，极性混乱；中分化DCIS的细胞核无规律，存在多形性，细胞沿腔面排列。因此，分化良好的DCIS，其ER和PR表达丰富；而低分化的DCIS缺乏两者的表达，多数HER-2阳性（Bobrow, et al,1994）。

在此之后，随着病理术语争论的出现，在Holland的提议基础上，不同的DCIS的分类标准大行其道。这一点在病理学专业上屡见不鲜。2003年，WHO采纳了新的分类法，该分类法与Holland分类法（Holland, et al,1994）十分类似。不同之处在于采用了新的术语，即DCIS/DIN导管上皮内肿瘤）Ⅰ、Ⅱ和Ⅲ。美国医保局（AFIP）乳腺癌办公室也采纳了该分类法（2009）。

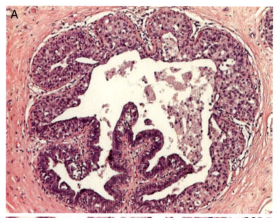

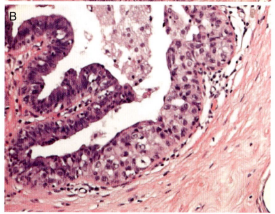

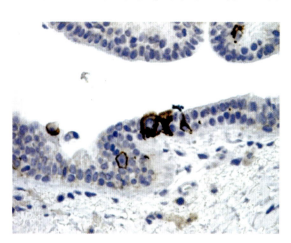

图6.1 *HER*-2阳性的树突样细胞沿着输乳管爬行。乳腺的深处为DCIS/DIN3，乳头为佩吉特肿瘤细胞，这些细胞位于二者之间

图6.2 A. 癌细胞在基底膜和腔面上皮间，以"地砖式"的方式播散；B. 癌细胞的核具有多形性（HER-2和E-cadherin阳性，此图未显示）。切片附近存在典型的DCIS/DIN3病灶

6.3 如何定义原位肿瘤？

1932年，Broders从组织学的角度定义了第1例原位癌。1941年，Foote和Stewart认为该病例是小叶原位癌。1934年，Bloodgood对毛刺样癌的定义为学术界所认同。1921年，Cheatle使用大切片技术指出，癌细胞最初存在于导管中。1933年，Dawson指出，绝大部分病例起源于终末、小叶间导管。1973年，Wellings和Jensen拓展了这一概念，他们发现，起源于导管或小叶TDLUs上皮的癌细胞，在基底膜内以一种非浸润连续性的方式增殖，造成了乳腺癌在导管内的播散。然而，在乳腺X线摄影普及以前，一些被诊断为3级DCIS/DIN3的病例同时伴有腋窝淋巴结的转移。有些学者因此定义乳腺的原发病灶为"浸润性毛刺样癌"。1950年，Stewart个人提出"只要发现毛刺样癌，就必然属于浸润性癌"的观点。1967年，Sirtori和Talamazzi认为，在乳腺癌中，原位癌几乎不存在。

目前的主流观点认为，原位癌周围必然有完整的肌上皮细胞层和基底纤维层，而浸润性癌周的基底纤维层不连续或为阶段性存在（Azzopardi, et al,1979）。按这种观点，会有例外情况存在。现已发现，当正常的乳腺向分泌腺转化时，会出现肌上皮成分的缺失（Cserni, 2008）。如果DCIS起源于此，那么，肯定会缺失这些结构。我们有一个DCIS的病例，其原位的性质确凿无疑（光镜结构和免疫组化都证实存在基底膜），但是，基底细胞的肌上皮分化情况却不明确（图6.3A~E）。1999年，Damiani设计了一个免疫组化的试验，评估"毛刺样癌"是原位癌还是浸润癌。他同时使用了3种不同的标志物（肌动蛋白actin、层粘连蛋白laminin和Ⅳ型胶原collagen），作者认为单独一种标志物并不能确诊，将标志物结合结构特征一起判断，就能够确诊原位癌的性质。尽管如此，在2个病例中，作者也未能明确病变的性质，只好定义为浸润待定。较大尺寸的囊内乳头状癌常无肌上皮层存在。这样的病灶从不发生淋巴结转移，被认为是等同于DCIS/DIN。因此，乳腺"原位"的概念看起来是指腺体内的增生性无转移病变，而非一定有形态学上的某种特征。这一定义同样适用于浸润性癌。包括动脉、静脉和淋巴管在内的脉管系统和神经，有时偶尔可被"良性"的腺管结构"浸润"，但是对患者的健康并无影响（Davies, 1973; Eusebi, Azzopardi, 1976; Taylor, Norris, 1967）。

肿瘤的导管新生是一个增生的过程，但是形态学上尚无定论。如果是DCIS，那么其特征是充满肿瘤细胞的新生导管呈指状突起，多数为低分化型（Tabár, et al, 2004）。生理状态下，怀孕时小叶中腺泡和腺管会出现增生，一些良性疾病，如腺泡型或导管周围型硬化性腺病时，也会出现类似的改变（Tanaka, Oota, 1970）。因此，新形成的大的腺管拥簇在一起，明显膨胀充满肿瘤细胞。绝大多数"新生"腺管有肌上皮层和（或）基底膜。在某些情况下，这一增生过程不完全，因此肌上皮成分和（或）基底膜缺失，呈现一种"浸润性毛刺样癌"的特征。一项小规模的包含11例标本的研究就发现了这种情况。这11例标本初诊为DIN3，HE染色下存在实质浸润的表现，于是行平滑肌肌动蛋白、层粘连蛋白和Ⅳ型胶原的IHC检测确诊了4例DIN3，5例是浸润性癌。然而，有2例在IHC后也无法确诊。这是因为"毛刺样"细胞巢周围的腺管染色呈现异质性的特点，总有某个标志物的阳性表达。最后，鉴于肿瘤细胞巢为球形或线形，类似原位癌时导管膨胀的表现，这2例被诊断为"膨胀浸润（blunt invasion）"（Koerner, 2009）。或许因为这一现象，1984年，Cowen和Bates提出，浸润性癌的诊断有时令人困惑，因为它总是表现出DCIS的特征。因此，原位癌的诊断，尤其是DCIS/DIN3的诊断，可能有时候会非常困难。免疫组化检查对诊断比较有帮助，但是大切片是必需的，因为在这种情况下，亚肉眼结构常与诊断保持一致。之

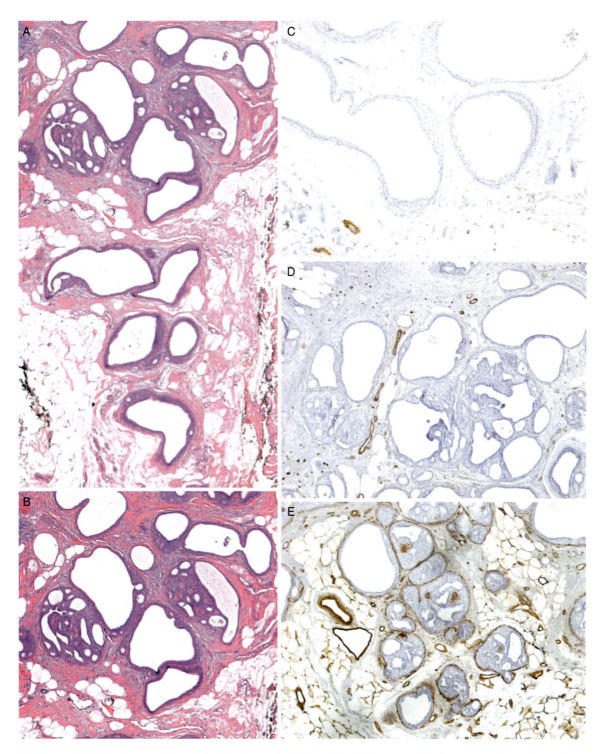

图6.3 A. 分化良好的DCIS的特征为扁平上皮的不典型增生和筛状结构。B. 细胞朝向一致；核单一。筛状结构明确。C. 角蛋白14免疫组化染色：基底细胞存在，但角蛋白14并未表达p63或平滑肌肌动蛋白也未表达，本图未显示）。D. 层粘连蛋白染色：腺体新生小管缺乏层粘连蛋白。E. Ⅳ型胶原染色：新生小管胶原染色阳性

前描述的导管新生化是一个尚未证实的猜想；然而，如果它的确存在，那么就能够解释为什么DCIS能够形成肿块。单个导管，即使极端膨胀，密布肿瘤细胞，也很难达到临床上触诊阳性的程度。相反，当几个膨大的新生导管互相挤压，里面同时充满细胞，临床上查体就可能会被发现。

6.4 单灶、多灶及多中心DCIS

1994年，Faverly等撰文指出，低分化的DCIS/DIN3都是单灶性，而分化好的DCIS/DIN1则是多灶性的。Tot（2007a）将DCIS分为3类：弥散型（24%），细胞沿导管分布；多灶型（40%），多个小叶发病，之间有正常组织；单灶型（32%），病变位于单个小叶或邻近小叶，之间无正常组织。Tot（2005,2007b）认为，同时或异时的原位多灶性病变多位于乳腺的同一个小叶。由此，他提出了乳腺的小叶疾病理论，即从出生时，乳房里病变小叶的基因背景就存在异常，而后数十年的基因改变的积累，足以使这个小叶的任一上皮组织发生癌变。

Foschini等（2006）在一项包含13例小叶上皮内肿瘤（Lobular Intraepithelial Neoplasia；LIN）（Tavassoli, Eusebi, 2009）的研究中，将同一个小叶内存在多处LIN病灶的情况定义为多灶性（multifocality）（图6.4），而位于不同的小叶中则定义为多中心性（multicentricity）（图6.5）（Foschini, et al, 2006；Tot, 2005）。这一观点也获得了Tot（2003）的认同。使用大切片技术对乳腺癌根治术后的病理标本进行研究后，发现6例标本（46%）中，癌灶的数目最少为2处，最多77处，平均值23.92处，平均大于20处。Foschini等（2006）也测量了LIN病灶之间的距离，他发现13例标本中有9例（69.23%），最小5mm，最大112mm，平均值35mm，平均大于20mm。由此看来，所有的

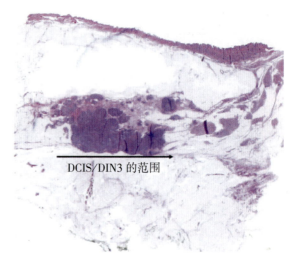

图6.4 DCIS/DIN3的范围：该病理完美呈现了单小叶中多灶性的特点。大组织切片，HE染色

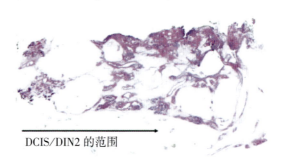

图6.5 DCIS/DIN1的范围：肿瘤至少跨越2个象限。这种情况可能是多小叶，也可能是多中心。大组织切片，HE染色

LIN病例都存在1个以上的病灶，部分病灶（30%）成簇分布，位于20mm的范围内，大部分病灶分散于整个乳腺的象限内。据估计，1个小叶约构成乳腺体积的2%~23%（Going, Moffat, 2004）。Foschini等（2006）观察到某些标本中，病灶间距最大达112mm。这似乎暗示了60%以上的LIN均起源于"优势"小叶，这样的推论简直令人难以置信。相比较之下，LIN起源于不同的小叶，但是表现出多灶和（或）多中心疾病的特征，这样的说法貌似可信。

Foschini等（2007）也研究了45例DCIS/DIN病例的大切片病理，其中，13例为DIN1，DIN1病灶的数目最少为1处（仅1例），最多可达100处以上（均值35.08处）；病灶之间的距离，最小12mm，最大55mm（均值35.42mm）；

13例中有10例（76.9%）病灶最大间距大于20mm。12例为DIN3，DIN3病灶数目最小为1处（仅1例），最大超过100处（均值24）；整体看，DIN3病灶数目小于DIN1，12例中4例（33.3%）病灶数目小于20处；病灶间距最小2mm，最大51mm，均值22mm；12例中5例（45.4%）的间距超过20mm。20例为DIN2，情况与DIN3十分类似。因此，似乎DIN1表现出广泛分布的趋势，多超过一个象限，因此应该多于1个小叶。而DIN2和DIN3成簇分布，可能位于一个小叶内。另外，与之前的观点不同，DIN1和LCIS之间的相似大于不同。

LIN和DIN1可能为多小叶同时出现，病灶相距甚远这一现象说明了可能某些小叶基因背景存在"构造异常（malconstruction）"，致癌因素在这些地方发挥了作用。然而，DIN3看起来更加局限化，并呈现单小叶的特征（图6.6），可能此时癌变的过程已经完成，"环境致瘤因素"会在局部进一步发挥作用。这样，推论就能自圆其说了。

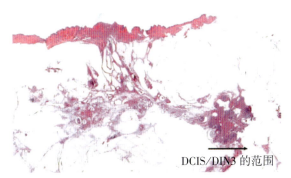

图6.6 单小叶、单灶性DCIS/DIN3。大组织切片，HE染色

6.5 总　结

绝大多数研究表明，DCIS1级（grade1）和LIN常为多中心（多小叶）疾病，而DCIS2级和3级常为单灶性或单小叶多灶性病变。大切片技术在常规病理中的应用，将会为我们带来更多的有关原位肿瘤的生长模式和程度的信息。

参考文献

[1] Azzopardi JG, Ahmed A, Millis RR. Problems in breast pathology. London：W.B. Saunders，1979.

[2] Bloodgood JC. Comedo carcinoma (comedoadenoma) of the female breast. Am J Cancer，1934，22：842-853.

[3] Bobrow LG, Happerfeld LC, Gregory WM, et al. The classifcation of ductal carcinoma in situ and its association with biological markers. Semin Diagn Pathol，1994，11：199-207.

[4] Braakhuis JMB, Leemans RC, Brakenhoff RH. A genetic progression model of oral cancer：current evidence and clini-cal implications. J Oral Pathol Med，1994，33：317-322.

[5] Broders AC. Carcinoma in situ contrasted with benign penetrating epithelium. JAMA，1932，99：1670-1674.

[6] Cheatle GL. Benign and malignant changes in duct epithelium of the breast. Br J Cancer，1921，8：306.

[7] Cowen PN, Bates C. The signifcance of intraduct appearances in breast cancer. Clin Oncol，1984，10：67-72.

[8] Cserni G. Lack of myoepithelium in apocrine glands of the breast does not necessarily imply malignancy. Histopathology，2008，52：253-254.

[9] Damiani S, Ludvikova M, Tomasic G, et al. Myoepi-thelial cells and basal lamina in poorly differentiated in situ duct carcinoma of the breast. An immunocy-tochemical study. Virchows Arch，1999，434：227-234.

[10] Davies JD. Neural invasion in benign mammary dyspla-sia. J Pathol，1973，109：225-231.

[11] Dawson EK. Carcinoma of the mammary lobule and its origin. Edinb Med J，1933，40：57-82.

[12] Egan RL, Mosteller RC. Breast cancer mammography patterns. Cancer，1977，40：2087-2090.

[13] Eusebi V, Azzopardi JG. Vascular infltration in benign breast disease. J Pathol，1976，118：9-16.

[14] Faverly DRG, Holland R, Burgers L. An original stereo-microscopic analysis of the mammary glandular tree. Virchows Arch A Pathol Anat Histopathol，1992，421：115.

[15] Faverly DRG, Burgers L, Bult P, et al. Three dimen-sional imaging of mammary ductal carcinoma in situ: clinical implications. Semin Diagn Pathol, 1994, 11: 193-198.

[16] Fechner RE. Epithelial alterations in the extralobular ducts of breast with lobular carcinoma. Arch Pathol, 1973, 93: 164-171.

[17] Foote FW, Stewart FW. Lobular carcinoma in situ. Am J Pathol, 1941, 17: 491-500.

[18] Foschini MP, Tot T, Eusebi V. Large-section (macrosection) histologic slides//Silverstein MJ (ed) Ductal carcinoma in situ of the breast. Lippincott, Philadelphia, 2002: pp 249-254.

[19] Foschini MP, Righi A, Cucchi MC, et al. The impact of large sections and 3D technique on the study of lobular in situ and invasive carcinoma of the breast. Virchows Arch, 2006, 448: 256-261.

[20] Foschini MP, Flamminio F, Miglio R, et al. The impact of large sections on the study of in situ and invasive duct carcinoma of the breast. Hum Pathol, 2007, 38: 1736-1743.

[21] Gallager HS, Martin JE. Early phases in the development of breast cancer. Cancer, 1969, 24: 1170-1178.

[22] Going JJ, Moffat DF. Escaping from Flatland: clinical and biological aspects of human mammary duct anatomy in three dimensions. J Pathol, 2004, 203: 538-544.

[23] Holland R, Peterse JL, Millis RR, et al. Ductal carcinoma in situ: a proposal for a new classifcation. Semin Diagn Pathol, 1994, 11: 167-180.

[24] Ingleby H, Holly C. A method for the preparation of serial slices of the breast. Bull Int Assoc Med Museums, 1939, 19: 93-96.

[25] Jackson PA, Merchant W, McCormick CJ, et al. A comparison of large block macrosectioning and conventional techniques in breast pathology. Virchows Arch, 1994, 425: 243-248.

[26] Koerner FC. Diagnostic problems in breast pathology. Saunders, Philadelphia, 2009.

[27] Mai KT, Yazdi HM, Burns BF, et al. Pattern of distribution of intraductal and infltrating ductal carcinoma: a three-dimensional study using serial coronal giant sections of the breast. Hum Pathol, 2000, 31: 464-474.

[28] Marucci G, Betts CM, Golouh R, et al. Toker cells are probably precursors of Paget cell carcinoma: a morphological and ultrastructural description. Virchows Arch, 2002, 441: 117-123.

[29] Ohtake T, Abe R, Kimijima I, et al. Intraductal extension of primary invasive breast carcinoma treated by breast conservative surgery. Cancer, 1995, 76: 32-45.

[30] Patchefsky AS, Shwartz GF, Finkelstein SD, et al. Heterogeneity of intraductal carcinoma of the breast. Cancer, 1989, 63: 731-741.

[31] Rosen PP, Oberman HA. Tumors of the mammary gland. Armed Forces Institute of Pathology, Washington, 1993.

[32] Sarnelli R, Squartini F. Multicentricity in breast cancer: a submacroscopic study. Pathol Annu, 1986, 21: 143-158.

[33] Sirtori C, Talamazzi F. Il carcinoma intraduttale della mammella non è mai un carcinoma in situ. Tumori, 1967, 53: 641-644.

[34] Slaughter DP, Southwick HW, Smeejkal W. Field cancerization in oral stratifed squamous epithelium; clinical implications of multicentric origin. Cancer, 1953, 6: 963-968.

[35] Stewart FW. Tumors of the breast. Armed Forces Institute of Pathology, Washington, 1950.

[36] Tabár L, Chen HH, Yen MF, et al. Mammographic tumor features can predict long-term outcomes reliably in women with 1-14mm invasive breast carcinoma. Cancer, 2004, 101: 1745-1759.

[37] Tanaka Y, Oota K. A stereomicroscopic study of the mastopathic human breast. II. Peripheral type of duct evolution and its relation to cystic disease. Virchows Arch A Pathol Anat Histopathol, 1970, 349: 215-228.

[38] Tavassoli FA, Devili P (eds). World Health Organization classifcation of tumors. Pathology & genetics. Tumours of the breast and female genital organs. IARC, Lyon, 2003.

[39] Tavassoli FA, Eusebi V. Tumors of the breast. American Registry of Pathology/Armed Forces

Institute of Pathology. Washington, 2009.

[40] Taylor HB, Norris HJ. Epithelial invasion of nerves in benign disease of the breast. Cancer, 1967, 20: 2245-2249.

[41] Tot T. The diffuse type of invasive lobular carcinoma of the breast: morphology and prognosis. Virchows Arch, 2003, 443: 718-724.

[42] Tot T. DCIS, cytokeratins, and the theory of the sick lobe. Virchows Arch, 2005, 447: 1-8.

[43] Tot T. Clinical relevance of the distribution of the lesions in 500 consecutive breast cancer cases documented in large format histologic sections. Cancer, 2007a, 110: 2551-2560.

[44] Tot T. The theory of the sick breast lobe and the possible consequences. Int J Surg Pathol, 2007b, 15: 369-375.

[45] Tsang WYW, Chan JKC. Endocrine ductal carcinoma in situ (E-DCIS) of the breast. Am J Surg Pathol, 1996, 20 (8): 921-943.

[46] Wellings SR, Jensen HM. On the origin and progression of ductal carcinoma in the human breast. J Natl Cancer Inst, 1973, 50: 1111-1118.

第7章 多灶性与弥漫性乳腺癌影像学表现的意义

Laszlo K. Tabar, Peter B. Dean, Tibor Tot, Nadja Lindhe, Mats Ingvarsson, Amy Ming-Fang Yen

7.1 概述

对无症状女性进行乳腺X线检查，通常既可以检出全部原位病灶也可以检出不可触诊的1~9mm及10~14mm的浸润性病灶。然而，在疾病的早期阶段或病灶尺寸较小时检出乳腺癌病灶并不能确保每一例患者都处于疾病体积尚小的时期。事实上，无论病灶尺寸大小，多灶及弥漫性乳腺癌几乎构成了乳腺癌的主体（Holland, et al, 1985；Tot, 2007）。研究发现，肿瘤的大小对于分辨单灶性病变与多灶性病变而言并无明显作用（表7.1）。

此外，多灶性或弥漫性乳腺癌通常发生率较高。以上这些均提示乳腺癌需要依赖多学科的综合诊断。

1. 放射科医生在筛查发现病灶，以及使用多种影像学检查手段确定诊断后，需要评估病变累及的乳腺体积。

2. 通过筛查发现的不可触诊的乳腺癌属于早期阶段，是一种外科疾病而非系统性病变，其早发现的意义在于能够通过外科手术将肿瘤完全切除。应使用影像学标示出的乳腺癌的全部范围引导外科手术。

3. 对于频繁发生的多灶性分布和小叶分布的乳腺癌，其诊断需要依靠病理学大切片技术以提供能与影像学资料相对应的足够的病变信息。高清晰度三维成像技术（如乳腺MRI及超声诊断）的应用，也暴露了传统的小尺寸组织切片技术的缺陷。后者不能确定影像学下的病变本质，会低估真正的病变程度，并且对影像学诊断做出"过度诊断"的错误判断。

4. 从风险效益与成本收益评估的角度，对筛查发现的1~14mm的乳腺癌进行辅助治疗是学术界反对的（图7.1~7.6）。图7.1是一项针对576例直径1~14mm的浸润性乳腺癌妇女的

表7.1 2005—2007年在Falun诊断的565例乳腺癌单灶性病变与多灶性病变的频率（根据肿瘤大小划分）

	单灶	多灶	全部
原位	29% (23/79)	71% (56/79)	79
1~9mm	37% (33/90)	63% (57/90)	90
10~19mm	46% (103/225)	54% (122/225)	225
20~29mm	36% (36/100)	64% (64/100)	100
30+mm	18% (13/71)	82% (58/71)	71
全部	37% (208/565)	63% (357/565)	565

L. K. Tabár
Department of Mammography, Central Hospital Falun, Falun, Sweden
e-mail: laszlo@mammographyed.com

调查研究，该研究发现，这些乳腺癌患者经过保乳手术加术后放疗后，其26年生存率约为88%。而另一项研究包含384例乳癌患者，经保乳手术后未经放化疗及内分泌治疗其26年生存率为89%（图7.2）。然而以上这些研究结论是通过将一些分散的研究进行汇总所得，反映了同样尺寸的乳腺癌内在的异质性。对术后残余乳腺行X线摄影，依据钙化特点可以将病例分类为预后差和预后良好两组。图7.3和7.4显示了这两组患者有无进行术后放疗的结局（图7.3、7.4）。如果把乳房X线摄影的5项参数共同纳入分类指标，可以更加精确地区分预后不同的两组病例，包括是否应接受辅助治疗（图7.5、7.6）。据此，我们可以得出辅助治疗方案对于触诊阴性、经筛查发现的直径1~14mm的乳腺癌患者而言，作用微乎其微甚至毫无意义。Cady和Chung曾在2005年表达过类似的观点：的确有必要减少对放疗与辅助性化疗的需求，因为这两项治疗措施即昂贵又具有毒副作用，尤其是在乳腺癌早期，如可治愈的T1a和T1b期（Cady，Chung，2005）。

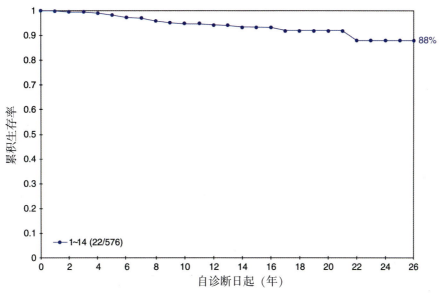

图7.1 576例连续诊断的浸润性乳腺癌患者（直径1~14mm）26年累积生存率。年龄范围40~69岁，经保乳手术治疗，辅以术后放疗（瑞典Dalarna地区）

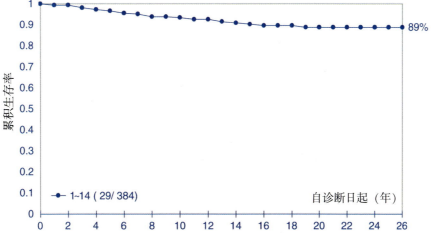

图7.2 384例连续诊断的浸润性乳腺癌患者（直径1~14mm）26年累积生存率。年龄范围40~69岁，经保乳手术治疗，未接受术后化疗、术后放疗或内分泌治疗（瑞典Dalarna地区）

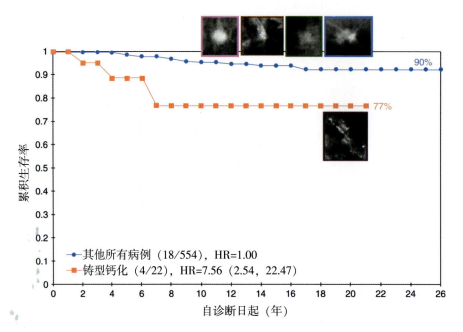

图7.3　576例连续诊断的浸润性乳腺癌患者（直径1~14mm）26年累积生存率（按照乳房X线摄影是否出现铸型钙化为分组指标）。年龄范围40~69岁，经保乳手术治疗，术后辅以放疗（瑞典Dalarna地区）

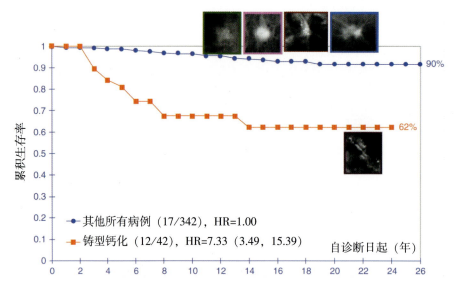

图7.4　384例连续诊断的浸润性乳腺癌患者（直径1~14mm）26年累积生存率（按照乳房X线摄影是否出现铸型钙化为分组指标）。年龄范围40~69岁，经保乳手术治疗，未接受术后化疗、术后放疗或内分泌治疗（瑞典Dalarna地区）

第7章 多灶性与弥漫性乳腺癌影像学表现的意义

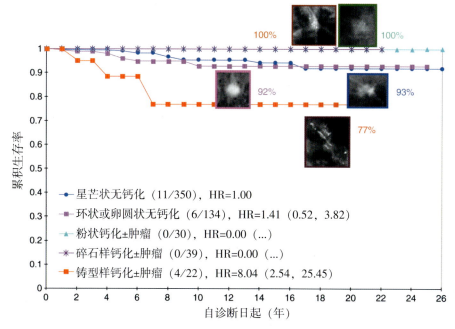

图7.5 567例连续诊断的浸润性乳腺癌患者（直径1~14mm）26年累积生存率（按照乳房X线摄影下5种典型特征分组）。年龄范围40~69岁，经保乳手术治疗，术后辅以放疗（瑞典Dalarna地区）

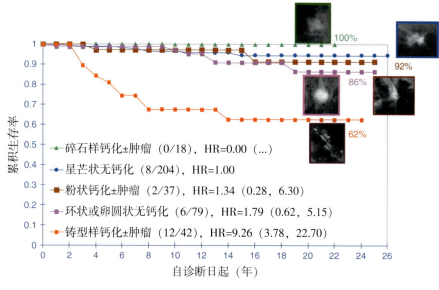

图7.6 384例连续诊断的浸润性乳腺癌患者（直径1~14mm）26年累积生存率（按照乳房X线摄影下5种典型特征为分组）。年龄范围40~69岁，经保乳手术治疗，未接受术后化疗、术后放疗或内分泌治疗（瑞典Dalarna地区）

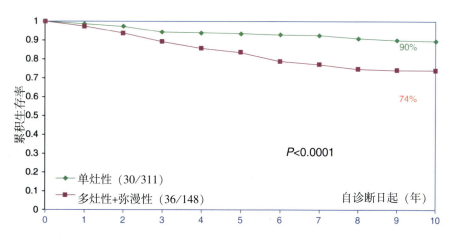

图7.7 1996—1998年311例连续诊断的单灶性乳腺浸润性癌患者（伴或不伴原位癌）与148例多灶性或弥漫性乳腺浸润性癌患者10年累积生存率比较（瑞典Dalarna地区）

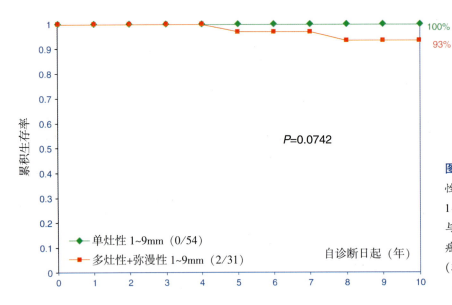

图7.8 1996—1998年单灶性乳腺浸润性癌患者（直径1~9mm，伴或不伴原位癌）与多灶性或弥漫性乳腺浸润癌患者10年累积生存率比较（瑞典Dalarna地区）

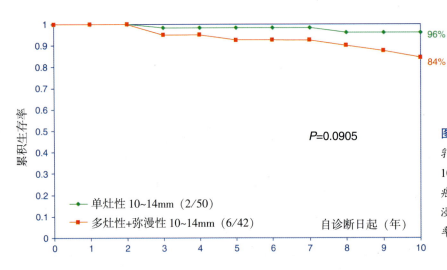

图7.9 1996—1998年单灶性乳腺浸润性癌患者（直径10~14mm，伴或不伴原位癌）与多灶性或弥漫性乳腺浸润性癌患者10年累积生存率比较（瑞典Dalarna地区）

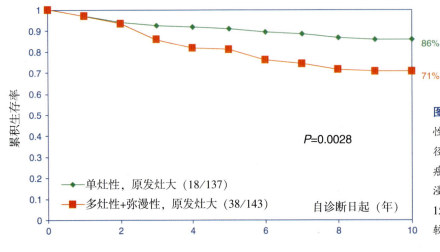

图7.10 1996—1998年单灶性乳腺浸润性癌患者（直径>15mm，伴或不伴原位癌）与多灶性或弥漫性乳腺浸润性癌患者（直径>15mm）10年累积生存率比较（瑞典Dalarna地区）

7.2 乳腺癌多灶性本质及影像学方法的选择

2家权威的医疗机构20年间先后出版了对乳腺癌疾病程度与分布范围的组织病理学相关的权威著作，著作中均一致表明多灶性和弥漫浸润性乳腺癌几乎占全部病例的60%（Holland, et al, 1985. Tot, 2007）。根据Tot新近基于对组织学大切片的研究发现：约40%的乳腺癌病灶为单发（不计尺寸）；20%为多灶性但仅局限于某一区域内，且直径<40mm；其余40%的病灶则或为弥漫分布或为多灶，且浸润范围或原位癌灶往往≥40mm。因此，虽然有点主观，但是，40mm的病灶范围现已被采纳成为实施保乳手术抑或是乳腺切除术的一个关键指标。

在过去的20年间，多种乳腺成像技术被广泛使用的原因在于：

- 乳腺癌的肿瘤异质性及其多病灶的特性。
- 在致密的乳腺组织中难以检测体积偏小的癌灶。
- 的确需要明确实际侵袭范围以确定合理的外科手术方案。

每种影像学方法都能够在一定程度上反映正常解剖构造与病理学病变，但仍各具适用范围，并存在相对的局限性。选择什么方法或哪几种方法联合应用于乳腺良性或恶性肿瘤的检查，取决于这些方法在以下方面的可视化程度：

- 潜在病变的性质。
- 组织病变的范围。
- 乳腺实质背景下可疑病变的情况。

在不考虑X线下乳腺实质分布模式时，乳房X线摄影技术能够很好地反映脂肪型乳腺的各种形式的病理变化，包括微钙化情况（Tabar, et al, 2005）。尽管大多数乳腺癌的X线片并不存在钙化灶，但是，该技术在检出直径<15mm的浸润性非钙化病灶方面具有很明显的优势，包括致密型腺体（Yen, et al, 2003）。乳房超声检查尽管在检查钙化性病灶时不够敏感，但由于病灶周围组织对检出浸润性病灶干扰较少的特点，因此已成为影像学诊断乳腺癌必要的、辅助性的工具。同时，超声检测也是经皮乳腺穿刺活检最便捷的方法。乳腺导管造影术对乳腺出血性或浆液性病变的病因诊断最具有意义，尤其是在乳房X线摄影和触诊阴性时。核磁共振成像检测是一种新的功能学成像技术，特别擅长反映乳腺整体病变的范围，也能够检测乳房X线摄影未能发现的同侧或对侧乳腺的病灶。其他功能学成像手段如放射同位素检测法等目前还处于试验评估阶段。

7.3 单灶性、多灶性及弥漫性乳腺癌的不同影像学表现与长期预后

乳腺癌多样的组织学特征是与其多样的影像学特征相对应的，包括乳房X线摄影、超声及核磁共振成像等。以下的典型病例的图片将对单一的影像学手段与多种影像学方法联合应用进行说明（详见例7.1~7.15）。

乳腺癌单灶性病变约占全部乳腺癌患者的40%，多为浸润性，并且外观呈毛刺样实性包块或圆形或椭圆形实性结节（例7.1、7.2）。我们的研究资料显示，全部乳腺原位癌中，单灶性病变占29%。在一些病例中，单一的末端小叶导管会并被癌细胞推挤出现扩张，伴中心部组织坏死及无定形钙化（例7.3）。有些缺乏钙化特征的单灶性乳腺原位癌病例，则会表现为实性肿物（例7.4、7.5）。多灶性或弥漫性乳腺癌病变占全部乳腺癌的60%，其中20%相对局限（例7.6~7.9），40%相对广泛（例7.10~7.15），其影像学特征均类似但程度不同，以40mm为界，此范围的界定是比较主观的。

例7.1　69岁无症状女性，X线摄影筛查。

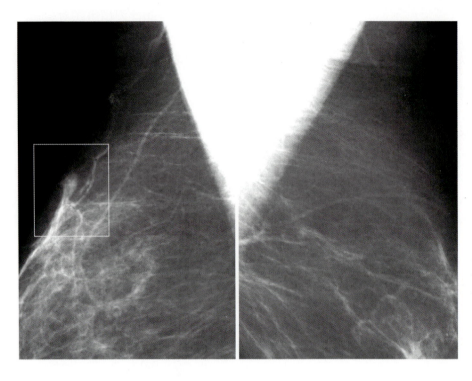

图7.1.1、7.1.2　分别为右侧和左侧乳腺斜位图，两侧均为脂肪型乳腺，右侧乳腺尾区示一较小的不对称密度增高区（矩形框内所示）

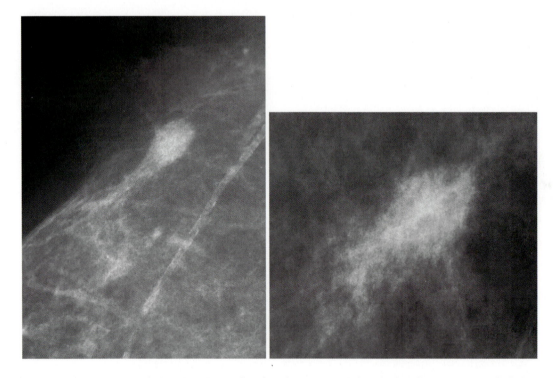

图7.1.3、7.1.4　右侧乳腺斜位放大图，可进一步观察该处微小的意义不明的病灶（1.3），微聚焦放大摄影图可见一个<10mm、孤立的、意义不明的无钙化的乳腺恶性肿瘤（1.4）

第 7 章　多灶性与弥漫性乳腺癌影像学表现的意义

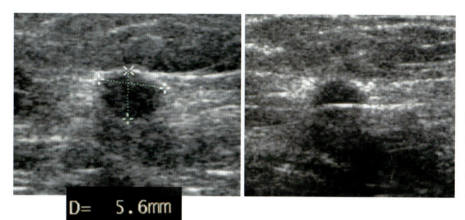

图7.1.5~7.1.7* 乳腺超声检查测量该病灶约6mm（1.5），该图像采自超声引导下14g空芯针活检时（1.6）

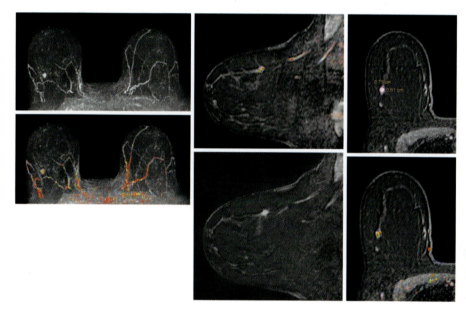

图7.1.8~7.1.13 乳腺MRI系列图证实病灶性质为孤立的

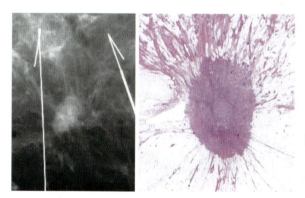

图7.1.14、7.1.15 手术标本X线摄影图（7.1.14）。病变位于标本的中央。低倍镜下组织学图片（7.1.15）显示为6mm×7mm的分化良好的浸润性导管癌

评论：该病例是典型的单灶性浸润性乳腺癌，这一类型占全部乳腺癌种类的40%。

---

*译者注：原书缺图7.1.7

例7.2 64岁无症状女性，X线筛查发现左侧乳腺内上象限一微小孤立、意义不明的病灶，要求进一步检查评估。

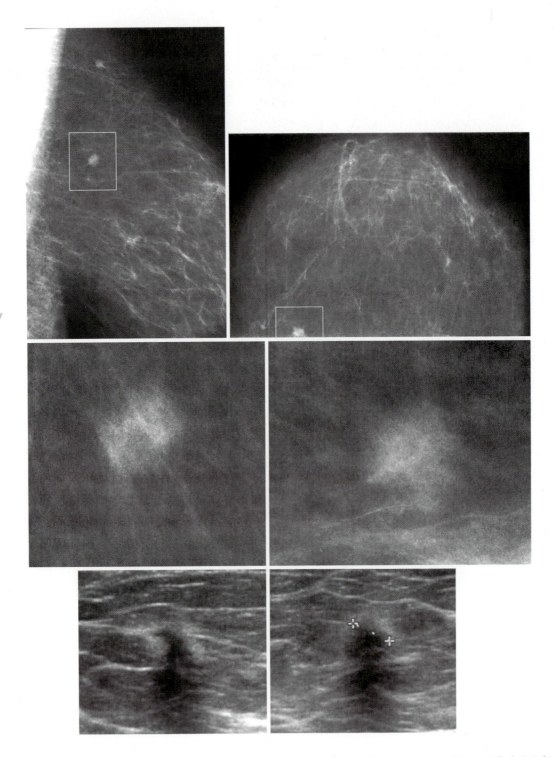

图7.2.1~7.2.6 左侧乳腺侧位（7.2.1）和头尾位图（7.2.2），内上象限可见一个<10mm的病灶，微聚焦放大摄影图（7.2.3、7.2.4）示一孤立的带有毛刺的乳腺恶性肿瘤，乳腺超声检查（7.2.5、7.2.6）证实了乳腺摄影的诊断

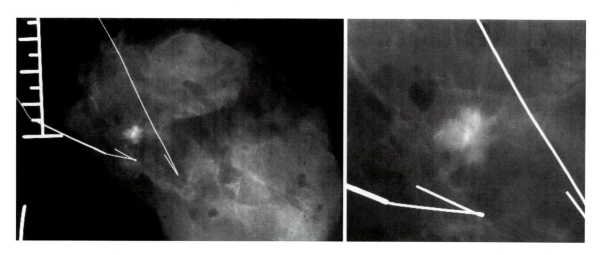

图7.2.7、7.2.8　术前导丝定位后，手术切除标本的X线摄影图

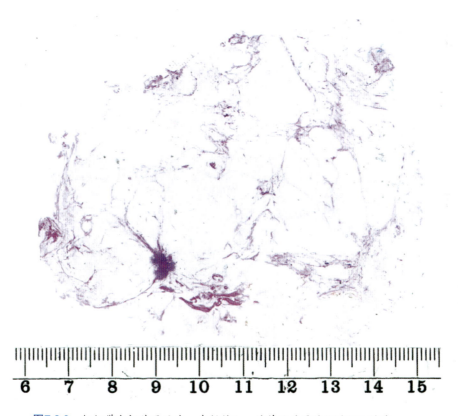

图7.2.9　组织学大切片显示为一直径约9mm的单独的星芒状浸润性肿瘤

评论：此病例是典型的单灶性星芒状浸润性乳腺癌。星芒状/刺状形态是1~14mm大小的浸润性乳腺癌在X线摄影上最常见的表现。

例7.3 54岁无症状女性，X线筛查发现左乳成簇微钙化，被要求复诊以进一步检查评估。

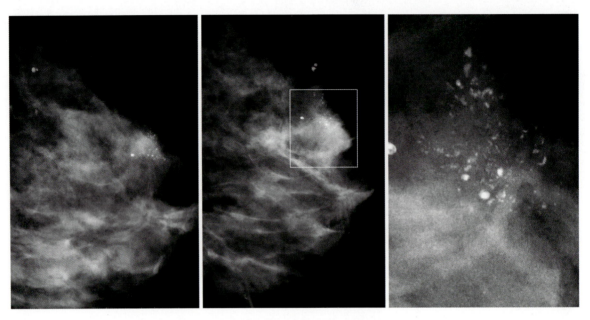

图7.3.1~7.3.3 左侧乳腺斜位图（3.1），侧位图（3.2），微聚焦放大摄影图（3.3），发现大小约15mm×10mm孤立、簇状的，形态、密度及大小均不相同的恶性特征的微钙化灶，未见可证实的肿瘤包块

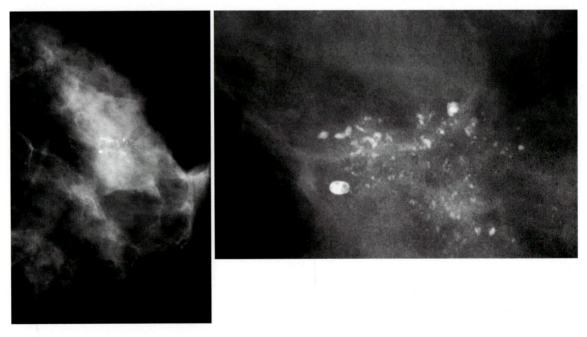

图7.3.4、7.3.5 左侧乳腺头尾位图（3.4）和微聚焦放大摄影图（3.5），发现一大簇碎石样和短铸型混合的X线摄影下恶性征象的微钙化灶

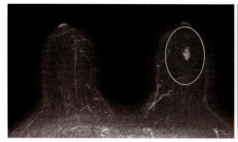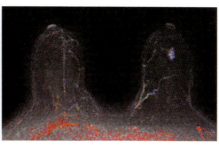

图7.3.6、7.3.7 乳腺MRI示：左侧乳腺外侧范围约15mm×10mm对比增强区，提示为恶性

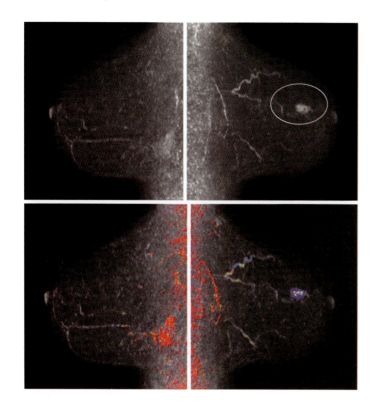

图7.3.8~7.3.11 乳腺矢状位MRI示：对比增强区位于外上象限，范围为13mm×10mm×7mm

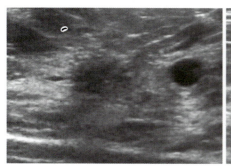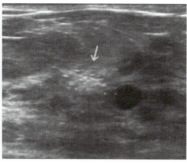

图7.3.12、7.3.13 与X线摄影发现恶性钙化的位置相符，超声检查发现呈低回声，约15mm意义不明的病灶，该病灶包含很多微小钙化，病灶旁可见一微小的单纯囊肿

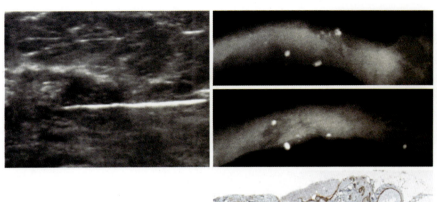
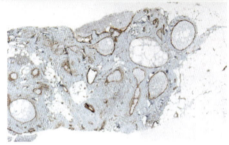

图7.3.14~7.3.17 超声引导下14g空芯针活检时图像（7.3.14），经皮穿刺活检组织X线摄影图（7.3.15、7.3.16）粗针穿刺标本的免疫组化SMA染色图片（7.3.17）

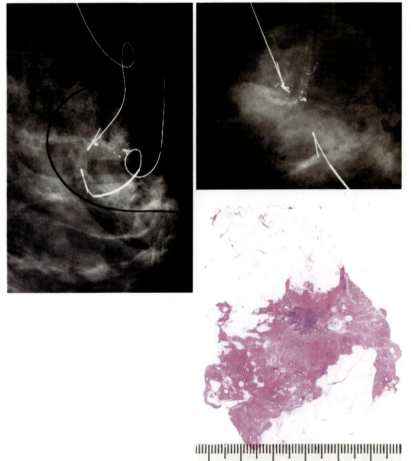

图7.3.18~7.3.20 使用导丝术前定位X线摄影图（7.3.18），包含微钙化的标本X线摄影图（7.3.19），组织学大切片图（7.3.20），病变范围约为15mm×10mm

第 7 章　多灶性与弥漫性乳腺癌影像学表现的意义

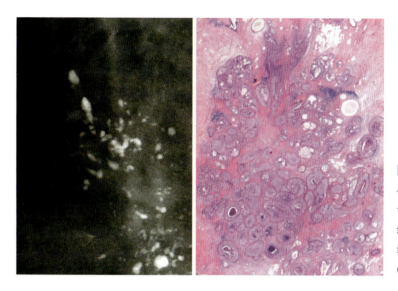

图7.3.21、7.3.22　一张标本切片的微聚焦放大摄影图，可见成簇的铸型样和碎石样的钙化灶（7.3.21）；组织学表现腺泡极度扩张，内充癌细胞，中央坏死和无定形钙化（7.3.22）

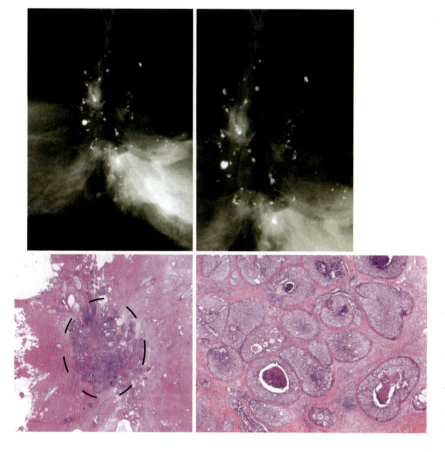

图7.3.23~7.3.26　标本X线摄影可见一大簇恶性特征的钙化（7.3.23、7.3.24）；组织学低倍镜和高倍镜显示范围约15mm×10mm的TDLU实性病变区，呈导管原位癌2级（7.3.25、7.3.26）

评论：该病例是一个典型的单灶性原位癌，局部的TDLU被肿瘤细胞充满，中央有坏死和不定形钙化。

例7.4 47岁无症状女性，X线筛查发现右侧乳腺乳晕后病灶，被要求复诊以进一步检查评估。

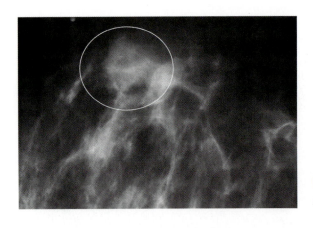

图7.4.1 右侧乳腺，头尾位，乳晕后可见一无钙化的环形低密度灶

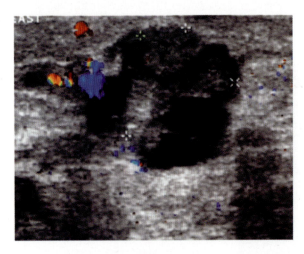

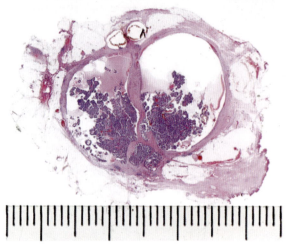

图7.4.2、7.4.3 超声检查（7.4.2）可见一囊内乳头状影；低倍组织学大切片影像（7.4.3）显示为囊内乳头状原位癌，外周为纤维性增厚包囊

评论：该病例是一个典型的单灶性原位癌，X线摄影发现了巨大包块；然而，超声检查显示存在囊内的乳头状结构生长，经组织学检查证实为囊内的原位癌。

第 7 章 多灶性与弥漫性乳腺癌影像学表现的意义

例7.5 64岁女性，X线筛查发现左侧乳腺下部一处微小的不对称密度增高区，被要求复诊以进一步检查评估。

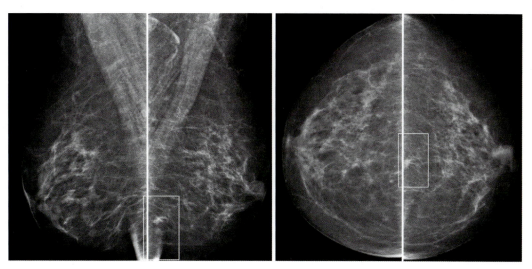

图7.5.1~7.5.4 右侧乳腺和左侧乳腺斜位（7.5.1、7.5.2）和头尾位（7.5.3、7.5.4）图，示左侧乳腺下部6点钟位置一处微小的非特异性不对称低密度区，其内未见钙化

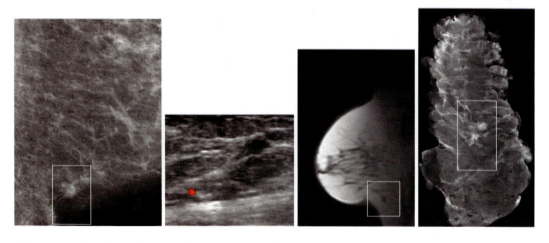

图7.5.5~7.5.8 斜位微聚焦放大摄影（7.5.5）、超声（7.5.6）、MRI（7.5.7）和标本X线摄影图（7.5.8）均可见该意义不明的恶性特征区域

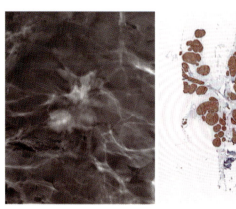
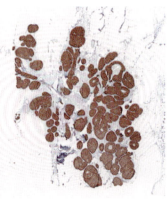

图7.5.9、7.5.10 标本切片的微聚焦放大摄影图可见一微小的意义不明的肿瘤（7.5.7）。对TDLU的组织学检查（对ER进行免疫组化染色）发现12mm、Grade2的原位癌（7.5.8）。组织学图片由Pia Boström, M.D., Department of Pathology, Turku University Hospital, Turku, Finland 惠赠

例7.6 71岁无症状女性，X线摄影筛查发现右侧乳腺微钙化，被要求复诊以进一步检查评估。

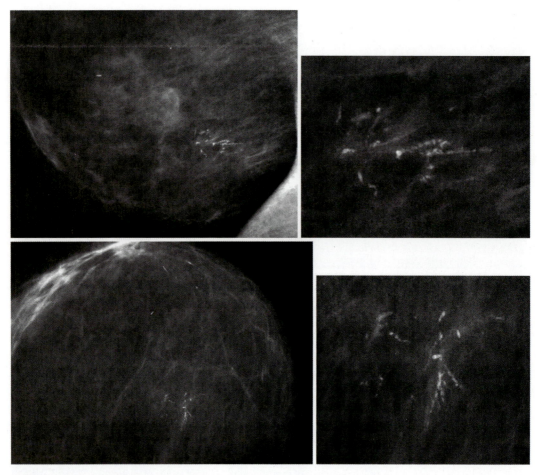

图7.6.1~7.6.4 右侧乳腺斜位（7.6.1）和头尾位（7.6.3）图像发现内下象限无肿瘤包块的簇状钙化，微聚焦放大摄影图（7.6.2，7.6.4）可见碎片状、斑点状铸型混杂的恶性特征钙化

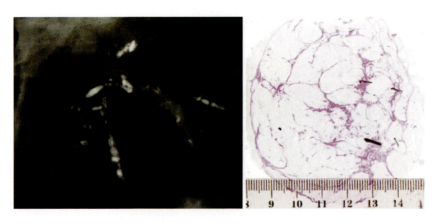

图7.6.5、7.6.6 标本切片微聚焦放大摄影图可见碎片状、斑点状铸型钙化（7.6.5）。手术切除后的大切片组织学（7.6.6）

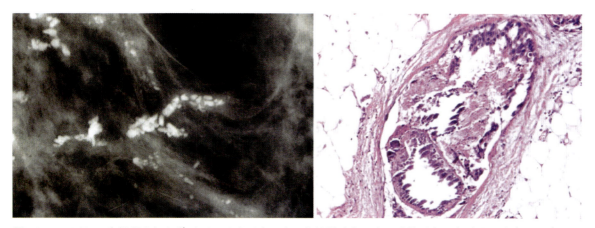

图7.6.7、7.6.8 X线摄影和组织学对照：无定形钙化与X线摄影图中斑点状的铸型钙化相对应，存在于含有癌细胞和坏死扩张的导管中

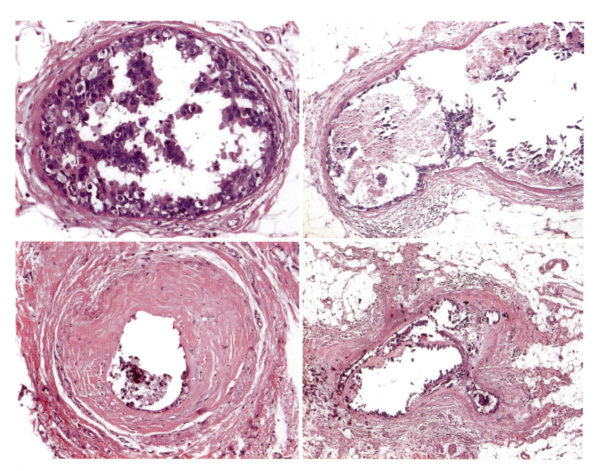

图7.6.9~7.6.12 组织学显示：组织学3级、微乳头状导管原位癌（7.6.9），其中一个扩张的导管内可见无定形钙化和坏死（7.6.10），横截面显示导管内不完全恶性细胞层，导管周围纤维化（7.6.11）及导管周围广泛的促结缔组织增生性反应（7.6.12），包含少量癌细胞和大量片段化的无定形钙化

最终组织学：15mm×10mm，组织学3级，原位癌，无明显浸润。

评论：此病例是典型的40mm以内的高级别原位癌。相应的乳腺X线摄影显示了铸型钙化。

例7.7 54岁无症状女性，X线摄影筛查发现右侧乳腺多发簇状碎石样钙化，被要求复诊以进一步检查评估。

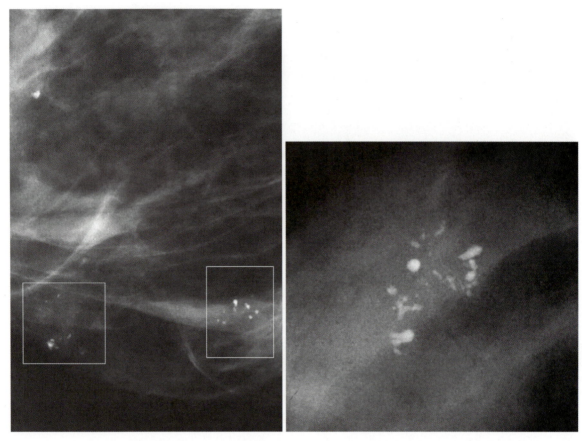

图7.7.1、7.7.2 右侧乳腺斜位图（7.7.1）示多发簇状碎石样钙化（矩形框内所示），无明显包块，（7.7.2）为其中一簇的微聚焦放大摄影图，这些钙化具有恶性特征

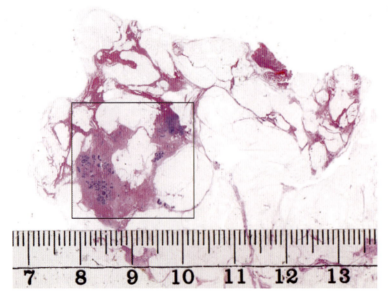

图7.7.3 大切片组织学显示矩形框内的多发性原位癌病灶

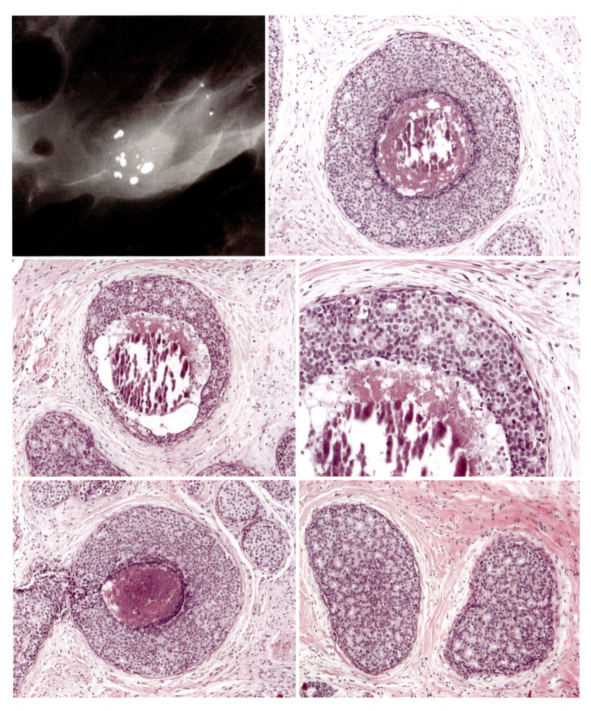

图7.7.4~7.7.9 伴有两簇碎石样钙化的标本X线摄影图（7.7.4）；HE染色显示组织学特点（7.7.5~7.7.9）为导管原位癌、组织学2级，瘤细胞充满腺泡，部分腺泡伴中心性坏死及无定形钙化

评论：本例中多簇、碎石样钙化提示为典型的多灶性、范围局限（<40mm）的中等级别原位癌。

例7.8　66岁无症状女性，X线摄影筛查发现左侧乳腺微钙化，被要求复诊以进一步检查评估。

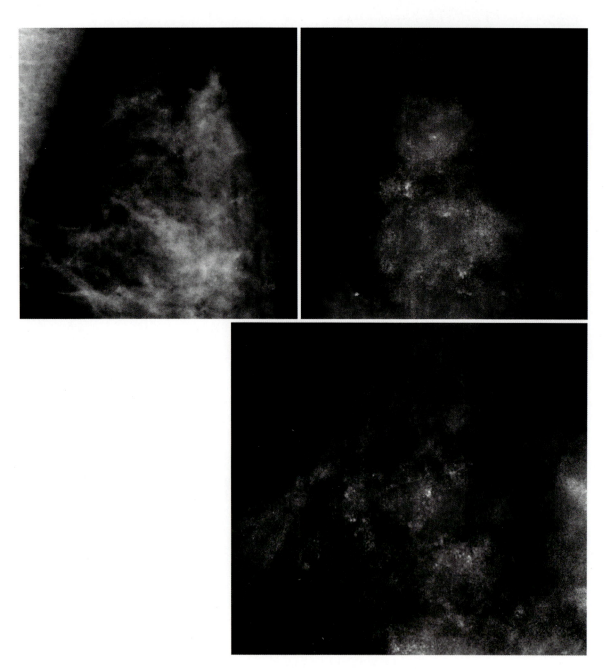

图7.8.1~7.8.3　左侧乳腺斜位图（7.8.1）示：腋尾区模糊钙化，微聚焦放大摄影图（7.8.2、7.8.3）可见多发簇状不伴有包块的粉末样、棉团样钙化

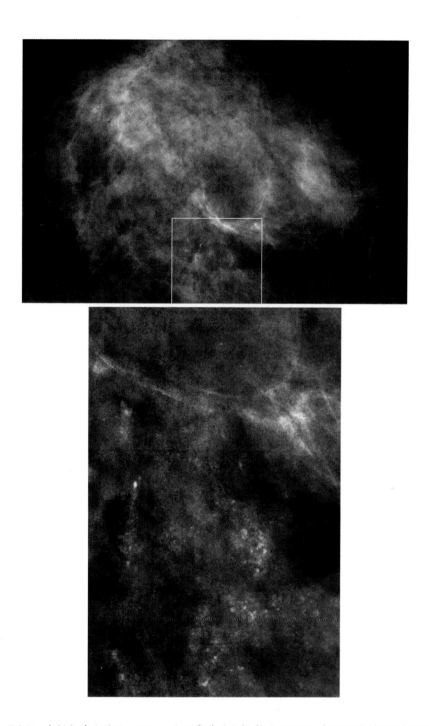

图7.8.4、7.8.5　左侧乳腺头尾位(7.8.4)和微聚焦放大摄影图(7.8.5)提示这些模糊的钙化邻近胸壁

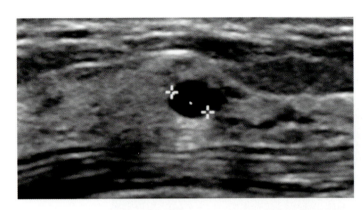

图7.8.6 超声检查未发现浸润性肿瘤，仅发现隐藏在致密纤维组织中的一个单纯囊肿

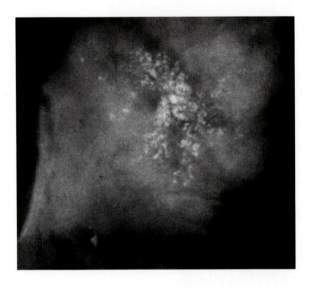

图7.8.7 带有射频功能的大孔径针经皮穿刺活检后标本的X线摄影图，该标本组织中含有一些钙化灶

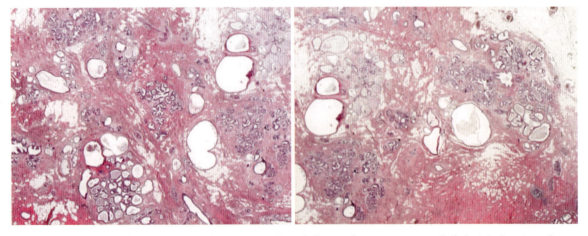

图7.8.8、7.8.9 经皮穿刺标本，低倍镜下显示几个末端导管小叶单位（TDLUs）呈导管内原位癌、组织学1级，局部呈现黏附和微乳头特征

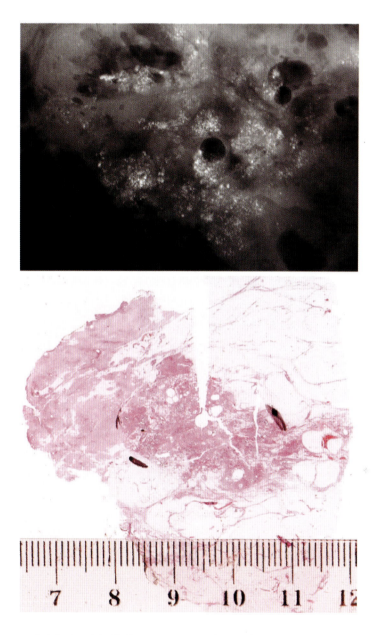

图7.8.10、7.8.11　手术标本X线摄影图（7.8.10）大切片组织学（7.8.11）显示与X线摄影相对应的钙化灶，范围30mm×20mm

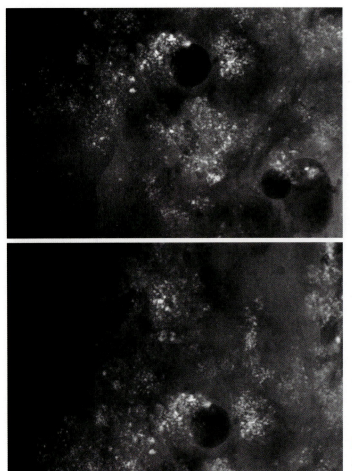

图7.8.12、7.8.13 手术标本的微聚焦放大摄影图示棉团样钙化灶

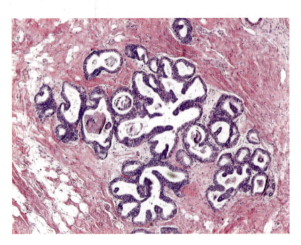

图7.8.14 组织学显示一根TDLU为原位癌、组织学1级，局部呈现黏附和微乳头特征

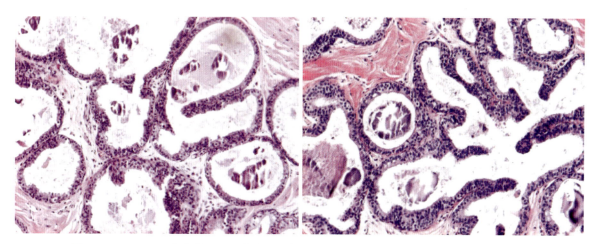

图7.8.15、7.8.16　高倍镜下组织学片显示腺泡扩张，充满原位癌细胞及腔内局灶性微钙化

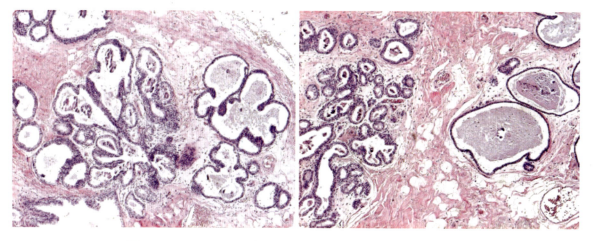

图7.8.17、7.8.18　组织学片显示囊性扩张的TDLUs伴分泌及微钙化

最终组织学：30mm×20mm的范围内为组织学1级，微乳头、筛状或黏性原位癌。无浸润性癌。

评论：此病例是典型的<40mm的低级别原位癌。相应的X线摄影提示粉末样、棉团样钙化。

例7.9 68岁无症状女性，X线摄影筛查发现左侧乳腺不对称密度增高，被要求复诊以进一步检查评估。

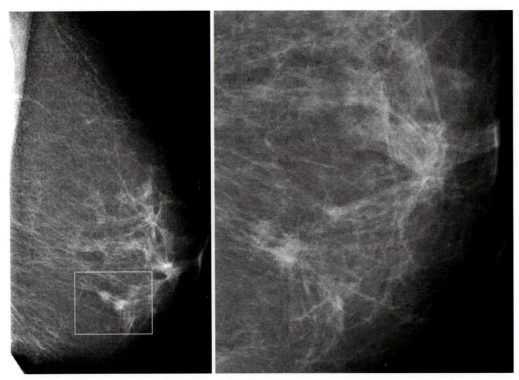

图7.9.1、7.9.2 矢状位（7.9.1）和微聚焦放大摄影图（7.9.2）示左侧乳腺下部两个相邻的毛刺样恶性肿瘤，未见有钙化

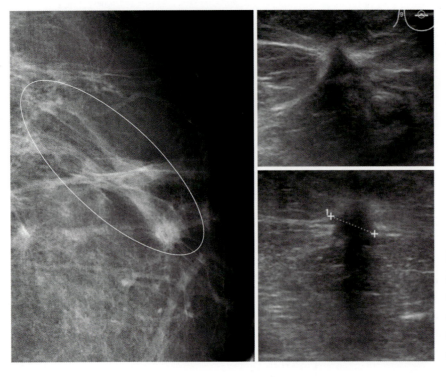

图7.9.3~7.9.5 头尾位微聚焦放大摄影图示（7.9.3）两个星芒状病灶相连，超声检查证实了（7.9.4、7.9.5）X线摄影的诊断

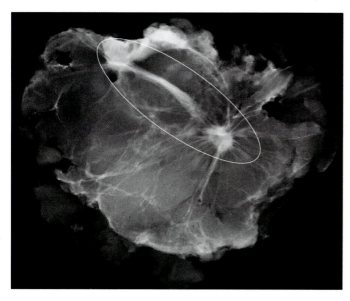

图7.9.6 手术标本X线摄影图显示这两个小肿瘤相互连接

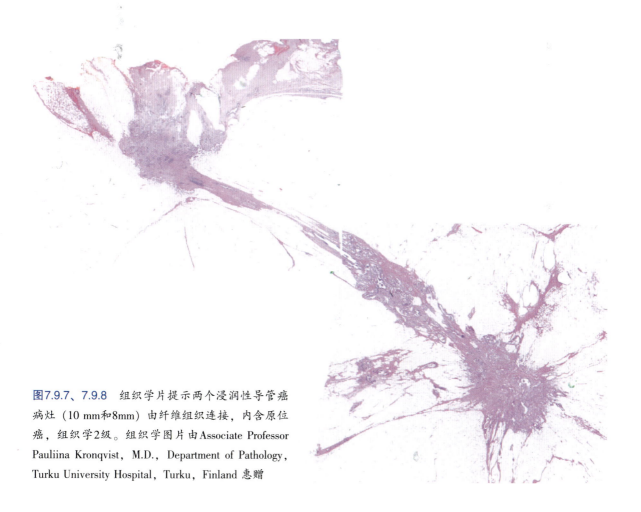

图7.9.7、7.9.8 组织学片提示两个浸润性导管癌病灶（10 mm和8mm）由纤维组织连接，内含原位癌，组织学2级。组织学图片由Associate Professor Pauliina Kronqvist, M.D., Department of Pathology, Turku University Hospital, Turku, Finland 惠赠

评论：此病例属于典型的多灶性浸润性癌，范围<40mm。

例7.10　86岁女性，发现左侧乳腺可触及的增厚，进行X线摄影检查。

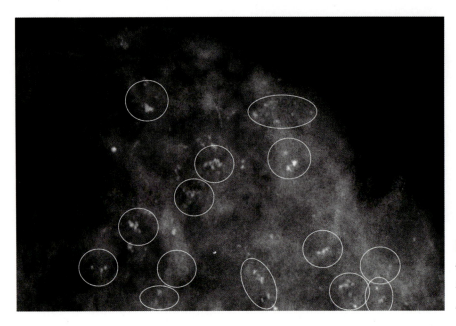

图7.10.1　左侧乳腺头尾位，图示纤维背景下不伴有肿瘤包块的多发簇状碎石样、铸型样钙化

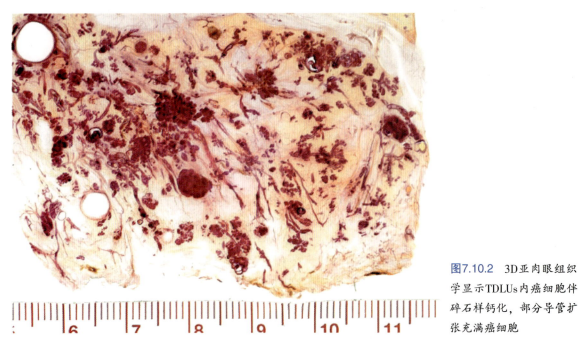

图7.10.2　3D亚肉眼组织学显示TDLUs内癌细胞伴碎石样钙化，部分导管扩张充满癌细胞

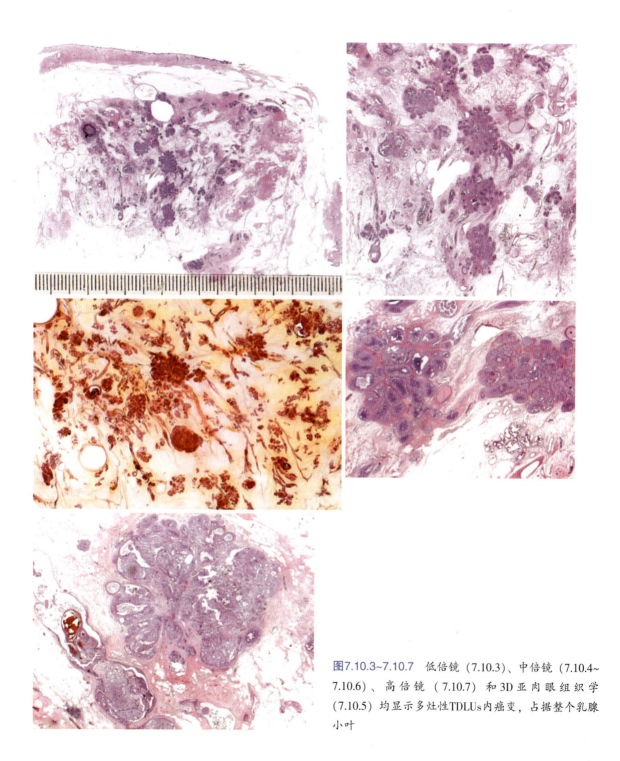

图7.10.3~7.10.7 低倍镜（7.10.3）、中倍镜（7.10.4~7.10.6）、高倍镜（7.10.7）和3D亚肉眼组织学（7.10.5）均显示多灶性TDLUs内癌变，占据整个乳腺小叶

组织学诊断：6cm×5cm的区域内密布多灶性原位癌，为实性或筛状和微乳头状结构。

评论：此病例是典型、广泛的（>40mm）原位癌，大量的癌细胞充满TDLUs，密布整个腺叶。导管内充满癌细胞、坏死碎片和无定形钙化，与X线片上检测到的碎石样和铸型钙化一致。

例7.11 58岁女性，X线摄影筛查发现右侧乳腺外上象限伴有微钙化的不均匀密度增高区，被要求复诊以进一步检查评估。

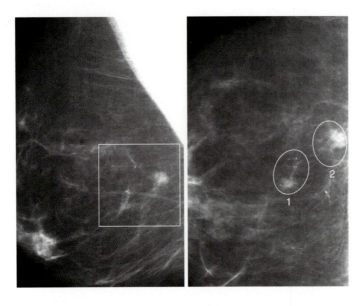

图7.11.1、7.11.2 右侧乳腺斜位（7.11.1）和矢状位图（7.11.2）示两个小的意义不明的伴有恶性特征钙化的恶性肿瘤

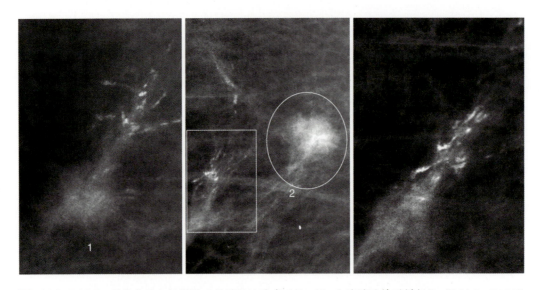

图7.11.3~7.11.5 微聚焦放大摄影图可见浸润性肿瘤（1#，2#）和伴随的铸型样钙化（7.11.3、7.11.5）

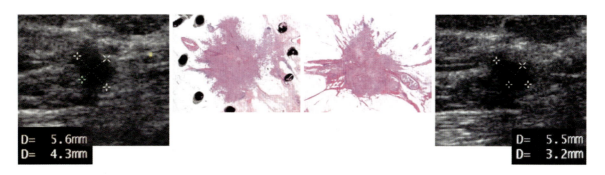

图7.11.6~7.11.11　超声检查图（7.11.6、7.11.10）可见小的浸润性肿瘤，低倍镜下的组织学图像（7.11.8、7.11.9）

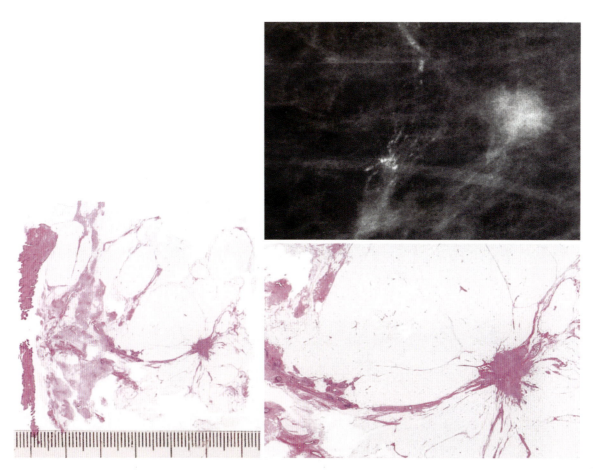

图7.11.12~7.11.14　浸润性肿瘤2#和伴随的铸型样钙化的微聚焦放大摄影图（7.11.12）及低倍镜大切片组织图（7.11.13、7.11.14）

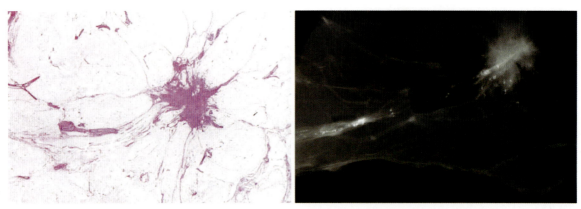

图7.11.15、7.11.16 浸润性肿瘤2#和伴随的组织学3级的原位癌的大切片组织图（7.11.15）和标本切片X线摄影图（7.11.16）的比较

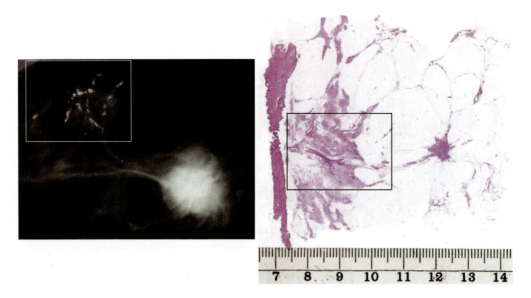

图7.11.17、7.11.18 另一个标本切片X线摄影图（7.11.17）与低倍镜大切片组织图（7.11.18）

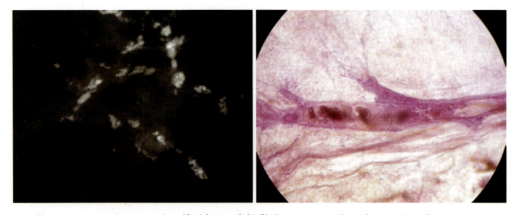

图7.11.19、7.11.20 斑点状铸型钙化X线摄影图（7.11.19）与亚肉眼3D组织图（7.11.20）

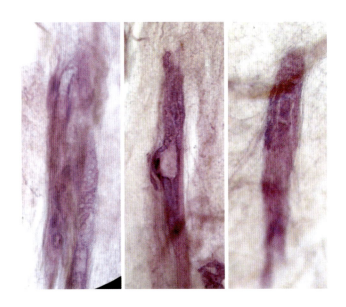

图7.11.21~7.11.23 3D组织学显示癌细胞累及的乳腺导管及形成实性和筛孔样的结构

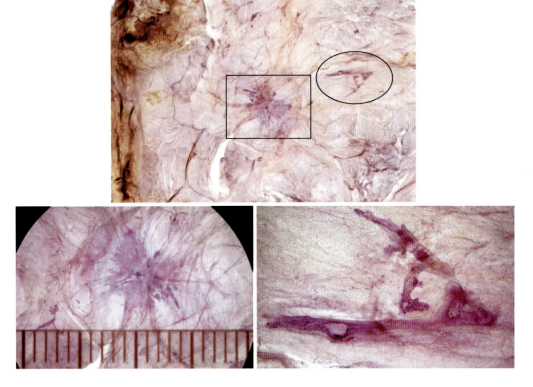

图7.11.24~7.11.26 大厚切片3D组织图显示了微小的浸润性癌灶（矩形框内）和原位癌成分（椭圆框；7.11.24）。以下分别为放大图像（7.11.25、7.11.26）

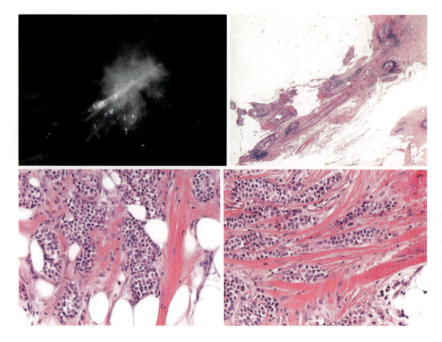

图7.11.27~7.11.30 手术标本切片X线摄影图（7.11.27）；组织学低倍镜显示导管原位癌，组织学3级（7.11.28），中分化浸润性导管癌（7.11.29、7.11.30）

最终组织学：两个中等分化的浸润性导管癌灶，面积约9mm×8mm和8mm×8mm。组织学3级的浸润性癌与组织学3级的原位癌共存，后者可见于浸润性癌灶中和周围。恶性肿瘤的总面积约60mm×50mm。5/13腋窝淋巴结转移，可见淋巴管侵犯（LVI）。

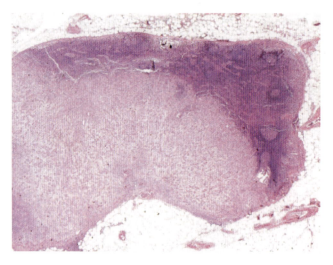

图7.11.31 淋巴结转移

第7章 多灶性与弥漫性乳腺癌影像学表现的意义

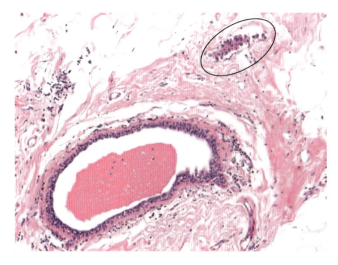

图7.11.32 淋巴管侵犯（H-E染色）

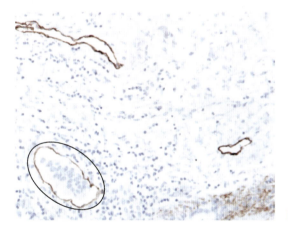

图7.11.33 淋巴管侵犯（免疫组化D2-40）

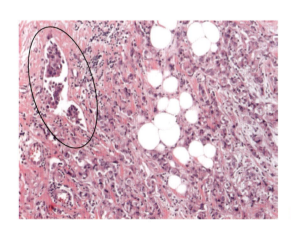

图7.11.34 淋巴管侵犯（H-E染色）

评论：此例广泛的、转移的恶性肿瘤侵犯绝大部分腺叶，其中心部分尺寸似乎在6~10mm，故TNM分期仍为T1b。对疾病的真实尺寸的评估很必要，会影响后续合适治疗措施的制订。

例7.12 66岁女性，最近一次X线摄影检查在20年前，那时就发现双侧巨大囊性病灶，已引流数次。

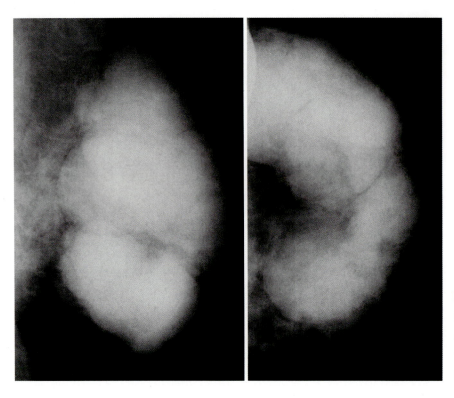

图7.12.1、7.12.2 左侧乳腺斜位（7.12.1）和头尾位图（7.12.2）。该片摄于20年前，示巨大囊性病灶，其被引流了数次

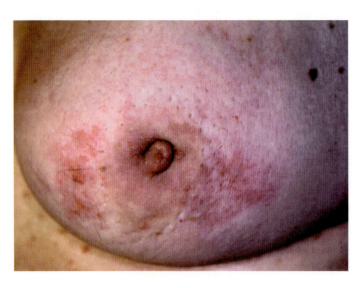

图7.12.3 本次检查前数周（X线摄影后20年），患者发现左侧乳晕及乳晕旁明显的外观变化，自觉左侧乳腺外上象限增厚

第 7 章 多灶性与弥漫性乳腺癌影像学表现的意义

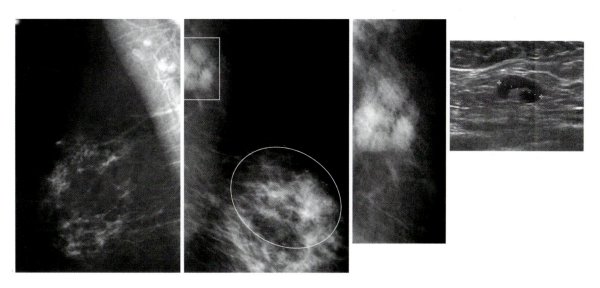

图7.12.4~7.12.7 右侧乳腺（7.12.4）及左侧乳腺斜位图（7.12.5），左侧腋窝淋巴结的微聚焦放大摄影图（7.12.6）和超声检查示左侧腋窝的病理性淋巴结

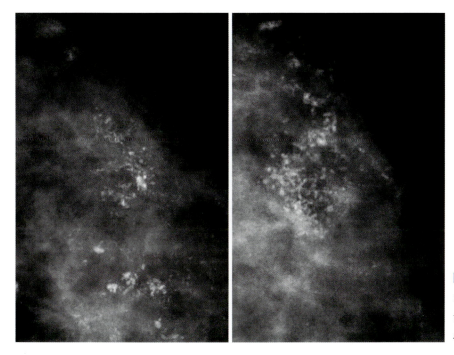

图 7.12.8、7.12.9 微聚焦放大摄影图示广泛的铸型样恶性特征的钙化，占据外上象限大部分

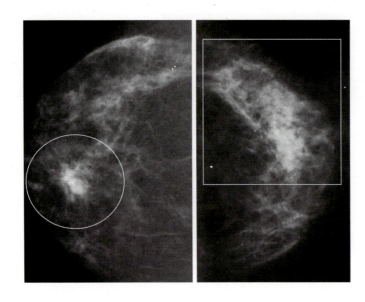

图7.12.10、7.12.11 右侧乳腺(7.12.10)及左侧乳腺头尾位图(7.12.11),示恶性特征的钙化灶位于左侧乳腺侧方(矩形框内所示),也见右侧乳腺内侧局部结构扭曲(圆圈内所示)

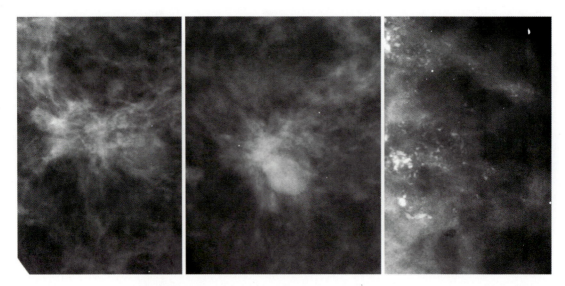

图7.12.12~7.12.14 右侧乳腺头尾位(7.12.12)、斜位图(7.12.13)的微聚焦放大摄影图可见结构扭曲,左侧乳腺头尾位放大图(7.12.14)

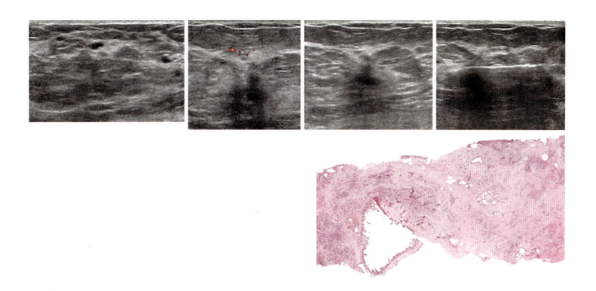

图7.12.15~7.12.19　对照微聚焦放大摄影图（7.12.12、7.12.13），超声检查提示右侧乳腺病变区为乳腺增生，而不是恶性肿瘤；左侧乳腺外上象限超声检查（7.12.16、7.12.17）提示若干浸润性癌存在，为超声引导下空芯针活检确诊为伴原位癌成分的浸润性导管癌（7.12.18、7.12.19）

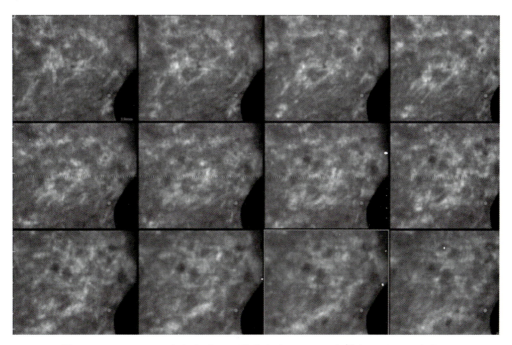

图7.12.20~7.12.22　左侧乳腺2mm厚重建的冠状位3D超声切面图，示多发不规则、低回声病灶，与浸润性癌表现一致

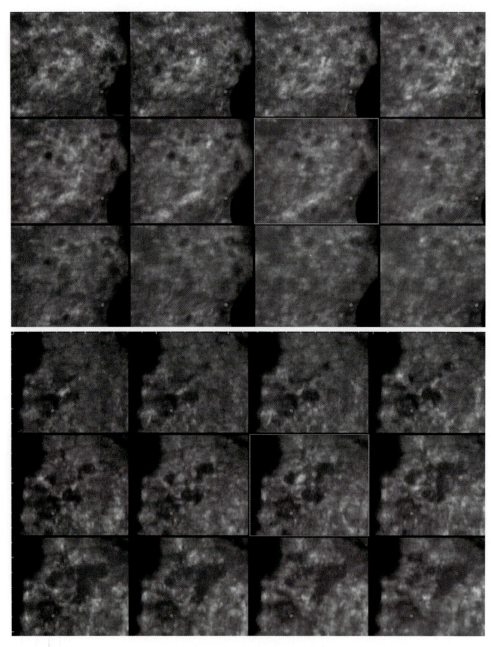

(续)图7.12.20~7.12.22

第 7 章 多灶性与弥漫性乳腺癌影像学表现的意义

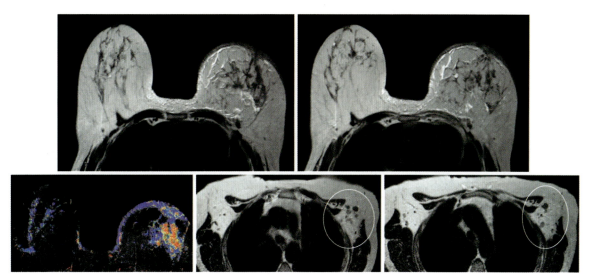

图7.12.23~7.12.27 乳腺MRI示乳腺外形改变，该乳腺很多区域发生广泛恶变，乳腺皮肤增厚是由于腋窝淋巴回流受阻

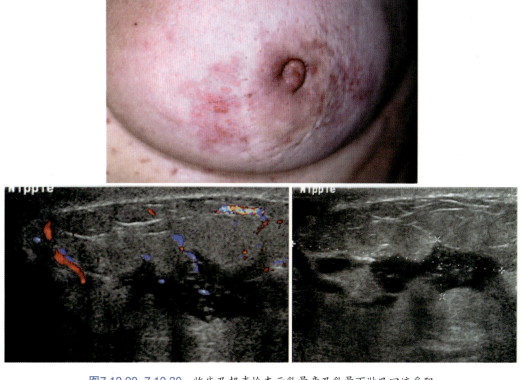

图7.12.28~7.12.30 临床及超声检查示乳晕旁及乳晕下淋巴回流受阻

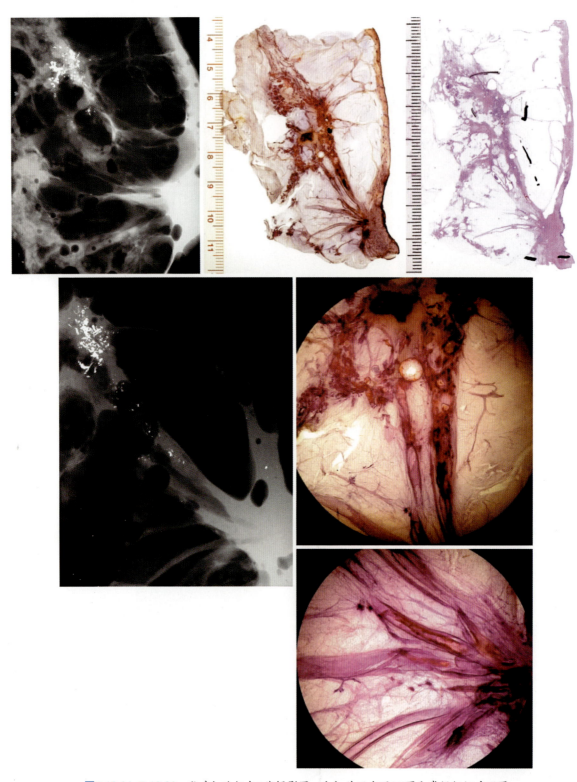

图7.12.31~7.12.36　乳房切除标本X线摄影图、大切片亚肉眼3D图和常规组织病理图

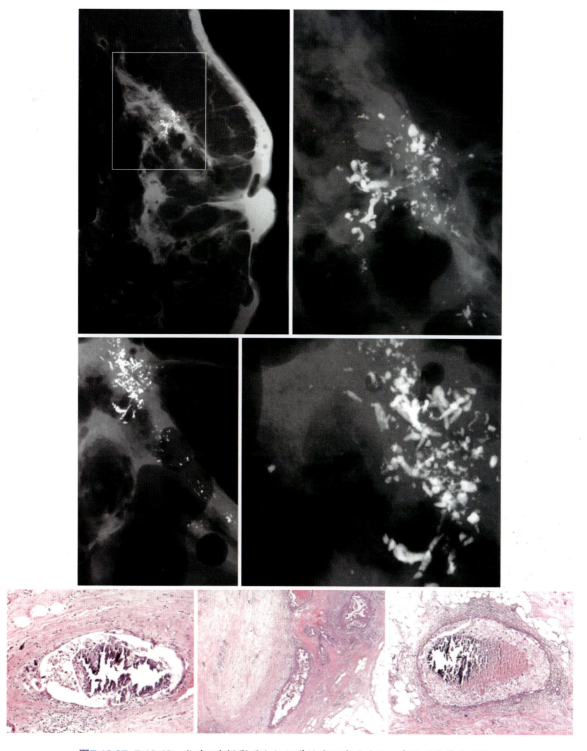

图7.12.37~7.12.43 乳腺X线摄影图和组织学检查证实为广泛、高级别导管内恶性变

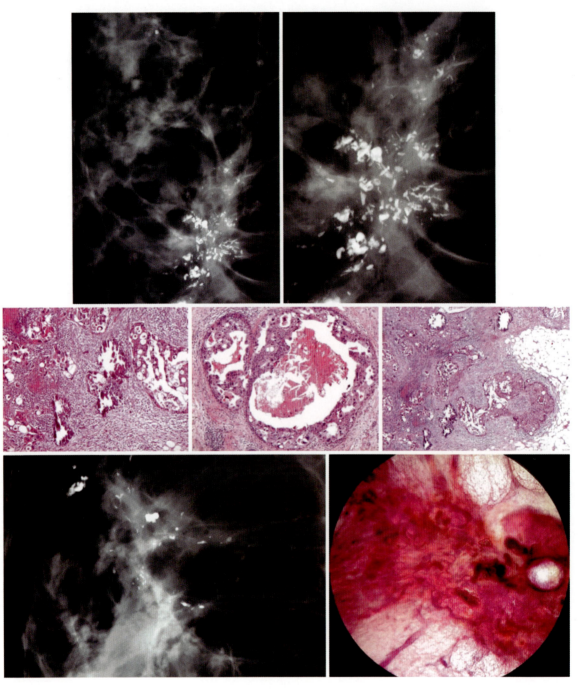

图7.12.44~7.12.50 乳腺切除标本另一切片的X线摄影图（7.12.44、7.12.45、7.12.49）示局部结构扭曲，与浸润性癌相符；组织学（7.12.46~7.12.48、7.12.50）示原位癌和浸润性癌混合存在

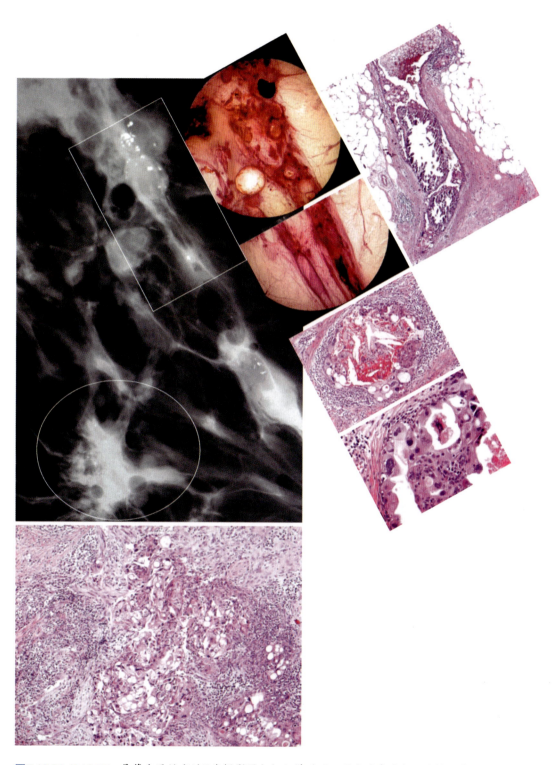

图7.12.51~7.12.57 导管内恶性变的X线摄影图与组织学对照。圈内伴有放射状结构的意义不明的密度增高区即为低分化的浸润性导管癌 (7.12.57)

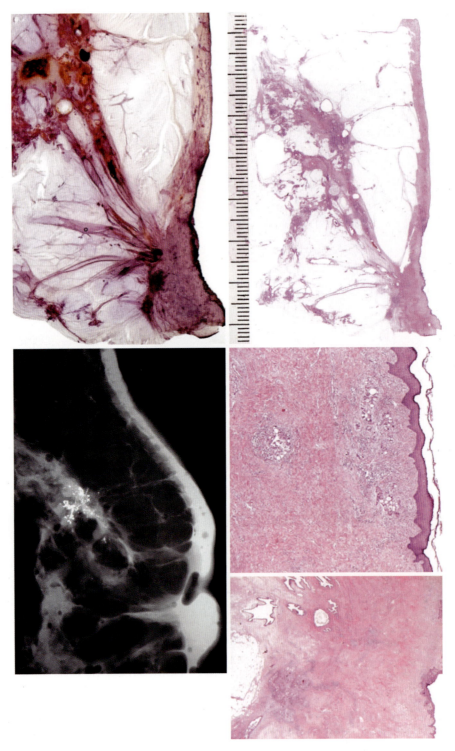

图7.12.58~7.12.62 广泛的恶性变累及皮肤和乳晕下组织

组织学：（左）乳腺多灶性低分化癌（5mm×5mm，3mm×3mm，1mm×1mm），伴组织学3级的原位癌，病变累及范围为70mm×60mm。总疾病范围：70mm×60mm pN6/7. LVI。

第 7 章 多灶性与弥漫性乳腺癌影像学表现的意义

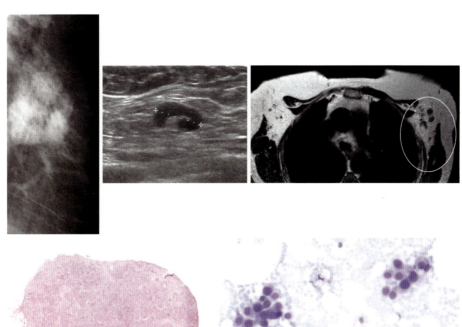

图 7.12.63 ~7.12.65 乳腺X线摄影、超声及MRI检查示腋窝淋巴结转移，细针抽吸细胞学和低倍镜下组织学均显示腋窝淋巴结转移癌

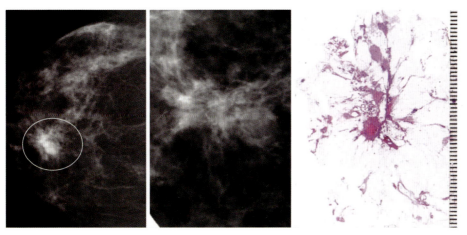

图 7.12.68 ~7.12.70 右侧乳腺头尾位（7.12.68）、微聚焦放大摄影图（7.12.69）提示结构扭曲部位。组织学（7.12.70）示放射状疤痕和纤维囊性变

评论：广泛的多灶性及弥漫性乳腺癌的诊断和治疗都很有难度。尽管医护人员已竭尽全力，但是，绝大部分患者的预后不佳不幸的是，在当前的分级系统下，此类病例的肿瘤负担被低估了。须使用多种影像学手段来精确评估真实的疾病范围。

例7.13 61岁女性，右侧乳头血性溢液，体格检查时未触及包块。

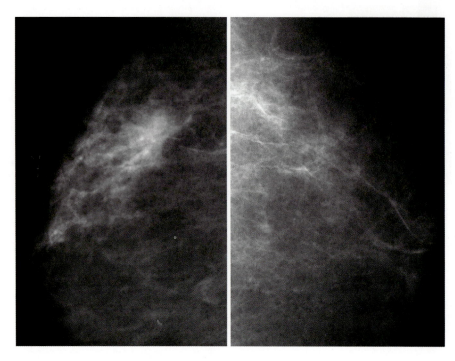

图7.13.1、7.13.2 右侧乳腺和左侧乳腺斜位图示：右侧乳腺上部存在不对称的密度增高区，无微钙化

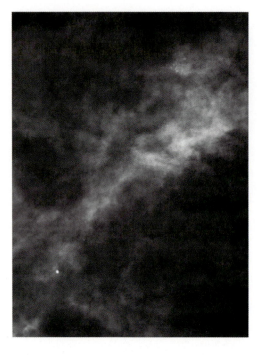

图7.13.3 右侧乳腺斜位微聚焦放大摄影图示：该不对称密度增高区存在一定程度的结构扭曲

第 7 章　多灶性与弥漫性乳腺癌影像学表现的意义　　137

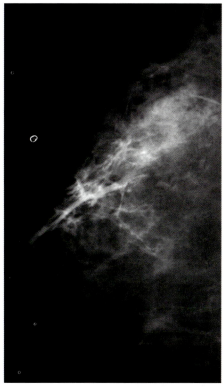

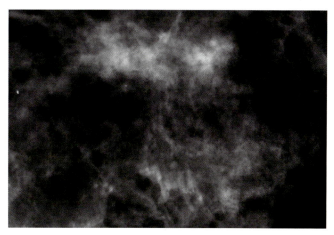

图7.13.5　标本切片X线摄影图示：扭曲扩张的导管

图7.13.4　右侧乳腺导管造影术示：主导管及其分支充满造影剂，近胸壁处较多异常的大导管分支

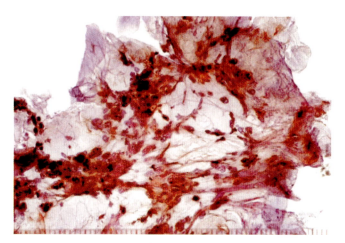

图7.13.6　3D亚肉眼组织学特点：大量异常的导管增生，密集紧实排列

图7.13.7　标本X线摄影图示增多、充满癌细胞、扩张的导管，同亚肉眼3D组织图

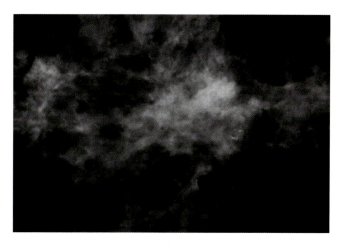

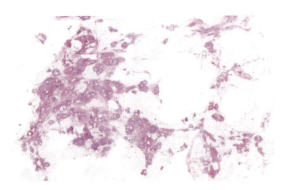

图7.13.8 低倍镜下观察薄切的大组织学切片，显示肿瘤化的新生导管密集紧实的排列

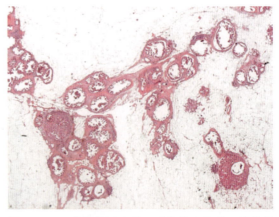

图7.13.10 高倍镜下观察：原位乳头状癌，导管壁增厚伴纤维组织增生

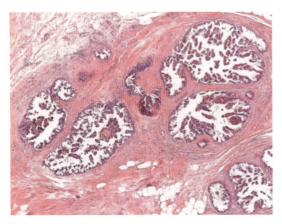

图7.13.9 中倍镜下观察导管内癌形成

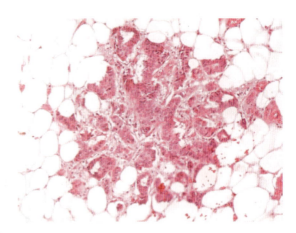

图7.13.11 广泛的微乳头状原位癌病变伴局部微小浸润

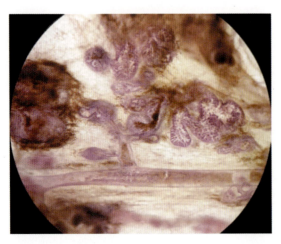

图7.13.12 3D亚肉眼组织学特征：导管内原位微乳头癌形成，伴分泌现象

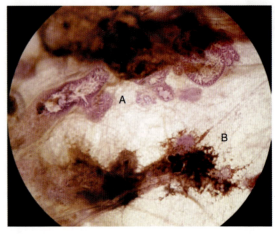

图7.13.13 原位癌灶（A）和局部小的浸润性病灶（B）

组织学：大量微浸润癌灶，最大者尺寸约5mm（中分化浸润性导管癌）。原位微乳头状癌面积较大（>70mm）。pN 0/2。

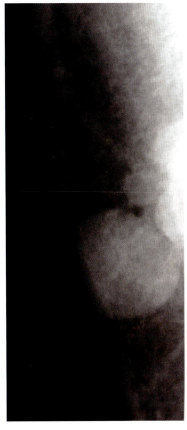

图7.13.14 乳房切除术后3年，斜位图示原术区肿瘤多处复发

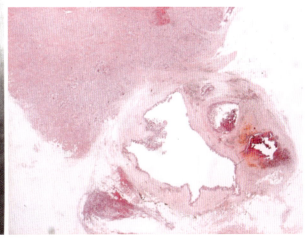

图7.13.15 组织学提示：复发病灶中浸润与原位成分并存

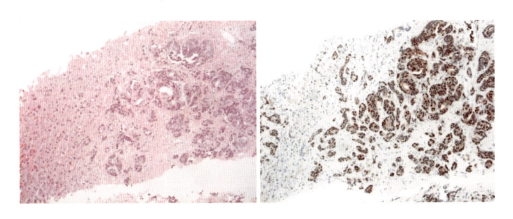

图7.13.16、7.13.17 治疗10年后，细针穿刺活检显示肝脏转移，再次治疗后1年患者死亡

评论：本例原发性肿瘤的临床分期为T1a期，但实际上肿瘤负担很广泛，几乎涉及整个腺叶。除了浸润性癌灶以外，整个腺叶内密布5mm以下的恶性微乳头病灶，伴导管新生。

例7.14 67岁女性，X线摄影筛查发现左侧乳腺外上象限不对称密度增高区，患者自觉左侧乳腺外上象限轻微皮肤回缩，被要求复诊以进一步检查评估。

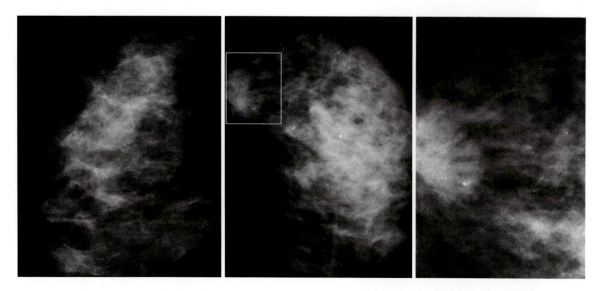

图7.14.1~7.14.3 右侧乳腺及左侧乳腺斜位图（7.14.1、7.14.2），矩形框区微聚焦放大摄影图（7.14.3），示带有毛刺的伴有恶性特征钙化的恶性病变

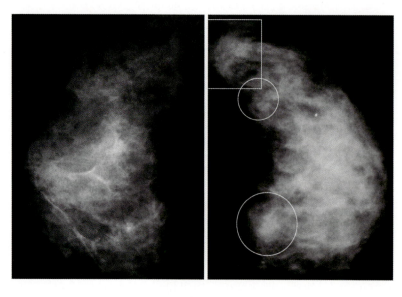

图7.14.4、7.14.5 右侧乳腺及左侧乳腺头尾位图，示带有毛刺的肿瘤位于左侧乳腺外上象限（矩形框内所示），另外见两个凸面的、边界不清、可疑恶性的病灶（圆圈内所示）

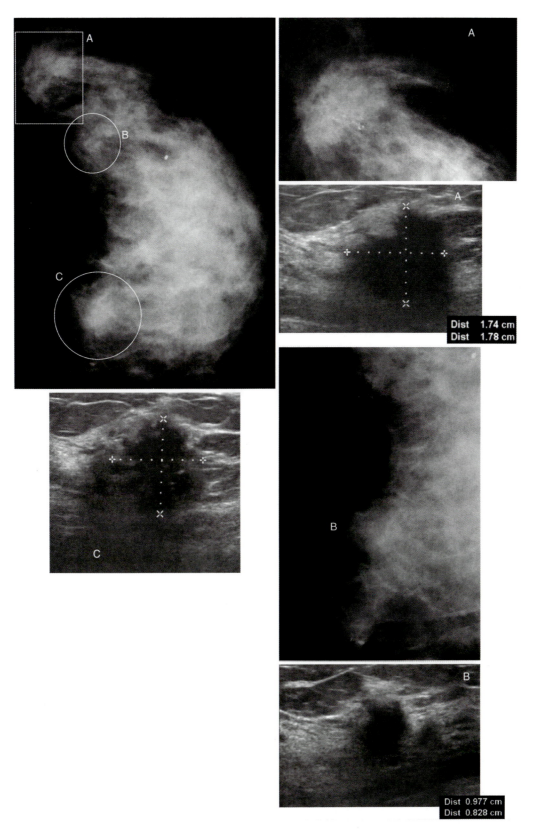

图7.14.6~7.14.13 左侧乳腺头尾位图（7.14.6），带有毛刺肿瘤（矩形框内A）的微聚焦放大摄影图（7.14.7）及超声检查图（7.14.8），包含第二个病灶（圆圈内B）的微聚焦放大摄影图（7.14.10），第二个病灶（圆圈内B）和第三个病灶（圆圈内C）的超声检查图

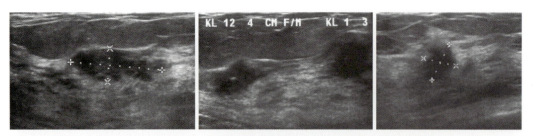

图7.14.14~7.14.16 便携式超声检查发现的左侧乳腺另一个癌灶

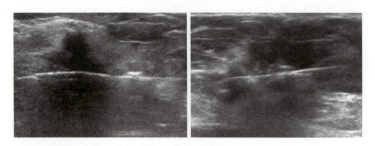

图7.14.17、7.14.18 两个单独瘤灶的14g空芯针活检

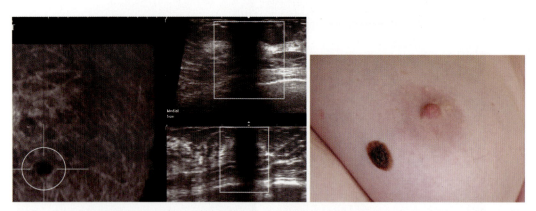

图7.14.19、7.14.20 皮肤层面的自动冠状位超声图像（7.14.19）示皮肤局部低回声改变，常规超声检查将会视其为声影（矩形框内所示），皮肤上大痣子（7.14.20）造成了这一影响

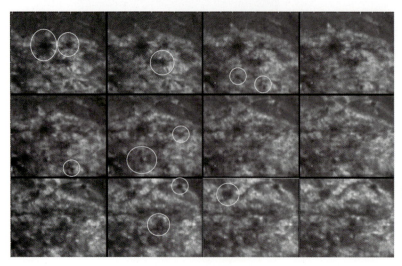

图7.14.21 一系列2mm厚的3D自动冠状位超声图可以多视角地发现许多低回声区癌灶，一些被圆圈标示出来

第 7 章　多灶性与弥漫性乳腺癌影像学表现的意义　　143

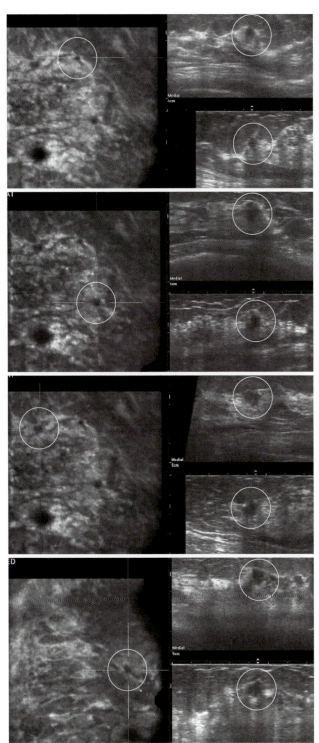

图7.14.22~7.14.25　十字准线表明3D冠状位超声图中所选的低回声区，常规正交轴位及矢状位图像与十字准线所示位置相符，可提供超声诊断

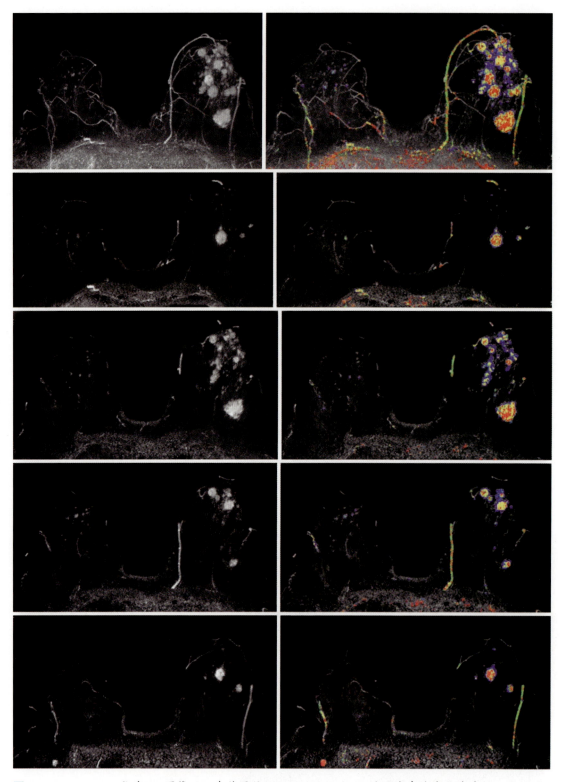

图7.14.26~7.14.35 乳腺MRI图像示：在范围约100mm×75mm×45mm的区域有许多乳腺癌灶。7.14.26、7.14.27示左图为不伴有伪彩的最大密度投影图（MIP），右图为伴伪彩的MIP图，7.14.28~7.14.35为左右侧不伴有和伴有伪彩的薄层MIP图

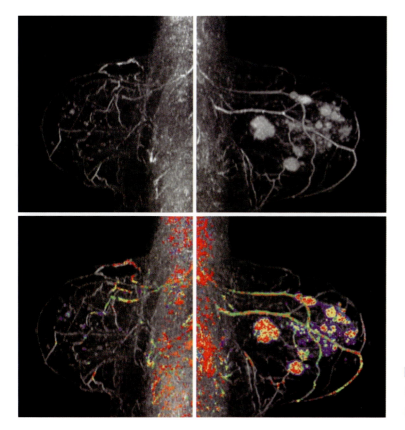

图7.14.36~7.14.39 乳腺MRI矢状位图像示：100mm×75mm×45mm的区域内多发癌灶

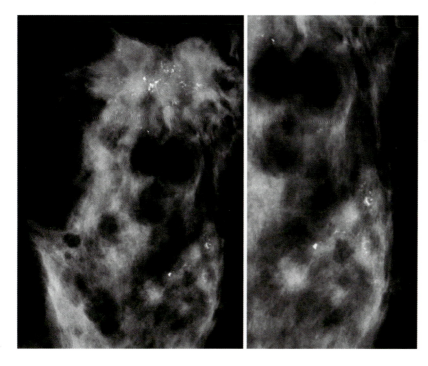

图7.14.40、7.14.41 两个乳房切除标本的X线摄影图示两个大的星芒状肿瘤中均可见铸型样钙化（7.14.40），但不伴有包块（7.14.41）

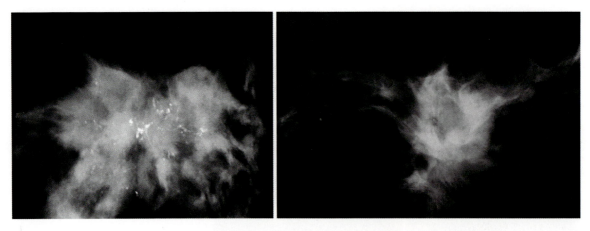

图7.14.42、7.14.43　大组织切片标本X线摄影放大图示许多癌灶中的两个最大的癌灶

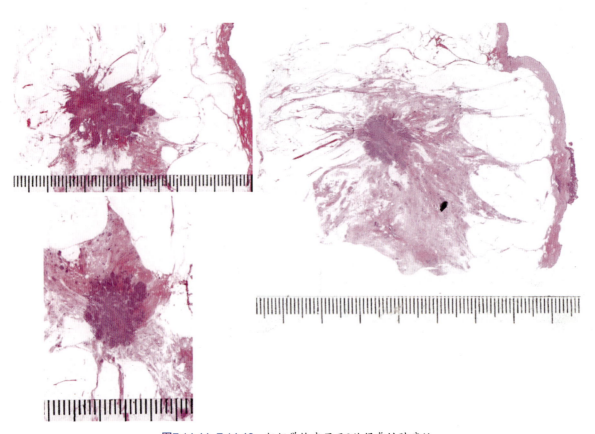

图7.14.44~7.14.46　组织学检查显示3处侵袭性肿瘤灶

组织学特征：多处低分化导管原位癌病灶，累及侵袭范围为180mm×60mm。浸润性病灶由大到小分别为：24mm×15mm，15mm×12mm，14mm×11mm。腋窝淋巴结（4/9）发现转移癌。

评论：本例是典型的多病灶、浸润性癌与原位癌并存。多种影像学与大组织切片检查证实在40mm的区域内，有大量的浸润性和原位性癌灶存在。尽管每个单独的癌灶尺寸较小，但多灶性浸润性乳腺癌的肿瘤负荷较大。

第7章 多灶性与弥漫性乳腺癌影像学表现的意义

例7.15 73岁女性，自觉左侧乳腺一质硬包块，要求行X线摄影检查。

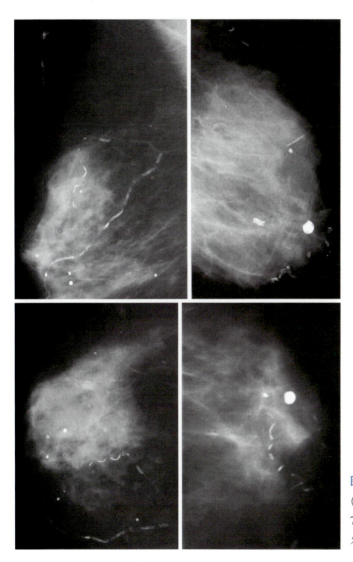

图7.15.1~7.15.4 右侧乳腺和左侧乳腺斜位（7.15.1、7.15.2）和头尾位图（7.15.3、7.15.4），由于广泛均质的纤维化不能通过触诊发现可触及的包块

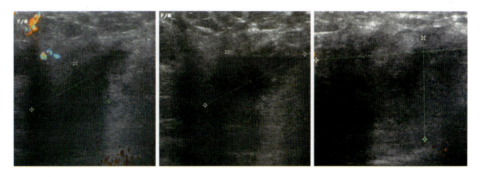

图7.15.5~7.15.7 乳腺超声检查发现一较大、不规则、低回声病灶，提示为恶性

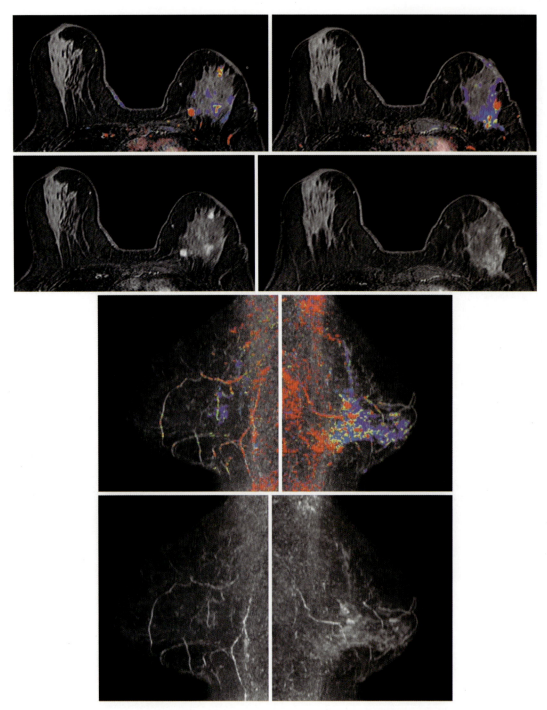

图7.15.8~7.15.15 一系列乳腺MRI轴位及矢状位图示：左侧乳腺由于广泛、弥漫性恶变致其明显变形

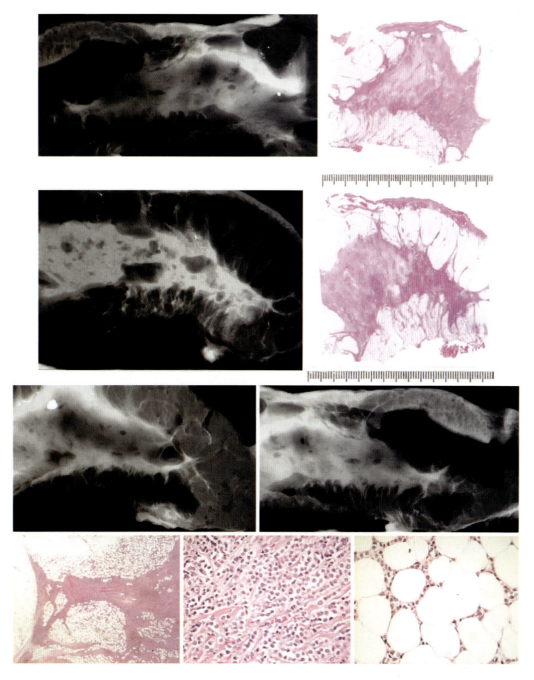

图7.15.16~7.15.24 放射学–组织学对照：标本切片X线摄影图与大切片组织图、低倍镜组织图

评论：浸润性乳腺癌是弥漫性浸润性癌的典型种类，即使能摸到包块，X线摄像技术还是会低估或遗漏病灶，然而，乳腺超声和MRI能够很好地发现这一类型的癌灶。

生存分析的研究结果显示，单灶性病变明显具有生存优势且与肿瘤的大小无关（图7.7~7.10）。以上数据量化了多灶性乳腺癌的恶性效应，且强调了检测出这一病变本质的重要性。多种术前的影像学方法包括乳房X线摄影、乳腺超声，特别是MRI对于检测乳腺癌单灶、多灶或弥漫性病变的性质和观察真正的病变范围提供了绝佳的机会。尽管多灶性病变的预后不良效果随肿瘤尺寸的增大而严重，但它仍是一个独立于尺寸的预后不良的因素。

7.4 区分乳腺癌单灶性病变与多灶性病变的现实意义

经典的TNM分期系统对于多灶性乳腺癌病例的主要依据是最大病灶的直径。据此，一个10mm×10mm大小的单一实性浸润性病灶与最大病灶直径不超过10mm的多灶性病变的分期是相同的。然而，实际上多灶性病变给机体带来的肿瘤负荷要远大于单灶性病变，因为多灶性病变的淋巴结转移率和淋巴管侵犯概率往往明显高于单一病灶（Chua, et al, 2001; Coombs, Boyages, 2005; Andea, et al, 2002; Tot, 2009）。Tot等的研究表明，无论单灶还是多灶性，乳腺癌淋巴管的侵犯（LVI）及腋窝淋巴结转移均与肿瘤的直径呈正相关，但是多灶性病变出现LVI与腋窝淋巴结转移的风险几乎是单一病变的2倍（表7.2）。

此外，单一的原位病灶的乳腺癌局部复发率仅为3%，而在多灶性或弥漫性原位病灶的复发率分别为13%和12%（有导管新生的病例复发率达17%，无导管新生者则为8%）（Tot, Tabar, 2005）。在实际临床实践中，不同肿瘤的组织学特征往往提示不同的预后及对应不同的治疗措施（Woo, et al, 2002）。事实上，高的LVI和腋窝淋巴结转移数目往往预后较差；Egan等的研究发现，多灶性病变的年死亡率约为15%，而单一病变为2.5%（Egan, 1982）。上述研究均在近期被Tot所证实，其发起了一项为期5年的随访研究计划，结果表明，单灶性原位病变，或直径<14mm的浸润性病变的年死亡率仅为1%（2/134），而多灶性病变中同等大小的病灶其年死亡率为5%（6/108）。以上数据（表7.3）均说明了利用多种影像学方法诊断多灶性病变的意义，尤其强调了乳腺MRI的作用。

对于弥漫浸润性乳腺癌病例，如巨大浸润性小叶癌相对于多灶性乳腺癌而言，其淋巴结转移率和远期预后则更糟糕。另一类在乳房X线摄影下显示铸型钙化的弥漫性浸润癌，其预后更是惊人的差。以上类型的肿瘤在TNM分期（1~9mm，10~14mm肿瘤直径）与预后方面存在诸多矛盾。而这类伴有新导管形成的浸润性癌会增加肿瘤负荷及明显的血管浸润，则可以很好地解释这些矛盾（Tabar, et al, 2007）。综上所述，尽管弥漫性乳腺癌有时在

表7.2 瑞典Falun中心医院诊断的704例乳腺癌患者淋巴管侵犯与淋巴结转移的频率

	脉管侵犯			淋巴结转移		
	单灶	多灶或弥散	总和	单灶	多灶或弥散	总和
1~9mm	13% (8/61)	17% (16/93)	16% (24/154)	3% (2/61)	14% (13/93)	10% (15/154)
10~14mm	15% (11/71)	27% (26/95)	22% (37/166)	11% (8/71)	29% (28/95)	22% (37/166)
15~198mm	33% (20/61)	43% (35/82)	38% (55/143)	26% (16/61)	37% (30/82)	32% (46/143)
20~29mm	26% (14/53)	51% (47/92)	42% (61/145)	23% (12/53)	53% (49/92)	42% (61/145)
30+mm	40% (8/20)	53% (40/76)	50% (48/96)	45% (9/20)	64% (49/76)	60% (58/96)
总计	23% (61/266)	37% (164/438)	32% (225/704)	18% (47/266)	39% (169/438)	31% (217/704)

表7.3 1996—1998年在瑞典Falun中心医院诊断的乳腺癌单灶性病变与多灶或弥漫性病变患者的死亡率比较（依据尺寸分类）

浸润癌成分 原位癌成分	单灶 单灶	单灶 非单灶	多灶浸润 任何情况	弥漫性浸润 任何情况	总和
原位	0% (0/35)	5% (2/43)	n.a.	n.a.	3% (2/78)
1~9mm	0% (0/52)	0% (0/14)	8% (1/13)	0/0	1% (1/79)
10~14mm	4% (2/47)	11% (2/19)	5% (1/19)	0/0	6% (5/85)
15~19mm	2% (1/55)	20% (2/10)	15% (4/27)	0/0	8% (7/92)
20~29mm	16% (9/57)	25% (5/20)	33% (11/33)	0/0	23% (25/110)
30+mm	24% (5/9)	20% (1/5)	25% (6/24)	26% (6/23)	25% (18/71)
未知	n.a.	n.a.	n.a.	n.a.	60% (26/43)
全部	6% (17/265)	11% (12/111)	20% (23/116)	26% (6/23)	15% (82/558)

译者说明：此表分别反应了癌灶中两种不同成分的癌组织，在不同病理类型（单灶、多灶或弥漫性）时，浸润癌还包括不同尺寸时，死亡率的不同

组织学上易与原位癌相混淆，但其侵袭的生物学特征往往类似于晚期乳腺癌，易局部复发，预后可能也会非常差。

部分患者由于未行手术切除或术前经新辅助化疗等原因，肿瘤大小无法评估。

7.5 结论：现有的TNM分期系统对于恶性肿瘤的评判存在弊端

现有的TNM分期系统仅将最大肿瘤病灶的直径作为一个独立的分期因素，而没有将多灶性病变这个因素考虑进来是存在缺陷的。事实上治疗计划的制订应该首先将肿瘤侵袭的范围作为第一要素，但是TNM并没有包含这一关键信息。多种影像学手段并用可以明确分析病灶的侵袭范围。评估肿瘤负荷的最佳方法应该就是描述所发生肿瘤的体积之和及相应的肿瘤组织所波及的范围（Andea, et al, 2004）。如果治疗之前能将上述因素都考量到位的话，则更能保证将全部肿瘤都切除干净。现有的乳腺癌手术治疗方案（肿块切除加术后放疗）有点过于教条，强调肿瘤直径往往导致了对单一病变的过度治疗和对其他多灶性病变的治疗不足。未考虑多灶性使得单灶性病变预后较好，而多灶性病变预后较差。为了能弥补这一缺陷，我们提出对肿瘤累及范围进行定量评估，采用总的肿瘤体积和肿瘤所累及的区域范围，将这一指标纳入肿瘤注册数据库，这样会为治疗措施的选择提供更为确凿的证据，为预后的推测提供更可靠的信息。

参考文献

[1] Andea AA, Wallis T, Newman LA, et al. Pathologic analysis of tumor size and lymph node status in multifocal/multicentric breast carcinoma. Cancer, 2002, 94: 1383-1390.

[2] Andea AA, Bouwman D, Wallis T, et al. Correlation of tumor volume and surface area with lymph node status in patients with multifocal/multicentric breast carcinoma. Cancer, 2004, 100: 20-27.

[3] Cady B, Chung M. Mammographic screening: no

longer controversial. Editorial. Am J Clin Oncol, 2005, 28: 1-4.

[4] Chua B, Ung O, Taylor R, et al. Frequency and predictors of axillary lymph node metastases in invasive breast cancer. ANZ J Surg, 2001, 71: 723-728.

[5] Coombs NJ, Boyages J. Multifocal and multicentric breast cancer: does each focus matter. J Clin Oncol, 2005, 23: 7497-7502.

[6] Egan RI. Multicentric breast carcinomas: clinical-radiographic-pathologic whole organ studies and 10-year survival. Cancer, 1982, 49: 1123-1130.

[7] Holland R, Veling SHJ, Mravunac M, et al. Histologic multifocality of Tis, T1-2 breast carcinomas. Implications for clinical trials of breast conserving surgery. Cancer, 1985, 56: 979-990.

[8] Tabar L, Tot T, Dean PB. Breast cancer: the art and science of early detection with mammography. New York: Thieme, 2005.

[9] Tabar L, Tot T, Dean PB. Breast cancer. Early detection with mammography. Carting type calcifcations: sign of a subtype with deceptive features. New York: Thieme, 2007.

[10] Tot T. Clinical relevance of the distribution of the lesions in 500 consecutive breast cancer cases documented in large-format histologic sections. Cancer, 2007, 110: 2551-2560.

[11] Tot T, Tabar L. Mammographic-pathologic correlation of ductal carcinoma in situ of the breast using two-and three-dimensional large histologic sections. Semin Breast Dis, 2005, 8: 144-151.

[12] Tot T. The metastatic capacity of multifocal breast carcinomas: extensive tumors versus tumors of limited extent. Hum Pathol, 2009, 40: 199-205.

[13] Woo CS, Silberman H, Nakamura SK, et al. Lymph node status combined with lymphovascular invasion creates a more powerful tool for predicting outcome in patients with invasive breast cancer. Am J Surg, 2002, 184: 337-340.

[14] Yen MF, Tabar L, Vitak B, et al. Quantifying the potential problem of overdiagnosis of ductal carcinoma in situ in breast cancer screening. Eur J Cancer, 2003, 39: 1746-1754.

乳腺腺叶超声

Dominique Amy

第 8 章

8.1 引 言

乳腺癌的影像学诊断是基于3种不同的技术：钼靶、磁共振成像（MRI）和乳腺超声检查（声像图）。钼靶的主要缺点是缺乏精确的解剖学参照。实际上，使用这种技术的放射科医生对含有纤维腺体的结缔组织和脂肪组织进行了整体分析，但乳腺腺叶不是普通钼靶的成像重点。乳腺MRI则基于依赖血管生成的对比增强成像，这样就没有将病变与腺叶解剖的关系联系起来。在放射科医生看来，传统的乳腺声像图的垂直和水平扫描只是钼靶结果的一个副本罢了。它没有提供解剖结构的观察，并且只能对乳房体积的一部分进行研究。一份声像图报告中从未出现过对腺叶、小叶、导管以及终末导管小叶单位（TDLUs）的描述。

作为这些观察的首个结果，第一个问题是乳腺是否是唯一的、影像图像上不依赖普通解剖知识来理解的人体器官；第二个问题是怎样检测以"毫米"（几毫米大小）级的病变，在不知道病变位置及发展情况的条件下如何去寻找它。为了解决这些问题，我们致力于引入乳腺模型的大型组织切片这个新概念（图8.1）。这个概念被称为乳腺导管超声成像，使用这种方法得到的准确和可重复性的结果给我们提供

D. Amy
Centre de Radiologie,
Aix-En-Provence, France
e-mail: domamy@wanadoo.fr

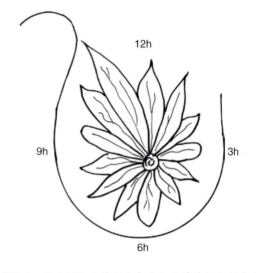

图8.1 乳头周围的腺体分布犹如雏菊花瓣遍布在每小时（顺时针）的位置

了一种乳腺成像的新方案，帮助我们提高了诊断的准确率，并且使我们对乳腺腺叶的形态和生理性变化有了更好的了解。

首先，考虑到腺叶的起源、大小以及形态，和本书之前讨论的内容，我们将强调其复杂性和多变性。随着我们对腺叶在乳腺癌自然发展早期阶段的形态学改变的了解增多，检测出"毫米"级病变的概率相应升高。癌症可能出现在哪里、它会如何演变以及用哪种方法检测，当我们了解了这些，一切都将变得简单明了。

经过多年使用乳腺导管超声成像进行常规诊断以及对上千例病例的分析，我们认为目前的诊断准确性已经得到了提高，尤其在检测多发性、多中心和弥漫性生长的肿瘤时。

对这些肿瘤的检出率明显优于钼靶检查或结合常规超声的钼靶检查，使用该方法，可以在早期间质反应缺乏时提早检测出肿瘤，这种间质反应是钼靶检测的重要指标。同时，应该认识到乳腺导管超声成像并不是一种解剖病理学技术，它并不能检测出所有的"毫米"级病变，少数病变依旧会被遗漏。

综合的影像学方法，结合钼靶与乳腺导管超声成像（以及多普勒超声、弹性成像、三维超声图像）才是如今最好的诊断早期乳腺癌的方法。乳腺MRI在一些明确的适应证上也是很有意义的补充。

8.2 解剖背景

图8.2A~C大型组织学图像的详细分析为我们提供了解剖结构与乳腺导管超声成像结果的基本比较。从表皮到胸壁，我们会发现乳头、乳晕和薄薄一层皮下脂肪组织下的其他皮肤结构（图像从左至右），接下来，我们可以看到浅筋膜浅层的线形连接结构（浅筋膜）。典型的脂肪瓣被Cooper韧带分隔，韧带连接于筋膜和乳腺腺叶的上表面。腺叶是一个非常明确的结构，在解剖面的左上方与乳头相连，于图像的右侧边缘结束（部分出现在图像中）。腺叶中也可看到导管轴和小叶团。Cooper韧带竖直穿过腺叶的下表面（以腺叶前表面的镜面模式），经脂肪组织到达筋膜深层（筋膜下）。

我们致力于将乳房解剖细节成像与优秀组织学切片呈现出的一样完美。我们询问过是否可以通过超声学技术全部或者至少一部分重构这个模型。乳房是一个特别适于使用超声检查的外部器官。然而，超声探查手法的选择是至关重要的。目前的问题是，我们应该从上到下、从内到外横纵向探查所有的乳房象限，还是在乳晕周围以径向重新探查腺叶和导管结构？哪一个超声探头是最适于分析不同腺叶并且最适于探查腋窝组织的？

8.3 乳腺导管超声成像

像很早之前描述的一样，乳房含有15~20个腺叶，如雏菊花瓣一样遍布在乳头的周围。由于没有任何一种成像技术可以展示这样的分布，在很长一段时间里这个描述只是纯理论性的。一些腺叶可解剖变异至14~16cm长，这说明只有使用尽可能长的超声探头才能显像所有的腺叶。由于已设计出9.5cm的专用探头，使用10MHz频率加上一个合适的水囊，使所有腺叶的成像都变成了现实。为了显像最大的腺叶，需要沿着导管轴和腋窝区域进行同心扫描和（或）变换探头运动。

使用这种方法，我们可以在一台超声仪器上同时成像所有的腺叶，无论其大小、形态以及在乳腺的位置。顺时针标记它们的位置使定位变得精确（如R.10表示右侧乳房10点钟方向，L.6对应腺叶在左侧乳房6点钟位置）。

这种超声表现提供了和大型组织学切片相同的分析乳腺组织的机会（图8.2）。从左向右由皮肤看到胸壁，乳头（内含一些乳腺管）出现在图8.2B~C的左上方，乳晕和乳房皮肤则在它的右侧。位于乳房悬韧带上的高回声纤维组织将浅筋膜和腺叶前表面相连接，形成了高回声的小圆锥。同样，Cooper韧带的深部穿过脂肪层将腺叶背面与胸大肌表面平行的深筋膜连接在一起。腺叶对应的是一块高回声区，在其内可见不同的导管轴，最大的在腺叶顶，最小都在腺叶底。腺小叶对应的小块低回声区主要位于导管前端。

组织学图像和超声图像的完美匹配说明乳腺导管超声成像是研究乳腺解剖的非侵入性方法之一。没有其他成像方式可以呈现出与之相媲美的信息。获得更多的经验、探索使用恰当设备的优势以及跟随Teboul医生的教学（Teboul, 2004; Teboul, Halliwell, 1995），使我们能够更好地理解乳腺腺叶形态学对于腺叶位置、年龄相关的生理学改变以及对因治疗、激素影响和病理条件下产生的变化。

第 8 章 乳腺腺叶超声

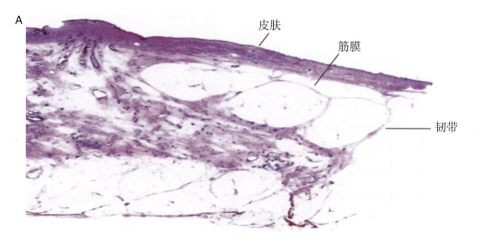

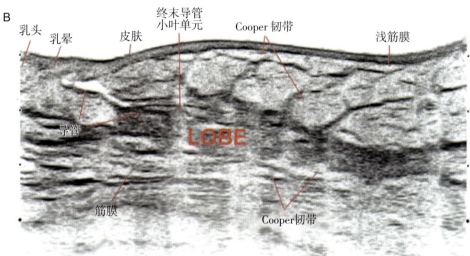

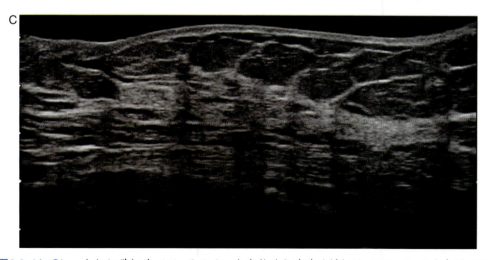

图8.2（A~C） 大组织学切片（A）显示了一个完整的乳腺腺叶横切面（Tibor Tot医生惠赠，Falun Sweden）。翻转（B）和原型（C）径向腺叶扫描的乳腺导管超声成像图像；注意超声图像和组织学图像（图8.2A）的完美相关性

我们同时也认识到，我们观察的结果与Tot医生（2007b）提出的乳腺癌的腺叶特点这一概念是一致的。

8.4 腺叶的形态学改变

乳腺腺叶解剖的声像图变化有很多，有些可能难以分析。严格和可重复方案的使用允许我们稳定地观察所有的腺叶，忽略它们的尺寸和位置，最大限度地降低技术上的困难，同时略微缩短检查时间。这种方案使得该方法不依赖于检查者的技巧；而且可以检查更大量的病例，但结果分析依赖于医生对解剖变异的透彻理解。

3个主要的腺叶回声类型：

- 大部分高回声纤维性腺叶，只包含很少可检测的上皮结构。
- 大部分低回声上皮性腺叶，包含非常少的结缔组织。
- 等回声腺叶，包含了同等量的上皮细胞和纤维组织。

年龄相关的腺叶形态变化也是多种多样的，其中有两个极端模式：

- 年轻女性的乳房腺叶含有丰富的腺体，以及极少量的脂肪组织（图8.3）
- 成年女性的乳房腺叶含有的实质组织和脂肪量则保持平衡（图8.4）

部分绝经前女性（图8.5）和大部分绝经后女性的腺叶会发生退化。随着退化的进行，腺叶结构可能会消失，只留下薄弱的结缔组织和腺叶的"骨架"（图8.6），或者二者可能会全部消失。了解以上内容后，就知道腺叶也具有各不相同的大小和位置。乳房内侧和下侧象限处的腺叶较小，较大的腺叶则位于外上象限，其中一部分甚至会到达腋下。

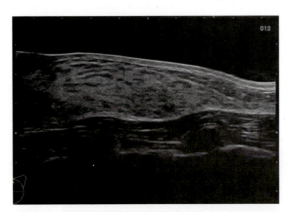

图8.3 一位年轻女性的乳腺大腺叶导管超声成像图显示了小叶和导管轴的生理性上皮增生的标志

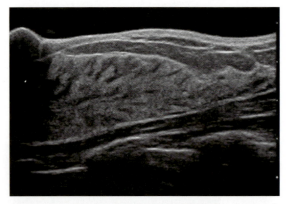

图8.4 一位成年女性的腺叶超声成像图，在高回声的腺叶背景下的低回声小叶和导管

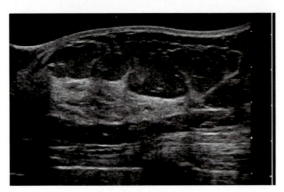

图8.5 图示一例绝经前女性的乳腺超声成像图，体积减小的小叶和增多的脂肪组织

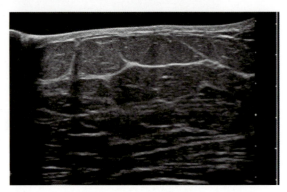

图8.6 超声图像显示整体的腺叶退化，可见在残余的高回声腺叶和一些Cooper韧带中的小导管轴

腺叶的起源也同样存在着变异。最大的腺叶位于外上象限，为青春期第一个发育的腺叶，而较小的腺叶则位于内侧象限，在年轻女性生命周期的晚期出现。相反，较小的腺叶在绝经期和绝经后最早消失，而位于外上象限、较早发育的腺叶则可存活更长时间。

就乳晕周围腺体的朝向和分布而言，也可以观察到腺叶另外的变异。其中大多数腺叶的分布以辐射状朝向乳头，但也有一部分是迂曲蜿蜒遍布乳头的，甚至可能会相互重叠。这些重叠的腺叶会造成叶间连接的假象，会导致高估或低估实际腺叶的尺寸。由于腺叶和乳头间的连接很短，在乳晕后区很难区分清楚不同的腺叶。然而，通过研究青春期乳腺和部分复杂绝经后女性的腺叶、以及男性乳腺发育，表明腺叶是完全独立并彼此分开的，每一个腺叶都是一个独立的个体。

乳腺导管超声成像是可视化腺叶解剖的一种理想的工具。然而，通常的导管和小叶因为尺寸小而常常不显影。导管和小叶内的上皮细胞的增殖导致结构局限性或弥漫性扩张，伴随着结构的畸变和声阻抗的改变，之后它们变成"可声波探测"：低回声对应的小叶和导管腔内容；这些结构的组织壁依旧不可见。病理反应会导致回声发生变化，这种变化将会取代上皮增生的声像图表现。

8.5 乳腺病理学中腺叶的影响

导管径向超声探查的主要目的是改良导管和小叶结构以及腺叶周围的结缔组织的普通超声模式。Nakama（1991）描述了Cooper韧带和浅筋膜内，恶性细胞与淋巴细胞、组织细胞和成纤维细胞一起向皮肤的迁移。这些结缔组织参与了早期癌症的发展（图8.7展示了这个概念）证实了Gallager医生在1969年12月所发表文章的结论，特别是他的第二条结论"乳房的结缔组织也受到致癌因素的影响"（Gallager, Martin, 1969）。Teboul（2004），

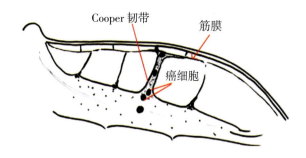

图8.7　本图说明癌细胞从TDLUs迁移到Cooper韧带、浅筋膜和皮肤

Teboul 和 Halliwell（1995），以及 Stavros（2006）同样描述了结缔组织和韧带参与了早期癌症的发展。他们还强调了乳腺癌在某些情况下的多灶性。多亏了Teboul（2004）精确的超声解剖学背景，他确定了导管-小叶终末单元的特性、位置以及它们在病理改变初期阶段的参与。他强调，如果我们需要研究上皮结构和结缔组织的早期病理改变，那么导管轴横截面和韧带轴的交叉区域则是我们应该关注的关键区域，导管-小叶终末单元就位于此。

这些观察方向是乳腺超声检查发展史上的重要标志：超声径向截面，小叶分析，导管轴的寻找，识别韧带的走向，以及分析筋膜和皮肤的变化。了解病变的起源与发展对分析结果至关重要。乳腺导管超声成像的概念从根本上改变了乳腺的检查方法。在乳房不同象限上使用正交回波投影系统时，检查医生不应该把重点放在寻找病变本身，而应该放在腺叶分析上（根据上文提出的既定方案）。病变通常都会在预期的结构和范围内被发现，病变发展也通常会遵循预期模式。

异常腺叶的研究应在与正常腺叶解剖结构对比下进行。所有的上皮病变（包括无回声的、液体和低回声的、实性）都与导管或小叶有关联，例如导管扩张、膨胀和乳头状瘤，以及小叶上改变。分辨导管和小叶的微小囊肿将成为可能。小叶间纤维腺瘤的定位也会变得显而易见。小叶内互相重叠生长了一些小纤维腺瘤，这解释了为什么大纤维腺瘤有分叶状轮廓。同样，由于上皮增生导致

的导管扩张的检查将成为惯例,以及在特定的TDLUs周围查找出多灶性病变也将成为常规。必须强调间接的韧带变化常与癌症有关,并且往往都是恶性的。这个微妙的早期超声迹象比与实质反应有关的放射学迹象出现早,同样也早于临床症状出现之前。

图8.8A~D展示了一位典型的病例。乳腺癌的初步诊断是由钼靶发现可触及结节开始。乳腺超声和MRI检查发现其他5个浸润性乳腺癌病灶。Di Marino教授(解剖实验室,Marseille医科大学)分析指出,多灶和多中心性肿瘤是乳房切除术的指征。同一所大学病理系的Rojat-Habib医生也用大型组织学切片记录过这种病例样本。他的病理组织学切片与一个10cm长的径向超声截面相对应。组织学切片和超声截面的对比揭示了这两种技术的完美呼应。对不同的导管轴的分析表明有导管扩张的迹象。在腺叶末端发现两个位于Cooper韧带连接中的癌灶(分别是"厘米"级和"毫米"级)。某些韧带很薄,因此难以进行组织学研究。在其他切面中,更多的肿瘤病灶被检测出来,在图8.8中未显示。像钼靶检查一样,乳腺导管超声成像对多灶性和多中心性病变提供了一个快速、准确、费用低廉的分析方法,此方法使得早期乳腺癌的诊断有了真正的进步。

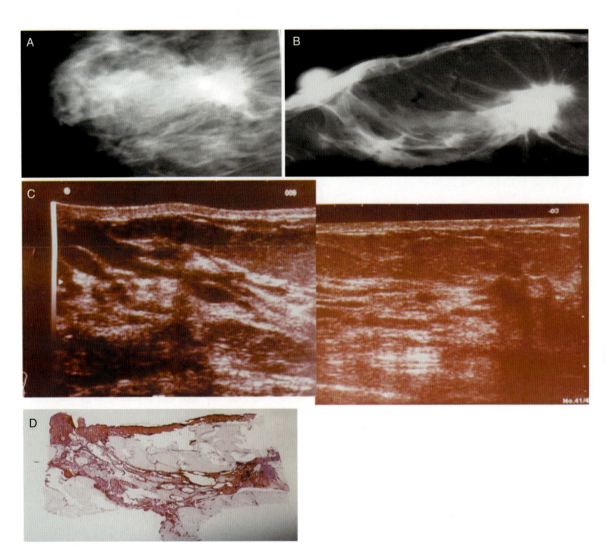

图8.8 X线钼靶(A、B)和超声(C)多灶性乳腺癌的图像。注意与大组织切片(D)的完美吻合(由Di Marino教授和Rojat Habib教授惠赠,Marseille France)

8.6 多灶性、多中心性和弥漫性病变

放射科对乳腺癌的成像已经进行了几十年，单发病灶最常见，有时可见多发病灶。区分多灶性和多中心性病变的要点在于两个病灶间的距离（4cm）。随着乳腺导管超声成像的普及，出现了一种对多发病灶的新定义。多灶性癌应该被定义为同一个腺叶内、沿着导管轴生长的癌变，而多中心性癌是在不同腺叶发生发展的（它们可以是单病灶也可以是多病灶）。这种定义是与组织学研究相一致的。

图8.9A~B展示了一个单灶性乳腺癌。多灶性癌对应的是低回声病灶，它沿着特定的TDLUs的导管轴发展（形似一串珍珠；图8.10和8.11）。它们的大小取决于生长时间，并且或多或少与间接地与解剖特点（韧带）或超声信号（后吸收阴影）有关。虽然乳腺导管超声成像识别了很多病灶，但由于新出现的极其微小的病灶几乎难以发现，所以，导管超声成像可能还是低估了病灶的真实数量。随着技术的进步和使用专用探头的数字化仪器的使用，随着检查方式的提高和相关知识的进步，多发性癌灶的检出已经可以实现。

多灶性和多中心性乳腺癌的检出率已从非常低的概率达到几年前的10%~20%，如今已惊人地升至45%（Tot，2007a）。这一数据令人惊讶，因为它与我们的传统观念不符。然而，这项数值已经被乳腺导管超声成像专家，特别是乳腺病理学家证实了真实性。似乎对我们而言，"病态腺叶理论"（Tot，2007b）反映了每天我们在"体内"所观察到的现实。

弥漫性癌灶代表单独并且特殊的一组病变（Tot，2003）。这些疾病本身就很难诊断，而且，如果超声下不能将它与上皮增生类病变相区分，那诊断就变得更为困难。这种特点往往反映了超声这种方法的局限性，结果通常导致诊断失败（图8.12）。

8.7 外科观点

乳腺超声检查报告应提供最大的信息量，包括病变存在与否、病变的性质、病变的数量和位置。对病变位置的精确描述（用精准

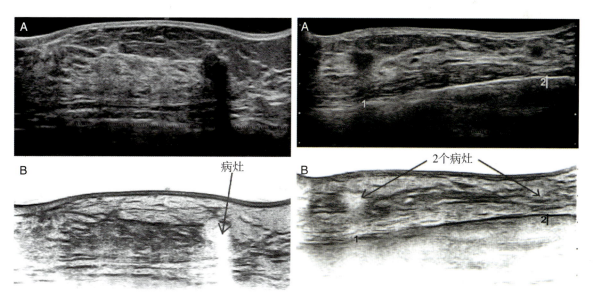

图8.9A、B 超声图像（A）和翻转超声图像（B）的几毫米大的单灶癌，位于Cooper韧带和其他腺叶的接触面

图8.10A、B 超声图像（A）和翻转超声图像（B）是一个近端和远端距离5cm的彼此位于同一腺叶的双癌灶

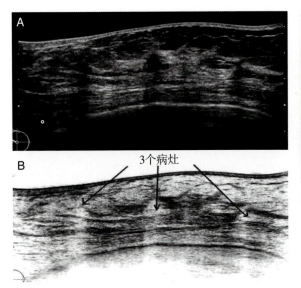

图8.11A、B 超声图像（A）和翻转超声图像（B）是一个病灶位于不同TDLUs的沿导管轴分布的多灶癌（形似一串珍珠）

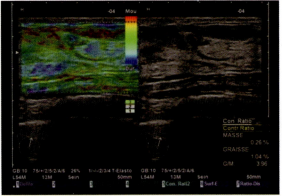

图8.12 弥漫浸润性小叶癌，在Cooper韧带中难以察觉，其相应的弹性评分为2分

的时钟定位法）有助于医生选择最好的治疗方法。值得注意的是，如果术前诊断信息不完善，那么术后可能出现的复发就不是外科医生的责任。因此，诊断医生的角色十分重要，他（她）给出的诊断信息可能会导致严重的结果。多亏了径向超声技术的发展（在术前、术后以及需要时在围术期进行检查），Dolfin教授（Dolfin，et al，2008）以及Durante教授（2006）等外科医生才能够设计出特定的腺叶切除手术方案。这绝对是乳腺外科的一项创新。放射科医生、外科医生、肿瘤学专家、治疗师和乳腺团队其他医生的紧密协作，一定会使乳腺癌的治疗效果达到最好。

8.8 总　结

我们认为乳腺导管超声成像是乳腺癌诊断的一项不可替代的创新与进步。这个技术理念是基于对腺叶解剖的分析，充分了解腺叶形态学和生理学变化以及乳腺内良性和恶性病变的表现而出现的。超声学和组织学的完美融合是乳腺导管超声成像诸多优点的最好证明。突出显示每个腺叶，可以进行单独恰当的分析（与传统超声是在一个象限内找寻一个单独的病灶形成对比）。以我们的经验来看，大多数乳腺含有的腺叶数为12~15个（少于Going和Mohun 2006最初描述的15~20个）。TDLUs和它们所在的区域需要特别留意，这是检查中一个重要的环节。结缔组织（如Cooper韧带、筋膜和皮下附件）的细微变化有助于发现早期乳腺癌，而传统的检查方法很难觉察（Amy，2005；Amoros，et al，2009）。

因为探头分辨率有限，以及特别设计的超声仪数量有限，现代超声学检查方法存在一定的局限性。因此，仍然有成千上万的乳腺小叶不能得到充分的检查。但事实上，能检测到它们表现出上皮增生或病理改变的迹象，我们还是满意的。我们检查过的接近一半的病例，无证是多灶性还是单灶性病变，都得到了组织学验证，这一点非常关键。未来的发展应着眼于乳腺癌亚型的准确分型，如导管、小叶和导管小叶混合等。

超声是否能检测到最早期的乳腺病变仍需商榷，但是，我们已经能够观察到病变过程中正常乳腺组分的形态改变。多灶性或多中心性病灶多认为是恶性细胞转移导致，这一现象的过程不能被超声图像所追踪记录。然而，所观察到的同一腺叶内不同大小和时间节点的病变也许是局部细胞转移导致（图8.13）。同一腺叶内相隔数厘米的早期双灶或多发癌灶（图8.10、图8.11），同样大小的病

第8章 乳腺腺叶超声

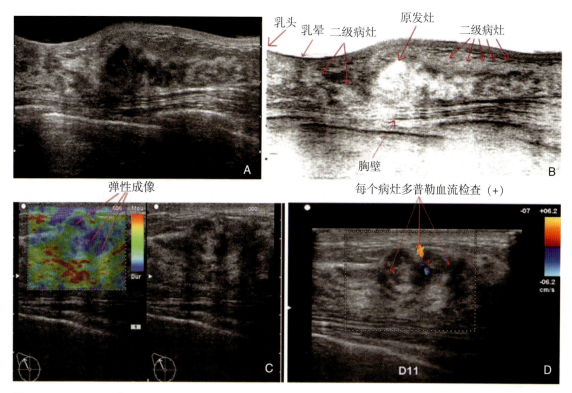

图8.13 （A~D）超声图像（A）和翻转超声图像（B）示一个病变乳腺腺叶有一个大的原发癌灶和分布于导管轴两侧的一些新病灶。C. 位于同一腺叶远端的每一个新的毫米级别的病灶，超声弹性成像评分4分。D. 多普勒血流检查（+）。

灶是否存在于同一个和（或）不同的腺叶内，这些发现使我们得出了一个结论，那就是恶性多灶性癌可能是独立起源的，这是它们同步或不同步恶性转化的结果。

本章及本书所提出的所有新概念为外科和医疗人员展示了全新、有趣的观点。多灶性、进行性和广泛性腺叶受累不应该采用与单发灶相同的方式来处理。对于早期和晚期乳腺癌应采取不同的治疗方法。

乳腺导管超声成像的的使用，加上大组织学切片、改良腺叶切除术、新的肿瘤学分子靶标或围术期放疗或冷冻治疗的使用，提高了乳腺癌的诊断水平。并且，只有这些手段之间的协同作用持续存在，未来的诊断才可能一帆风顺。现在，多学科的交叉比以往任何时候都重要。每一个学科的进步都依赖其他学科的发展。

以超声学为例，新的仪器（数字化仪器、专用探头的多普勒超声、弹性成像、新一代三维重建）也提供了最好的诊断数据。但是，有奉献精神和有能力的人才源源不断的参与也是至关重要的。乳腺导管超声成像已称为乳腺专科治疗中心必不可少的部分。有了上述这些方法，我们就能为患者提供最有价值的治疗措施，使其达到最佳康复。

参考文献

[1] Amoros J, Dolfn G, Teboul M .Atlas de Ecografa de la Mama. Ananke, TorinoAmy D（2005）Millimetric breast carcinoma ultrasonic detection// Leading Edge conference Pr. Goldberg B. USA, 2009.

[2] Dolfn G, Chebib A, Amy D, et al. Carcinome mammaire et chirurgie conservatrice. 30eSeminaire Franco-Syrien d'Imagerie Médicale. Tartous, Syrie, 2008.

[3] Durante E. Multimodality imaging and interventional techniques. IBUS Course Abstracts. Italy: Ferrara, 2006.

[4] Gallager HS, Martin JE. Early phases in the development of breast cancer. Cancer, 1969, 24: 1170-1178.

[5] Going JJ, Mohun TJ. Human breast duct anatomy, the 'sick lobe' hypothesis and intraductal approaches to breast cancer. Breast Cancer Res Treat, 2006, 97: 285-291.

[6] Nakama S. Comparative studies on ultrasonogram with histological structure of breast cancer: an examination in the invasive process of breast cancer and the fxation to the skin//Kasumi F, Ueno E (eds) Topic in breast ultrasound. Shinohara, TokyoStavros T (2006) Breast ultrasound. Philadelphia: Lippincott: 1991.

[7] Teboul M, Halliwell M. Atlas of ultrasound and ductal echography of the breast. Blackwell Science, Oxford, 1995.

[8] Teboul M. Practical ductal echography. Medgen. Spain: S. A. Madrid, .2004.

[9] Tot T. The diffuse type of invasive lobular carcinoma of the breast: morphology and prognosis. Virchows Arch, 2003, 443: 718-724.

[10] Tot T. Clinical relevance of the distribution of the lesions in 500 consecutive breast cancer cases documented in large-format histologic sections. Cancer, 2007a, 110: 2551-2560.

[11] Tot T. The theory of the sick breast lobe and the possible consequences. Int J Surg Pathol, 2007b, 1: 68-71.

乳腺癌病灶在腺叶中的分布：乳管内镜检查及手术

第9章

Willima C. Dooley

9.1 引言

乳管内镜是一项不断发展的外科技术，它是一种能最早获得乳腺癌癌前病变和恶性病变的新方法。在过去的40年中，临床内镜技术得到了迅速发展，使研究人员和临床医生能够接触到许多有恶变风险的上皮组织。在1990年代，随着亚毫米级内镜的出现，这项技术终于可以用来检查乳腺导管上皮细胞了。经过不到20年的临床应用，我们就已经能直接观察解剖结构以及解剖结构与乳腺癌发生的关系。无论是单灶性还是多灶性，乳腺癌似乎只在单一的导管树中出现。新生血管存在与否及程度高低似乎与病变出现在导管-小叶树不同的区域有关。目前我们的活组织切片技术还十分落后，但随着技术的进步，能够从基因上记录从癌变起源到导管树内浸润的整个过程的能力会越来越强，它也许会成为许多能进一步了解乳腺癌发生原因的光明大道中的一条。

9.2 乳管内镜的早期历史

早在1990年代，冈崎及他的同事开始尝试使用第一台直径<2mm的内镜，并将它应用于病理性乳头溢液的诊断与治疗中（Okazaki, et al, 1991; Okazaki, et al, 2007）。随着直径1mm内镜的出现和技术的提高，开通乳头乳管入路并且找到病变位置，如乳腺导管腔内息肉或其他病变的成功率不断提高（Shen, et al, 2000; Shao, Nguyen, 2001; Matsunaga, et al, 2001; Yamamoto, et al, 2001a; Yamamoto, et al, 2001b）。东方女性的异常乳头溢液是乳腺癌比较常见的一种症状，这种新技术提供了一种表面定位活检的方式，但空气进入导管导致图像质量差以及强光折射等限制了这一新技术的使用。此外，由于大多数病灶在当时只能通过开放手术活检取材，所以乳管内镜只被看作乳腺影像异常时的钢丝定位类技术。

然而，学术界终于认识到导管对于癌症和观察癌症时解剖学改变的重要性。Love医生和她的同事使用日本内镜技术，开始在美国尝试进行第一例试验（Loveand Barsky, 1996; Love, Barsky, 2004）。这直接导致了对内镜冲洗乳腺导管内增生性病变细胞能力的认可，也是现代乳腺导管灌洗术的起源。我当时参与了一个未经评估的导管灌洗试验。我所在的机构在进行乳腺导管灌洗实验时，很快发现可以从一个固定的导管孔内灌洗出明显恶性或者说可疑恶性的细胞。尽管当时我们使用了最好的成像设备，但是，依旧无法更准确地识别细胞的来源。我在当时现有的亚毫米镜范围内搜寻，发现了一家美国制

W. C. Dooley
Division of Surgical Oncology, Department of Surgery,
The University of Oklahoma Health Sciences Center,
Oklahoma City, OK, USA
e-mail: william-dooley@ouhsc.edu

造商。通过使用亚毫米镜和在灌洗试验中开发出的盐水扩张导管的方法，能够确定每一个病例中我感兴趣的病变位置（Dooley, 2000）。那些病理性乳头溢液的患者接受了导管镜观察，并进行了手术，这立刻向乳腺专业的外科医生展示了导管镜在诊断和治疗方面的潜在价值（Yamamoto, et al, 2001a）。

9.3 乳管内镜在乳腺癌应用中的经验教训

当刚开始在那些溢液导管明确的早期乳腺癌中常规使用乳管内镜时，我很快学会识别一些重要的乳腺解剖结构，及确定导管树中癌细胞浸润的导管位置（Dooley, 2002; Dooley, 2003）。首先是导管的解剖和管道分布，如同Love医生在她的著作里描述的一样，大多数外上象限的病变都会与一个大的导管小叶复合体有关，这个复合体在乳头乳晕处有一个开孔，一般位于8点到2点钟间。临床或影像学确诊的>2cm的病灶几乎不含溢液导管在内，很难在乳房按摩或压迫时被发现，除非导管内广泛增生。一般来说，那些周围明显存在增生性声晕改变的病灶，最容易确认溢液的导管。空芯针穿刺活检或切开活检难以在乳头表面准确辨识产生液体的小叶导管单位开孔。

一旦目标导管被选中进行内镜检查，我都会选用局部麻醉药物进行导管扩张。在局部麻醉的作用下扩张最大的小叶单位的导管分支，通常都是乳腺增生最厉害的导管。镜检最大的分支将会以最快的方式发现癌灶或者癌前病变。小分支则很少被发现有显著的增生变化。通常浸润性癌会导致导管皱缩关闭，镜检解除液体梗阻后，查体可及的或超声可见的肿瘤就会发生移动。一些浸润性肿瘤可出现严重的溃疡性病变，但这是比较罕见的。有40%的早期乳腺癌从原发灶区域向管腔内生长，并明显超出影像学或临床上确诊的癌灶边界为1cm以上的范围（Dooley 2002）。大多数病例含有明显、广泛的导管内成分（EIC），但有些只有多灶性不典型导管增生（ADH）或普通导管增生。不幸的是，如果完整切除相关区域，内镜下导管内增生的视觉表现与最终病理结果并不完全相符。

一般情况下，导管内增生分为以下几类，大型海绵状病变伴有明显的茎通常是孤立的乳头状瘤（Shen, et al, 2000; Khan, et al, 2002; Dooley, 2005; Moncrief, et al, 2005; Sauter, 2005; Sauter, et al, 2005; Valdes, et al, 2005），导管壁出现断裂或皱褶的导管只发生在更大或更中央的导管，这些异常改变通常是低级别的导管原位癌（DCIS），或者柱状或复杂性导管增生。乳腺外周的导管内增生，且局部充血证实有血管生成，这种病变很可能是ADH或DCIS（伴固体或粉刺样坏死）。这些类别的病变，只有在离导管树非常远的位置才会出现外生性生长。偶尔，在大的导管内可见固定的充血斑，数量极少且非常分散，与ADH并存。通常情况下，如果在一片区域内病灶数量众多，则当整块区域被切除后，会有很大概率被诊断为DCIS。有些患者伴有白色的形似海葵的小叶状生长物，极为罕见。这些可能是微乳头状瘤、微乳头状增生或者微乳头状DCIS。如果再次复发，病变的多样性会大大提高DCIS的诊断概率。组织学分级为3级的浸润性导管癌似乎总是位于某个独立的远端小分支。相比之下，组织学1级的导管、小管和胶质类病变似乎更多的位于大的中央导管主干处。

为了进行保乳手术，在乳管内镜的引导下，我对增殖活跃的位置进行了标记，切除了已知的癌灶和所有与之有关的腔内生长的组织（Dooley, et al, 2004）。大多数乳腺癌为外周性的，所有可见的增殖活跃的组织都局限在某一个导管分支内，沿着这个分支可以轻松的切除至乳腺的边缘。一些乳腺癌伴随的增生性改变位于同一个腺叶的不同导管分支内。通常情况下，不同导管分支内的增生程度和类型都有明显的不同。因此，我认为，干细胞分散遍布在整个小叶单位中，病变的始动事件是一致的，但是不同部位后续的驱动事件可能不同。我见过许多患者在乳腺X线成像和MRI成像上为多病灶或多中心性。我观察过1 500例以上的早期乳腺癌病例，通过乳管内镜，我可以发现位于同一腺叶-导管树内的彼此互不连接的病灶，盖莫例外。这可能是支持另一种乳腺癌模型的重要证据（Okazaki, et al, 1991; Dooley, 2002; Kapenhas-Valdes, et al, 2008），比如腺叶理论。

我在内镜引导下完成的部分乳腺切除术，切除了包含原发灶在内的同一腺叶-导管树的所有病变分支。通过对这些患者的随访，我发现在没有淋巴-血管侵犯（LVI）的患者中，这种手术已经能够将局部复发率降低到传统保乳患者的1/10。现在，经我治疗的这一亚类保乳术的患者的局部失败率，实际上类似那些无LVI的接受乳腺癌改良根治术的患者。

德国乳管内镜专家已经能够重现类似于我在乳腺癌保乳切除术中得到的结果（Hünerbein, et al, 2006a; Hünerbein, et al, 2006b; Hünerbein, et al, 2007; Grunwald, et al, 2007; Jacobs, et al, 2007a; Jacobs, et al, 2007b）。美国的团队还不能重现我的结果，并且我相信他们都犯了经典的假设错误（Louie, et al, 2006; Kim, et al, 2004）。这些团队认为，如果常规病理检查没有发现导管原位癌或浸润性癌，那么乳腺中其他增殖活跃的组织是不重要的。过去的病理研究表明，术后切缘阳性，如ADH或普通导管增生对于局部复发并无影响，这个理论基础似乎合情合理。遗憾的是，病理学家并没有审视整个导管树上的表皮，而仅仅是检查一鳞半爪。因此，常规病理学就大大低估了共存的增生性疾病，从而混淆了其他系列的研究结论。很多时候，我发现并镜下拍摄病变后，必须请我的病理学专家同事多次取样，才能使我的视觉发现在组织学上被充分的说明。

近期更多的研究表明，性质不良的散在ADH的广泛分布可能是以后同侧乳腺癌的原因，这说明我基于内镜的研究的假设可能更接近于事实。

9.4 总　结

基于腺叶假说的数据日益丰富，这将大大改变我们使用的乳腺局部病灶切除术的方法。当乳腺的某一个区域存在问题时，切除受影响的整个腺叶单位或亚单位或许是正确的。这不能完全归因于单纯的病理距离测量就可以证明乳腺肿瘤局部切除术范围足够，我们需要从基因水平确认腺叶中致癌改变的程度，从而发展出解剖上最合理的局部切除术。

参考文献

[1] Dooley WC. Endoscopic visualization of breast tumors. JAMA, 2000, 284: 1518.

[2] Dooley WC. Routine operative breast endoscopy for bloody nipple discharge. Ann Surg Oncol, 2002, 9: 920–923.

[3] Dooley WC. Routine operative breast endoscopy during lumpectomy. Ann Surg Oncol, 2003, 10: 38–42.

[4] Dooley WC. The future prospect: ductoscopy-directed brushing and biopsy. Clin Lab Med, 2005, 25: 845–850.

[5] Dooley WC, Spiegel A, Cox C, et al.Ductoscopy: defning its role in the manage-ment of breast cancer. Breast J, 2004, 10: 271–272.

[6] Grunwald S, Heyer H, Paepke S, et al. Diagnostic value of ductoscopy in the diagnosis of nipple discharge and intraductal proliferations in comparison to standard methods. Onkologie, 2007, 30: 243–248.

[7] Hünerbein M, Raubach M, Gebauer B, et al. Intraoperative ductoscopy in women undergoing surgery for breast cancer. Surgery, 2006a, 139: 833–838.

[8] Hünerbein M, Raubach M, Gebauer B, et al. Ductoscopy and intraductal vacuum assisted biopsy in women with pathologic nipple discharge. Breast Cancer Res Treat, 2006b, 99: 301–307.

[9] Hünerbein M, Dubowy A, Raubach M, et al. Gradient index ductoscopy and intraductal biopsy of intraductal breast lesions. Am J Surg, 2007, 194: 511–514.

[10] Jacobs VR, Paepke S, Ohlinger R, et al. Breast ductoscopy: technical development from a diagnostic to an interventional procedure and its future perspective. Onkologie, 2007a, 30: 545–549.

[11] Jacobs VR, Paepke S, Schaaf H, et al. Autofuorescence ductoscopy: a new imaging technique for intraductal breast endoscopy. Clin Breast Cancer, 2007b, 7: 619–623.

[12] Kapenhas-Valdes E, Feldman SM, Boolbol SK. The role of mammary ductoscopy in breast cancer: a review of the literature. Ann Surg Oncol, 2008, 15: 3350–3360.

[13] Khan SA, Baird C, Staradub VL, et al. Ductal lavage and ductoscopy: the opportunities and the limitations. Clin Breast Cancer, 2002, 3: 185–191.

[14] Kim JA, Crowe JP, Woletz J, et al. Prospective study of intraoperative mammary ductoscopy in patients undergoing partial mastectomy for breast cancer. Am J Surg, 2004, 188: 411–414.

[15] Louie LD, Crowe JP, Dawson AE, et al. Identifcation of breast cancer in patients with pathologic nipple discharge: does ductoscopy predict malignancy. Am J Surg, 2006, 192: 530–533.

[16] Love SM, Barsky SH. Brest-duct endoscopy to study stages of cancerous breast disease. Lancet, 1996, 348: 997–999.

[17] Love SM, Barsky SH. Anatomy of the nipple and breast ducts revisited. Cancer, 2004, 101: 1947–1957.

[18] Matsunaga T, Ohta D, Misaka T, et al. Mammary ductoscopy for diagnosis and treatment of intraductal lesions of the breast. Breast Cancer, 2001, 8: 213–221.

[19] Moncrief RM, Nayar R, Diaz LK, et al. A comparison of ductoscopy-guided and conventional surgical excision in women with spontaneous nipple discharge. Ann Surg, 2005, 241: 575–581.

[20] Okazaki A, Okazaki M, Asaishi K, et al. Fiberoptic ductoscopy of the breast: a new diagnostic procedure for nipple discharge. Jpn J Clin Oncol, 1991, 21: 188–193.

[21] Okazaki A, Okazaki M, Watanabe Y, et al. Diagnostic signifcance of mammary ductoscopy for early breast cancer. Nippon Rinsho, 2007, 65 (Suppl6): 295–297.

[22] Sauter E. Breast cancer detection using mammary ductoscopy. Future Oncol, 2005, 1: 385–393.

[23] Sauter ER, Ehya H, Klein-Szanto AJ, et al. Fiberoptic ductoscopy fndings in women with and without spontaneous nipple discharge. Cancer, 2005, 103: 914–921.

[24] Shao ZM, Nguyen M. Nipple aspiration in diagnosis of breast cancer. Semin Surg Oncol, 2001, 20: 175–180.

[25] Shen K, Lu J, Yuan J, Wu G, et al. Fiberoptic ductoscopy for patients with intraductal papillary lesions. Zhonghua Wai Ke Za Zhi, 2000, 38: 275–277.

[26] Valdes EK, Feldman SM, Balassanian R, et al. Diagnosis of recurrent breast cancer by ductoscopy. Breast J, 2005, 11: 506.

[27] Yamamoto D, Shoji T, Kawanishi H, et al. A utility of ductography and fberoptic ductoscopy for patients with nipple discharge. Breast Cancer Res Treat, 2001a, 70: 103–108.

[28] Yamamoto D, Ueda S, Senzaki H, et al. New diagnostic approach to intracystic lesions of the breast by fberoptic ductoscopy. Anticancer Res, 2001b, 21: 4113–4116.

从现在起消灭乳腺癌——设想在乳腺癌细胞转移前发现防御、治愈的方法

第10章

Richard Gorden

"在乳腺癌的研究领域很少出现令人震惊的新发现,该领域取得的研究进展往往是通过'锦上添花'——也就是一点点的小进步积累而得(Freya Schnabel,个人通信,1998)"——Lerner(2001)。

10.1 概 述

蒂博尔·托特(Tibor Tot)提议将我的工作成果融入计算机断层扫描成像技术(CT)中。这种技术不同于广泛使用了长达一个世纪的传统的X线摄影技术(Strebhardt, Ullrich, 2008),它可以提高乳腺癌转移前的诊出率,及时阻止肿瘤发生转移。自1977年以来,该技术就被用于诊断乳腺癌。我曾经是一个理论生物学家,这个职业在我生活的国度里被认为是一个奇怪的职业。自从细胞膜双层结构发现者、《理论生物学》杂志(JTB)创刊人、曾担任位于布法罗(Buffalo)的纽约州立大学理论生物学中心主任的James F. Danielli辞世以来,理论生物学这个分支学科便遭到忽略(Danielli, 1961; Rosen, 1985; Stein, 1986)。Danielli的精神及其研究成果一直是支撑我不断进步的力量,那种感觉正如Louis Pasteur的终身助手描述有关Louis Pasteur奇妙的生物学精神一样(Duclaux, 1920)。在我的研究生涯中,长时间不能得到Danielli的陪伴,这将毫无疑问地使我的研究成果更像自说自话,承担着自传性质文章所具备的所有风险。我将尽全力对读者坦诚,也对自己坦诚。如果我们把包括CT在内的每项具体的科学活动看作一根游丝,那么科学就是由这些游丝织成的一张大网,而我将沿着自己最了解的那根丝爬过这张网。然而,当我在文中用到"我"这个字眼时,实则,我指的是"我和我亲爱的同事们"。我的人生轨迹与许多人交汇,他们使我的人生旅程更加丰富多彩,使我的科学研究取得成功。这些人包括"世界线"先生(My World Line 是George Gamow先生的自传)(Gamow, 1970),我们俩于1968年左右一起在科罗拉多波尔德分校Boulder旁听了一门气象课程;也包括他的儿子Igor,后来我们一起在Woods Hole和波尔德进行研究,模拟须霉的生长过程(Ortega, et al, 1974)。

10.2 3D电子显微镜

1968年,我在伍兹霍尔海洋生物学实验室(Woods Hole Marine Biological Laboratory)第一次见到了后来成为我博士后导师的(哥伦比亚大学生物科学系)Cyrus Levinthal,他引导我接触了"由投影重建图像"的概念(Levinthal, 1968)。Cyrus巧妙地向我提出问题:如何从一系列斜置的电子显微图像中完

R. Gordon
Department of Radiology, University of Manitoba,
Winnipeg, Manitoba, Canada
e-mail: gordonr@cc.umanitoba.ca

整地获得一个蛋白质分子的立体结构，但是他没有告诉我是否有其他人正在进行这项研究。第二年夏天，我在伍兹霍尔海洋生物学实验室学习了胚胎学的相关课程。我最开始的研究领域正是胚胎学（Gordon，1966），至于它是如何与乳腺癌及Tot进行交汇的，我将在本书的结语部分进行介绍（Gordon，2010）。每年夏天，伍兹霍尔就成了一个各种智力活动的汇聚地，我于1969年夏天在那里学习时，还听过Albert Szent-Györgyi的一个关于香蕉皮、氧化还原反应以及癌症的演讲（Szent-Györgyi，1960，1972）。后来，在一次散步漫谈中，shinya Inoué给我讲述了Györgyi在获得诺贝尔奖后的一个小故事，他向美国国立卫生研究院（NIH）提出了拨款申请，申请上只有一句话"我希望找到治愈癌症的方法"，结果申请遭到了拒绝（Inoué, et al，1986）。我作为加拿大负责研究基金会的会员（Forsdyke，2009），一直致力于使科学民主化，并且力图阻止同行评审制度遏制创新的情况发生（Gordon，1993；Poulin, Gordon，2001；Gordon, Poulin，2009a，b），这件事即种下了我的心锚。事实上，同行评审正是导致我对乳腺癌研究进展缓慢的最大肇因，同时还迫使我的研究更多地停留在理论层面，而不能使用实际设备在患者身上进行实验来论证这些理论。这也是我在文题中使用"设想"一词的原因。

为了降低我的记忆选择难度，简化我的思维过程，我将按照年份顺序介绍我与乳腺癌相关的研究论文，通过这些论文来阐述我对乳腺癌的研究成果，并在回顾过程中对这些文章进行点评。

1968—1969年，我与Cyrus Levinthal合作，在一台昂贵的计算机上共同完成了一项研究。这台计算机的速度可能比不上现在任何一种安装在各种笔记本电脑以及智能手机上的便携计算器，因此，能用那台计算机重新构建数字数组，勉强形成像素为10×10的图像，我已经很满足了。我研究平行投影，通过研究，我觉得平行光束的排列就好比日本枯山水园林中精心耙制的鹅卵石阵列（图10.1）。这个想法大概是在我参加由Arron Klug和Levinthal共同发起的研讨会前或者过程中产生的。这次研讨会上，Klug介绍了由射线投影定理奠基的傅里叶重建技术，这也是我第一次知道还有其他人在进行这项研究。Klug的资历远比我深，这使得我除了对该项目本身充满兴趣外，还存有一种竞争的欲望，更加重视该项研究。我们在后来还曾发生争论。

当时流行一种方法，通过对晶体形成的X射线衍射进行傅里叶变换，来分析晶体结构（Perutz，1990，1998）。血红蛋白分子结构发现者Max Perutz便是该方法的拥护者。可是，在那时，蛋白质分子很难结晶，而结晶是该方法中十分重要的一个步骤。Levinthal的目标是在无需结晶的条件下，通过3D电子显微镜进行观察，解开蛋白质分子结构之谜。Klug的研究显然继承了结晶学的思想，他想通过射线投影来实现重建。Ramachandran也是这么认为的（Ramachandran, Lakshminarayanan，1971）。然而，我却不这么想。也许是因为我十几岁时在芝加哥一家艺术机构上课时，一位到访的日本艺术家对我的影响太深刻了（日本枯山水园林带给作者的影像；图10.1）。

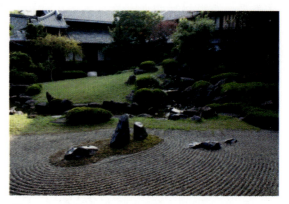

图10.1 日本枯山水园林的鹅卵石被精心耙制，这一点与投影很类似 [引自Wikipedia（2009），已获得GFDL（GNU Free Documentation License）+creative commons 2.5的授权]

10.3 寻找影像

在使用CT技术时，我们始终面临着如何找到合适影像的问题。合适的影像指的就是可以确切显示已知人体组织结构，而更重要的是合理地显示出未知结构（禁止活体解剖）的图像。那时还没有如3D动画、渲染、分形学这样的可以生成复杂图像的方法，而现在我们可以方便地使用这些技术。我在纽约试图接触一些最初的卫星云图，我猜测这些照片能粗略地代表直径在30nm左右的蛋白质电子显微照片，因为它们质地相近。拍摄显微照片时，常将蛋白质置于醋酸铀中，并用四氧化锇（这是我在列文托实验室里学会使用的一种固色剂）进行染色。在那短短的一学年时间内，我还在Eugene S. Machlin的实验室里学习了核乳胶的相关知识，了解到了它在放射能照相领域的应用——追踪单个已发射的粒子（Machlin, et al, 1975）。此外，我还尝试使用场离子发射显微镜观察维生素B的结构。这种显微镜的功能很强大，氦粒子沿着金属针尖的尖端与荧光屏之间产生的放射状电场加速到达荧光屏，在荧光屏上产生与表面原子一一对应的辉点，形成尖端表层原子的清晰图像。每个尖端表层原子都在没有光的情况下被放大了100万倍，此时通过光电倍增管即可真实观测到这些原子。当我还在芝加哥大学读本科时，曾在Albert V. Crewe的实验室里观看过单个铀原子以及原子扩散的电子显微图片（Wall, et al, 1974；Isaacson, et al, 1977），他在之后引用过我的关于CT的研究成果（Crewe, Crewe, 1984）。回顾往事，我发现像观察单个原子运动这样的"亲力亲为"的实验经历使我在日后的研究中习惯于每次建立单一量子（粒子或光子）的图像。

直到我前往位于布法罗（Buffalo）的理论生物学中心，与和我一样对形态发生学感兴趣的Robort Rosen共事后，我才解决了排列的问题（Goel, et al, 1970）。Rosen给予了我充分的学术自由，让我可以探索自己感兴趣的知识。当时因为无法区分"计算机中心"与新概念"计算机科学"，我向计算机科学助理教授Gabor Herman询问如何得到计算机的时间，同时也与他探讨了我一直致力于研究的重建问题。1周后，他也开始研究这个问题。所以我决定与他合作。

在计算机科学领域，排列有序的比特位取代了精心耙制的鹅卵石，它们的计算结果被加到给出的投影之上，通过蒙特卡洛仿真（Monte Carlo）获得三维投影数据，从而重建图像。我们很快提交了第一篇论文（Gordon, Herman, 1971）。

当时由于受到美国民权运动的影响，我选择了由Judith Carmichael拍摄的一位叫"朱蒂"的黑人女孩的影像作为测试样本。朱迪思的丈夫杰克是我1968年夏季博士后研究课题的主办人（Gordon, et al, 1972），他凭借一根光度计创立了一个相关的实验室。我将这份影像移动了2 500个位置，并读了2 500次电压表，最后得到了一张50×50像素的图像，这也是第一张令我满意的作品。脸部影像的拍摄最为容易，因为我们的面部很容易产生各种扭曲，这也使得假象易于辨别。

尽管一系列日趋复杂的乳房电脑模拟影像逐渐进入人们的视野（Taylor, Owens, 2001；Bakic, et al, 2002a、b, 2003；Bliznakova, et al, 2002, 2003, 2006；Taylor, 2002；Hoeschen, et al, 2005；Reiser, et al, 2006；Zhou, et al, 2006；Shorey, 2007；Han, et al, 2008；Li, et al, 2009），我还是更倾向于真实的东西（O'Connor, et al, 2008）。最终，事实证明，也许最好的X射线影像是能反映乳房原子级组成的3D图，因为X线的吸收和散射主要是原子运动产生的现象，而不是分子运动。正是因为这个原因，这种3D影像与核磁共振成像（MRI）的效果不相上下，但是却与超声波或电阻抗断层成像（EIT）及核磁共振波谱分析（MRS）观测的效果不尽相同，因为后面这些方法研究的都是分子性能。我建议用岩相分析法得到这样的"原子乳房影像"。我们可以对一具尸体的乳房进行解剖,将组织平面一层一层剖去或者进行蚀刻处理,做出剩下样本暴露表层的图像,就可以得到所需的3D数据。在解剖过程中,需要对样本进行冷藏或冷冻处理,以保证人体组织的活性,这样做还可以避免样本遭到细菌腐蚀。为了解原子组成并且进行蚀刻处理,理想情况下,应将暴露的表层置于一个大型次级离子质谱分析仪(SIMS)中,对整个表层的每个体素都进行分析,得到其原子组成(Hallégot, et al, 2006)。体素的尺寸必须低于下一步中将用到的任何一种3D乳腺成像方式的目标分辨率(见下文)。

10.4 ART的诞生

Robert Bender(Bender, Duck, 1982)以一名研究生的身份加入了理论生物学中心,我们成为了好朋友。我一直对蛋白质合成十分感兴趣。本科时,我曾与Victor Fried一起就读于芝加哥大学生物物理学系(Haselkorn, Fried, 1964),之后我们又一起在俄勒冈州大学就读研究生,正是他在芝加哥大学关于蛋白质合成的研究成果激起了我对该课题的兴趣。蛋白质合成的问题归根结底是讨论核糖体到底是什么,以及它们是怎么工作的。我曾进行过一项关于核糖体与信使RNA一起运动的蒙特卡洛仿真实验(Gordon, 1969)。Bender与David Sabatini(Sabatini, 2005)取得联系,从他那里得到了一系列核糖体的电子显微镜图像。与此同时,大概是受到了我与Terrell L. Hill合作完成的统计力学方面的研究论文的影响(Gordon, Herman, 1971),我意识到基于蒙特卡洛法的投影重建有一个确定的平均值,可以通过一组联立线性方程来表示,这种新方法需要一个名字。

Bender和我都很喜欢说双关语。他先想出"快速代数重建算法(Fast Algebraic Reconstruction Technique)"这个名字,我将其简短为ART(艺术)。我对这个首字母缩略形式表示的名字十分满意,因为我曾经受到一名艺术家的栽培(Gordon, 1979a)。后来,Boris K. Vainshtein(1972,个人交流;Vainshtein, 1971)告诉我ART在俄语中同样适用(我与忧思科学家委员会其他成员一起在苏联参加"被拒绝移民者"研讨会时,他还告诉我他也是犹太人)。之后,我将我的首个PET(正电子发射成像术)算法命名为"储存显像管快速代数迭代重建算法(ARTIST)"(Gordon, 1975c, 1983a)。ARTIST算法收集产生的一致信号(一组同时发射的γ射线/一对光子向相反的方向运动)。这是我第一次公开涉足单量子运动成像领域,仅通过1 000次实验数据便得到了一张貌似可信的重建影像。后来Barbara Pawlak用密度估计法对该算法进行了改进,使其变得更加复杂(Pawlak, Gordon, 2005, 2010)。详见下文。

10.5 追寻诺贝尔奖的青年

我们觉得自己离成功只有一步之遥——我们即将揭开核糖体的结构及功能之谜,那样将能获得当时分子生物学的最高奖项——所以从事这项研究工作时,我们一直有一种紧迫感。那时我才20多岁,满脑子只想着自己,我在脑海中一遍遍彩排自己拿到诺贝尔奖时的获奖感言,抑或是幻想自己狂妄地拒绝接受奖项的场景,至于拒绝的原因,我已经记不清了,大概是跟我当时反对、抗议越南战争有关。事实上,早些时候,以防我被应征入伍,Hill和我制订了一个迂回计划,让我前往瑞典与物理化学家Hugo Theorell一起工作。后来,在我的本科指导顾问Aaron Novick的帮助下,我躲过了征兵(Novick, Szilard, 1950)。

但是Bender和我遇到了一个问题:怎么展现我们的研究成果呢?我掌握了一种在一次印刷品的半米宽色带上套印的技术(overprinting to the point of once slicing across a half-meter-wide ink ribbon) (cf. Gordon, et al, 1976)。套印会使链式打印机停止工作，导致在同一位置打印多个字母，因此这种技术早已被淘汰。通过这种技术的打印结果不尽如人意，图片质量太差。Bender在位于纽约罗切斯特(Rochester)的施乐公司(Xerox)总部找到了一台标准的电脑图片打印机，不巧的是，它只能识别纸带。所以我们开着Bender的车从布法罗前往渥太华(Ottawa)，在国家研究委员会将磁带转储为纸带，然后又开车到施乐公司，停留了一晚上，读取纸带并打印出了我们的图片。Bender的车冷却器坏了，我们一路上必须不停地给它加水。

研究结果最终以两篇内容连续的论文形式呈现。论文发表在了丹尼利的《理论生物学杂志》上，介绍了ART的原理，以及其在研究核糖体中的应用（Bender, et al, 1970; Gordon, et al, 1970）。我们的研究还提供了一些早期蒙特卡洛仿真的图像，这些结果随后公布（Gordon, Herman, 1971）。在撰写论文的过程中，我突然意识到这种方法同样适用于X线，所以我在介绍ART原理的论文题目中加了"……和X射线照片"几个字。这种想法非常幼稚，当时我的实验室里根本就没有进行放射线摄影术实验的条件。这便是我医学生涯的开始：

"在采用放射线摄影术拍摄身体部位的领域内（Kane, 1953）有一种新趋势——将X射线源与胶片结合，这样做可以保证只保留人体内某个平面的影像是清晰的，而将其他部位影像都进行模糊处理，便于观察。如果取而代之，运用我们的方法，那么X射线可以只照射那些感兴趣的平面，而它上方或下方的组织都不会被拍摄到。之后通过光度计读取荧光屏，并将得到的密度数据直接传输到一台小型计算机上，1min后，计算机将通过计算得到重建图像，呈现在一个电视显示屏上。实际上，我们的方法可以在无需剪辑的条件下快速呈现横断面影像。因为X线摄影中经常出现非平行光，所以这种方法被归类为非平行光方法。"(Gordon, et al, 1970)

我们的成果并没有引起研究核糖体的电子显微学家们的注意。例如，我们本可以继续研究，重建核糖体内组成部分的结构（Nomura, 1987），得出一个3D立体的核糖体图，指出每个结构的具体位置。然而，理论生物学中心倒闭，我的同事们都各奔东西，现实条件迫使我们不得不终止这个项目。我在Hill的帮助下转移到了国家卫生研究院（NIH）。Hill在1972年来到了这里，成为了关节炎、代谢和消化疾病研究所数学研究分支的一名"专家"。在我与Marcello Barbieri（Barbieri, et al, 1970）一起研究关于核糖体的数组时，我提出的在NIH引进一套用作平板扫描仪的密度计设备（现在仅需50美元）的提议遭到了否决。尽管当时我已经年过30，但我在NIH仅仅是一个鲁莽的年轻人，并且找不到合适的工作。

10.6 降低CT剂量

这个研究还得出了重要的放射学结论，该结论与使用电子显微镜有关。通过观察一系列连续的实验结果不难发现，核糖体的数目明显减少，这说明电子束会破坏核糖体（Bender, et al, 1970）。我在高中时曾写过一篇关于第一次核爆的论文，这篇论文使我对电离辐射有了一定认识。加之前面所说的观察结果，我直接得出了CT辐射剂量相关影响的结论（Gordon, 1960）。

从剂量角度来说，基于X线断层摄影术进行图像重建，影像的范围越小越好。从另一方面来说，如果给定剂量，就要着手解决拍摄范围最大化的问题，如下：

总剂量=每个视图的剂量×视图数目

这又将我们带回了之前所说的量子成像问题。要想获得最佳效果，就要得到大量的附有噪声的视图，同时保证每个视图上只附着有少量光子（如ARTIST算法所述，极限情况下，每个视图只附有一个光子或者一个其他量子；Gordon, 1975c, 1983a）。但是，这需要一种噪声敏感性低于ART以及滤波反投影（FBP）的新算法。因此，如何确定最佳视图数目仍是一个待解决的问题。现在，这个问题多被看作是应用普遍的压缩成像技术或压缩传感问题的一个分支（Candes, Wakin, 2008; Ramlau, et al, 2008; Romberg, 2008; Sidky, Pan, 2008; Carron, 2009; Pan, et al, 2009; Yu, et al, 2009）。

目前，医学实践活动并没有制订更好的算法来减少CT剂量（Gordon, 1976b），而是仍然倾向于通过调整患者的拍摄体位、曝光程度、准直参数来达到既定目标（Vock, 2005）。这将所有的责任都推给了放射线研究者（Imhof, et al, 2003）。科学家们一直觉得CT算法是数学领域内一个讳深莫测的不解之谜（Pan, et al, 2009），这大概就是导致CT算法无人问津的原因。CT生产厂家唯一的商业秘密可能就是没有尽力降低CT剂量。政府则试图通过制订相关物理法律来解决这个问题（Krotz, 1999）。

我的大多数研究都集中在一些低噪视图上，ART算法很适合处理这些视图，并且其处理效果远远超过滤波反投影（FBP）技术（Herman, Rowland, 1973; Barbieri, 1974; Gordon, Herman, 1974; Barbieri, 1987）。因为我们所设计的第一台皮肤显微检测仪（Nevoscope）太过简陋，我曾经在检测黑色素瘤的主要预后因素——色素痣的深度时，只利用了3张视图就制作出了一幅CT图像（Dhawan, et al, 1984b）。显然，只用3张视图并不是最优选项，但是我的直觉告诉我在乳房X线摄影术中，选择10~30张视图就足以达到很好的效果（Wu, et al, 2003; Sidky, et al, 2006; Herman, Davidi, 2008; Pan, et al, 2009; Qian, et al, 2009; Jia, et al, 2010）。如果我的想法正确，那么将会是一个CT扫描机的结构，即很可能会配置一个由若干X线光源组成的固定阵列，指向检测阵列（Gordon, 1985b），实际上这已经是乳腺断层X射线影像的原型设计（Qian, et al, 2009）。梅奥诊所的动态空间再现器（Mayo Clinic Dynamic Spatial Reconstructor）由28个旋转的X线源组成（Altschuler, et al, 1980），所以我推测的这些数字是合理的。仪器不能活动的部分能够节约部分成本，但是这并不足以抵消X线光源的额外花费。

从有限的斜置角度中，我们还得出另一个结论：事实上，不用进行180°的角度变化，也可以重建图像，但是重建得到的图像分辨率具有各向异性，也许能进行修正。后来，这个结论被用于调整电子显微镜的倾斜物台。之后，我们通过皮肤显微检测仪相关的研究工作找出了修正分辨率的方法，这将在接下来的内容中进行描述。

10.7 用更多的方程式取代数据

CT技术可以用联立线性方程表示的事实使我们更加清楚地认识到，还可以开发更多的方程式帮助我们合理地重建图像。而将这些重建图像与原始影像进行比较，更能证明这一点。也就是说，当我们重建一张大小为n×n、像素为n^2的图像时，我们可以采用m投影，其中m远小于n。相比之下，克鲁格的傅里叶重建法需要填满重建图像的傅里叶空间，这就要求以密集的角度间隔采集统一的视图样本。这种技术充满争议：

"DeRosier和Klug（DeRosier, Klug, 1968）曾提出了一个通过电子显微图、采用傅里叶重建得到物体三维立体结构的方法。可惜的是，他们的方法有太多局限性，只能适用于高度对称的物体（对这种类型的物体来说，一张视图就可以代表其他很多不同角度的视图）。如果想要重建一个直径为250埃的核糖体，并保持30埃的分辨率，那么就需要在±90°的倾斜范围内，从30多个不同的角度拍摄该核糖体的电子显微图。如果用普通的电子显微镜拍摄这么多图片，核糖体的表层将附上一层显微镜内腔上的灰尘，破坏核糖体。我们所呈现的是一种全新而且直接的重建方法——ART。相比傅里叶重建法，它具有以下几个突出优点：①ART法适用于结构完全不对称的物体；②只需要5~10张视图，ART法即可获得丰富的物体结构信息；③由于拍摄只需要较小的角度变化范围（正负30°），所以普通倾斜置物台即可满足拍摄要求；④如果用Control Data 6400处理器进行图像处理，每个部位的计算只需要大概30s；⑤数据需要的存储空间小，所以可以使用小型计算机；⑥ART算法可直接适用于宏观X射线摄影，并且与其他现有的放射线摄影术相比，ART只需极少量射线……傅里叶重建法要求在180°的角度变化范围内拍摄30张不同角度的视图，这样才能在8×8的栅格上确定坐标，而我们的方法显然要好得多，我们只需要在60°的范围内拍摄5张视图即可（得到50×50像素的图像）"（Gordon, et al, 1970）。

Klug向Danielli提交了一篇供杂志发表的文章，驳斥我们的观点。这篇论文还以预印本的形式在全世界刊印。Danielli当时正为因他的好友Maurice H. F. Wilkins（Wade, 2004）辞世被迫退出DNA结构的研究感到十分难过（尽管他已经与Francis Crick、James Watson一起获得了诺贝尔奖），Klug在这方面与他有相同的感受。然而，Danielli唯一的举动就是将Klug的论文发表时间推迟了1个月，给予我们充分的时间撰文在《理论生物学杂志》上反驳他的观点。与此同时，Klug也重新提交了一份语气柔和的版本。鉴于预印本已经在全世界发行，我们引用原文进行反驳。Klug提到"ART算法和科学"（Crowther, Klug, 1971），我们有力地回应称"ART算法就是科学"（Bellman, et al, 1971）。我们还采取了一些非语言的手段进行反击。我们截取了《时代周刊》中一幅Klug的照片，将其进行图像重建。合成的图像中，一位在这段小插曲发生前曾陪Bender拜访过Klug的时尚模特惹恼了Klug，使他身心憔悴。并且因为Bender、Klug和我都是犹太人，在图片中，线粒体成了大卫之星的形状。最后，论文的首席作者S. H. Bellman化身成为Lewis Carroll所创作的史诗《斯纳克之猎》中的鸣钟者。我最初用FORTRAN Ⅱ语言编写我们SNARK项目的电脑程序时（Herman, 2009），经常出现错误，导致黑屏。而Bellman就如同我们的福星，总能帮助我们解决问题（Carroll, 1876; Bellman, 1970）。

回顾往事，我们的做法推迟了Klug获得诺贝尔奖的时间（Klug, 1983），他在研究病毒结构方面做出了很大贡献，得这个奖实至名归。同时，尽管我们还很年轻，但我们也得到了他的尊重，在多年后见面时，他的态度仍十分诚恳。Klug甚至还发表过一篇关于ART的研究文章（Crowther, Klug, 1974）。很显然，除了他自己的实验室外，没有人采用他那复杂而又需要大剂量的傅里叶重建法，而ART则作为一种常见的重建手段，得到推崇。

10.8 使ART算法得到重视

后来，数学家们指出，ART算法只是Kaczmarz提出的解决联立线性方程的一般方法中的一个特例，或者说至少从ART的线性结构方面来看是这样（Kaczmarz, 1937; Groetsch, 1999）。而他的理论早于ART的问世，这在一定程度上挫伤了我们肆无忌惮的气焰，使我们不得不谦虚一些。然而，非线性积极约束（相当于说患者不能发射X射线）被证明具有重要意义，甚至对平行光领域光谱去卷积都有影响（Jansson, 1984, 1997）。此外，Geoffrey Hounsfield独立发明了一种类似于ART的算法。他的公司EMI所设计的第一台商业扫描打标机就采用了这种算法（Hounsfield, 1973, 1976）。

1970年代的计算机运行速度都很慢，其计算速度是制约患者周转量的一大因素。当时，计算机断层X射线摄影仪（CAT），也就是后来所说的CT扫描仪，标价高达100万美元，这也使得计算机计算速度成为了业界关注的重点。那时，ART算法耗费的计算机时间是FBP算法的10多倍，而且有人正在研究一种专门为FBP算法设计的高速计算机，其硬件连接满足快速傅氏换算法（FFT）的要求（Cooley, Tukey, 1965）。

FBP算法最初是由物理学家Allan Cormack（Cormack, 1963, 1964）和X射线晶体学家G. N. Ramachandran发明的（Ramachandran, Lakshminarayanan, 1971; Subramanian, 2001）。Niels Henrik Abel在1830年左右提出了阿贝尔积分（Houzel, 2004），而Radon在此基础上提出了拉东变换（Radon, 1917），FBP算法就是对拉东方程式的一个数学解答。我们现在可以将阿贝尔积分方程看作是圆柱对称物体CT影像的数学形式（Gorenflo, Vessella, 1991）。事实上，阿尔贝方程一直应用于研究圆柱火焰的结构（Daun, et al, 2006），而现在，它已经被CT技术所取代（Chen, et al, 1997）。Cormack和Hounsfield（1980）一起获得了诺贝尔奖。其实，有一个被轻视的团队早在Hounsfield之前就设计并制造出了CT扫描仪（Kalos, et al, 1961）（图10.2）。

在Paul Lauterbur所撰写的第一篇关于MRI的论文中，就运用了ART算法（Lauterbur, 1973）。这篇论文帮助Lauterbur获得了诺贝尔奖。但是后来，其结论却被归结于傅里叶法。ART算法的应用十分广泛，在医学领域它被

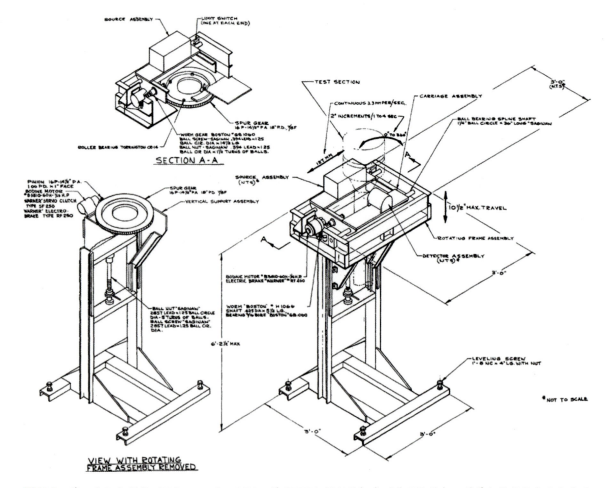

图10.2　第一台CT扫描仪（Kalos, et al, 1961），早于EMI扫描仪的概念（美国能量部，科学与技术信息办公室及Malvin H. Kalos授权）。很不幸，现实中的原型机未能保存下来

用于心脏成像（Nielsen, et al, 2005）、超声衍射层析成像、金属伪影抑制、局部区域重建（Wang, et al, 1996, 1999）、正电子发射断层扫描技术（PET; Matej, et al, 1994）以及三维计算机断层扫描痣和黑色素瘤原位（Nevoscopy）（Maganti, Dhawan, 1997）；在非医学领域，它应用于研究日冕（Saez, et al, 2007）、电离层（Cornely, 2003; Wen, et al, 2008）、等离子物理（Kazantsev, Pickalov, 1999; Wan, et al, 2003）、质子断层扫描（Li, et al, 2006）、晶粒边界（Markussen, et al, 2004）、贝纳德花纹（Bénard patterns）（Subbarao, et al, 1997a）、热不均匀流体（Mishra, et al, 1999）、无损检测（Subbarao, et al, 1997b）、光谱学（Song, et al, 2006a、b）、示踪气体浓度分布（Park, et al, 2000）、厚切片电镜观察（Jonges, et al, 1999）等。过程层析成像技术中也采用了ART算法（Fellholter, Mewes, 1994; Lee, et al, 2009; Zhang, et al, 2009），使用该技术时，被测物场的图像会随着物场的快速变化而实时变化。单纯地从数学角度来看，可以说ART算法使喀茨马茨（Kaczmarz）方法得到了更广泛的应用。

尽管FBP算法的高速使得ART算法在医学领域逐渐褪色，但我从来没有放弃过对ART算法的研究，因为ART算法具有功能多样、所需投影数较少等优点（Herman, Rowland, 1973; Barbieri, 1974, 1987; Gordon, Herman, 1974）。这些优点对于减少CT剂量、乳腺CT检查具有至关重要的作用，这也成为我日后研究工作的重心。对于很多学者来说，研究ART算法仅限于进行学术实验。关于ART算法的学术研究论文多达700多篇，还有一些相关的研究书籍出版（例如Marti, 1979; Herman, 1980; Eggermont, et al, 1981; Trummer, 1981, 1983; Andersen, Kak, 1984; Byrne, 1993, 2004; Watt, 1994; Garcia, et al, 1996; Mueller, et al, 1997, 1998; Marabini, et al, 1998; Guan, et al, 1999; Mishra, et al, 1999; Kak, Slaney, 2001; Donaire, Garcia, 2002; Kaipio, Somersalo, 2004）。坦白地说，这其中大部分作品都在阐述一些令人头大的数学问题。因为Feldkamp的FBP算法无法应对随着探测器行数从2行（Hounsfield 1973）增至320行（Pan, et al, 2009）而逐渐增大的X线源与探测器阵列间锥面角（Feldkamp, et al, 1984），ART算法以"锥面光ART"的身份重新得到了关注（Donaire, Garcia, 1999; Nielsen, et al, 2005）。ART算法可以处理任何几何形状（Gordon, 1974），它也可以在并行计算机上工作。1970年代（Gordon, et al, 1975），我曾设想在早期配置64位处理器的Illiac计算机上运行它（Fitchett, 1993; Garcia, et al, 1996; Rajan, Patnaik, 2001），但是后来随着一系列新理论的研发（Byrne, 1996; Censor, Zenios, 1997），它在并行计算机上运行的性能远远超出了我的期望，这当中也有我的贡献（Martin, et al, 2005）。

10.9 出售ART算法并改进CT技术

我和Bender向电子显微学家们展示了我们的研究成果（Gordon, Bender, 1971a），并且尽力将我们的理念推销给雷神（Raytheon）、友达光电（Optronics）、施乐（Xeror）等知名公司，想将其推广至医学成像领域，但是却没有公司接受我们的想法。我们回想起来，Hounsfield之所以取得成功，是因为他（Hounsfield, 1973）与一名神经外科医生（Ambrose, 1973, 1974）一起进行研究（并且不需要筹措研究经费）。所以，我们及我们之前组建的数学家小团队一直无法涉足医学领域的原因就是因为我们的团队中没有医生（Kalos, et al, 1961）。尽管我们已经认识到了团队中有医学内部人员的重要性，我们还是不清楚这么做的原因，但是我们学会了这么做。

当我还在NIH工作时，曾有幸前往瑞士

(Gordon, Bender, 1971b; Gordon, 1972)、维也纳（Gordon, et al, 1971）和墨西哥（Gordon, Kane, 1972）。我在墨西哥拜访了晶体学家 Boris K. Vainshtein。Vainshtein 设计了采用胶片的简单光学添加剂重建方法，该方法在数学上与传统断层成像及螺旋断层成像法一致（Takahashi, 1969），但是却得到了一个重要的观测结论：三维 CT 点扩散函数（PSF）曲线要比二维（Vainshtein, 1971）的陡得多，若用 r 表示到图像上任意一给定点间的距离，其点扩散函数分别是 $1/r^2$ 和 $1/r$（使去卷积更加容易）（图10.3）。该结论日后在 CT 技术中得到了应用，但是我们对其应采取谨慎的态度。因此，只要是根据数据进行逐平面重建或者是逐断层重建，任何领域的 CT 都需采用比需要更多的 X 线剂量（Gordon, 1976b）。

我曾参与过两门有关 CT 技术的授课（Gordon, Bender, 1971c; one with Z.H. Cho），这两门授课都没有通过正式审核，也并不太成熟（随着 EMI 扫描仪的应用日益广泛，这些课程随后变得流行起来）。所以，取而代之，我发表了一篇文章（Gordon, 1974），引导读者学习 CT 知识，并详细阐述了相关算法（Gordon, Herman, 1974），文章大受欢迎（Gordon, et al, 1975）。随后，我接连举行了一场会议（Gordon, Lauterbur, 1974）及一个研讨会（Gordon, 1975b），讨论 CT 技术广泛的应用前景。在研讨会上，我们还首次列出了关于投影重建技术的综合文献目录（Gordon, 1975a）。我曾是一个天文学业余爱好者，我曾环游世界，观摩全球的射电天文站。我惊喜地发现，射电天文学观测领域中所用到的很多图像重建算法的数学理论与 CT 技术相同（Gordon, 1978b），射电天文学家也为医学 CT 技术做出了很多贡献（Bracewell, 1977）。因为我曾经是一位天文学爱好者，所以我很高兴以这种方式结束我的工作。我将 CT 技术与大脑本身的功能进行类比，大脑在对视网膜观察到的图像进行重建时，视觉感

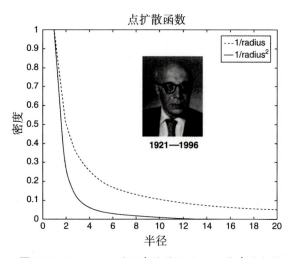

图 10.3 Vainshtein 的观察结果显示，3D 重建的点扩散函数较 2D 重建更陡峭（Micheal J.A. Potter 制图）。半径的单位不够客观，但是两条曲线的比值很客观

受野扮演的就是射线的角色（Gordon, Hirsch, 1977; Gordon, Tweed, 1983）。这样阐述能够使那些对 CT 技术感兴趣的人更容易接受（Gordon, Rangaraj, 1981）。

我曾在"投影重建"会议上发言（Gordon, 1975c），介绍自己关于每次从一个光子或粒子的角度出发重构图像的看法。也就是说，在进行下一步工作之前，扫描仪每次只会记录一个量子的运动，进而改变图像。这种想法适用于正电子发射断层显像（PET）。当时最常见的做法就是将普通的 CT 算法勉强应用于 PET 之上，将射线看作是两台检测器之间穿越患者的一个光带，记下在这个光带内发生的符合事件的次数。最终，由于这些统计数据存在巨大的泊松分布波动及普通 CT 算法对噪音具有较强的敏感性，得到的重建图像噪声较大，并附有条纹。检测器的宽度要足够大（1~2cm），从而降低空间分辨率。这不仅仅是因为检测器造价昂贵，也是因为小型检测器可能会得到高噪数据，致使普通的 CT 算法无法进行处理。但是在专为 PET 设计的 ARTIST 算法中，我着力估计在重合线上正电子湮灭的位置。这种方法类似于物理方法，选择的位置受到之前放置点位置的引导。Barbara Pawlak 后来完善了该方法，这种方法在

统计学中被称作密度估计（Pawlak, Gordon, 2005, 2010; Pawlak, 2007）。新型深度互动（DOI）检测器可以在检测器内部定位每条γ射线，从而确保重合线的宽度比检测器的宽度更窄（Shao, et al, 2008）。

ARTIST概念也间接提出了一种X线CT技术的新手段，即散射光子不应该被舍弃（Bradford, et al, 2002），而是应该使用能量鉴别探测器将它们逐一记录，作为辅助资料，用于3D重建及组织结构数据分析（正如我在射线天文学中所学）（Garmire, et al, 2003; Porter, 2004）。这样可以重建两幅图像：吸收系数图像和电子密度图像（Van Uytven, et al, 2007, 2008）。后来，通过准直及过滤技术，该手段的研究工作取得了更大的进展（Alpuche Avilés, et al, 2010）。

10.10 来自传统断层摄影术的挑战

在这个节骨眼上，非常有必要回头审视一下传统断层摄影术。传统断层摄影术采用胶片，与CT技术相比，具有更高、更好的空间分辨率。事实上，Hounsfield和Ambrose第一次拍摄的脑部CT图像效果还不如1940年代采用旋转断层摄影术拍摄的脑部影像(Takahashi, 1969)。第一台标准的乳腺CT扫描仪（Chang, et al, 1977, 1978），因为其体素（1.56mm×1.56mm×10mm）相较于拍摄对象0.1mm的直径过大，致使冲洗出的图像将微钙化放大了24 000倍。尽管有人说这没什么大不了的（Nab, et al, 1992; Karssemeijer, et al, 1993; Pachoud, et al, 2005），但是我们在数字化乳腺摄影中尚且没有达到胶片那样的高分辨率，更别说CT了（Chan, et al, 1987; Nickoloff, et al, 1990; Brettle, et al, 1994; Kuzmiak, et al, 2005; Yaffe, et al, 2008）。只有拍摄小动物的微计算机断层扫描技术的分辨率能达到这个标准，因为微CT扫描仪远小于拍摄人体部位的CT扫描仪，而总的辐射剂量也是影响CT分辨率的一个次要因素。在1970年代后期，研究者们尝试直接将正弦图记录在胶片上，来逾越空间分辨率的限制（Gmitro, et al, 1980）。但是，当时胶片扫描仪，即后来所说的测微密度计，价格特别贵，并且技术人才紧缺，所以这个依托旧工具的方法并没有使我们有新的突破。由此，我得出了一个简单的规律：如果你可以在乳房X线摄影图像中看出结构，那么肯定也能在3D CTM中看出。没有CT扫描仪可以到达这个目标。

10.11 欠定方程

我在芝加哥大学数学系攻读本科学位时，曾上过由Alberto Calderon执教的一门线性代数的课程（Christ, et al, 1998）。因此，我非常清楚我们用ART算法研究CT技术是一种大胆的举措，它可以帮助我们开发更多的方程式，通过欠定方程组解决问题。Hounsfield则认为这是"不可能的"（1974, personal communication），正是由于他这种想法的限制，他放弃使用自己发明的类似于ART的算法（Hounsfield, 1975）解决超定的问题。超定问题的出现是因为得到了比需要更多的投影。EMI公司承袭了Hounsfield的这种思想，在商业医学扫描仪概念上一直混淆不清，直到最近才将ART算法与FBP算法区分开来，所以他的这种态度也是导致对患者使用高CT剂量的根本原因。想要得到相同质量的重建图像，使用较少投影数的ART算法所用的剂量远小于与FBP投影数持平的超定ART算法。

这种错误思想造成的后果就是在为人体拍摄CT影像时，大大增加了辐射剂量（Huda, 2002; Linton, Mettler, 2003; Dawson, 2004; Prokop, 2005; Bertell, et al, 2007; Colang, et al, 2007）。我在几年前进行过一项粗略的计算，将在下文中进行介绍。普通的乳腺X线摄影术中，采用的辐射剂量多为

2mGy，超过了其他任何一种3D成像技术（Spelic，2009）。因此乳腺CT可以在减少CT剂量方面做出表率。然而，如果我们把罹患毛细血管扩张失调的女性排除在X线检查之外（Hall，et al，1992；Ramsay，et al，1996，1998），那么，其他人的平均值就将增加。例如，Boone做了一个实验，证明使用行常规人体部位CT扫描的高能X线束（120~140 kVp）（Chen，Ning，2002）行乳腺CT扫描时，为得到高质量、高分辨率（$0.3×0.3×1.2mm^3$）的下垂乳房CT图像所需的平均乳腺辐射剂量（MGD）与进行将乳房压缩至5cm（Boone，et al，2003）的双视图乳房X线摄影所需剂量相同。这个实验如果不是凑巧得出的最佳结论，那么便给我们未来的研究带来了希望。同步加速器辐射以体积为$0.047×0.047×0.3mm^3$的体素为基本单位，通过衍射增强成像（DEI-CT）进行逐层重建，在未来有可能使辐射剂量降低10倍以上（Fiedler，et al，2004）。

"欠定"方程面临的问题并不是无法得出答案，而正相反，它们有无数个答案。这使得分析结论有出错的可能，如果生成或选择了"错误的"解决方案，将会给患者带来危险。这并不是一个业内人士共享的秘密，因为CT和病理学之间的相互关系本来就有缺陷（Turunen，et al，1986；Zwirewich，et al，1990；March，et al，1991；Murata，et al，1992；Bravin，et al，2007），我们还不能完全解答为什么、什么时候CT会错过一些病理特征。事实上，Kennan Smith就是为了解决这些疑问才开始研究CT的（1980年，个人交流）。他的一个神经病学家朋友有一位患者，他确信这位患者长有肿瘤，可是CT检查却显示阴性（cf. Herman，Davidi，2008）。凯南后来得出了不确定性原理（Smith，et al，1977；Gordon，1979c；Leahy，et al，1979；Hamaker，et al，1980；Gordon，1985b）："一组有限的X线图像其实什么都说明不了"（Smith，et al，1977）。他认为有限的X线图像可以被实在的事物或者先验的局限性所推翻（Smith，et al，1978）。他的结论后来得到了证实（Clarkson，Barrett，1997；Clarkson，Barrett，1998）。最近有新的理论呼应这个结论："只要有其他的限制，辅助专家从一个成像方程的零空间内选择出一张'好的'图像，欠定方程的体系就是可以解决问题的"（Pan，et al，2009）。

EMI公司所采取的理念和做法，使其从商业CT行业的垄断者变成一个彻头彻尾的破产者，我亲眼见证了这一切。1974—1978年，我在NIH工作，同时也担任乔治·华盛顿的客座教授。当时，Hounsfield曾与我碰面，我们签署了一项合约。他同意我从位于乔治·华盛顿大学的头部CT扫描仪中获得一手材料。我发现数据中存在一个系统性错误，对于平行射线来说，投影数据中，头部几何中心的反向投影应该在中心相交，但是这些数据中并非如此，而是形成了直径为几毫米的环形包络。我把这个发现告诉了Hounsfield，并提出我有一个简单的纠错软件，我想将改正过的数据重新输入他们的电脑，看看图片质量是否得到提高，但是他却没有回应我。后来，我加入强生公司技术服务部（原名俄亥俄核公司）的阵营，反驳EMI公司1976年对于该公司侵犯专利权的指控（Strong，Hurst，1994）。我们证明了强生公司的研究成果有一部分取得了线性代数的授权，并且完整的扫描仪设计早就已经是共享资源（Kalos，et al，1961）（图10.2），然而令所有芝加哥专利辩护律师感到遗憾的是，强生公司最终选择了庭外和解。Cormack总结到：

"EMI公司为对付那些被它指控侵权的美国对手，制订了一套策略，其秘诀就在于利用法律系统漏洞将从指控到审判的时间拖得越长越好。这样可以避免专利被宣布无效的风险。但是，遗憾的是，虽然这样的策略取得了成功，EMI公司却并没有良好的工业生产能力及市场营销能力，不足以维持英国在CT扫描仪生产方面的领先地位"（Cormack，1994）。

10.12 超空间漫行

早在研究电子显微镜学时,我就开始尝试解决欠定方程的问题(Gordon,1973)。如果我们在观察单个蛋白质分子的相关实例之前就能得到先验,则任何一张由两个不相连部分组成的图像都是一个错误方程分析的先验。现在,我已经远离模式识别领域了,将解读图像的工作留给放射学研究者们去完成,我的工作则是为他们提供质量最高、最易解读的图像。因此,我想出了一种方法激励放射学家们研究CT图像,并在某种程度上对其进行验证,看看CT图像中通过欠定方程重建的病变征象是真的还是人为分析产生的。ART方程存在多种结果,数学家们称这些结果所在的集合为超平面,所以我准备开启一场"超平面上的智力之行"。这将使放射学家们开始学习解剖学及其他各种病理学知识,这些知识将为他们提供相关的先验信息,帮助他们更好的观察那些阳性征象,但同时又不仅依赖于这些征象做出判断。我选择了一张ART算法重建的图像,抹去了其中的一个特征,这样得到的新图像并不再符合欠定方程,但它可以作为重启ART算法的原始图像,之后它又会汇聚到超平面之上,只不过是在另一个位置。如果这个特征消失,我们则可以认为它与人为分析有关,因为X线数据与特征是否存在始终保持一致。也就是说,我们将发现有两种重建结果,一种包含这个特征,另一种则没有,后者导致我们怀疑这个特点是否真实存在。从另一个方面来说,如果特征重新出现,我们就能更加坚信它是真实的。尽管这个工作看上去很麻烦,但是现代模式识别项目(Gavrielides, et al, 2002; Nandi, et al, 2006)可以自主推进这个研究的进程,为每张CT图中的病理特征绘制一张"信心地图"。将这种高度非线性模式识别法与最新发明的统计反演法做比较是一件十分有趣的事情,后者根据包含不同白噪声矩阵的样本,将得出不同的方程答案(Kaipio, Somersalo, 2004)。

10.13 人体CT剂量

X线的主要缺点就是它可能引发癌症。因此,我们必须采取屏蔽措施,最起码要保证我们检测、治愈的癌症应比由X线检测引发的多(Bailar,1976)。所以我们必须强制寻找各种办法提高图像质量与X线剂量的比率,并且控制辐射总量及皮肤受照剂量在可以接受的范围之内(Gordon,1976b)。只有尝试将CT的X线辐射剂量降到最低,我们才能知道这样做是否可以得到大小为2~4mm(见下文)的目标影像。

如果考虑到在一般的放射学中发生的现象,我们将会更加重视将图像质量与X线剂量比率最大化的问题。受到电离辐射的人群中,15%是因为接受医学治疗(Ron,2003)。1999年,德国所有放射学检查手段中CT所占比率仅为5%,然而其辐射剂量却占总X线辐射剂量的40%(Kalender,2000)。在美国,从1990年中期至2002年,CT检查比率由4%增长至15%,辐射剂量占有率由40%增长至75%(Wiest, et al,2002)。这意味着,平均下来,CT研究辐射剂量是其他非CT X线检查手段的16倍。在CT技术得到普遍应用后,截至2002年,人均X线辐射剂量较之前已经增长了4倍。

计算过程如下。设:

D_i = i 时间的CT剂量

N_i = i 时间的CT检查次数

d = 非CT辐射剂量

n = 非CT放射检查次数

T_i = i 时间总人群辐射剂量

根据Wiest等人的计算,我们得出:

$D_1/(D_1+d) = 0.4$ 第一时间段(1990年中期)

$N_1/(N_1+n) = 0.04$

$D_2/(D_2+d) = 0.75$ 第二时间段(2002)

$N_2/(N_2+n) = 0.15$

据此:

$D_1/N_1 = 16d/n$

$D_2/N_2 = 17d/n$

我们假设n与d不变,得出的结果是一致的。我们还得到:

$D_2=3d$

所以

$T_2=D_2+d=4d$

有人可能会想,CT技术的应用使得那些非CT放射线检查的数量减少了,所以n与d这些数字应该有所降低。然而,事实上,这些数字反而还有微弱的增长(Rehani,2000)。

CT X线技术的应用迅速普及(Prokop,2005),CT已经成为人们曝光于X线下的主要因素(Hatziioannou, et al, 2003),其中儿科CT尤为令人担忧(Linton, Mettler, 2003)。相比于成人,儿童对放射线更为敏感,更有可能因照射X线罹患癌症(Brenner, et al, 2001),特别是乳腺癌(Li, et al, 1983; Rosenfield, et al, 1989; Donnelly, Frush, 2001; Berdon, Slovis, 2002; Brenner, 2002; Linton, Mettler, 2003)。对于经期前的女人也同样如此,因为此时她们体内含有大量增殖的细胞(Ferguson, Anderson, 1981; Vogel, et al, 1981; Going, et al, 1988; Dabrosin, et al, 1997; Dzendrowskyj, et al, 1997)。这就意味着应该在女性来月经期间拍摄CT,这时体内增殖的细胞数目最少(Bjarnason, 1996)。从另一方面看,有说法称乳腺癌手术应该在月经期间进行,这种说法被证明是谬论(Kroman, 2008; Thorpe, et al, 2008; Grant, et al, 2009)。在经期间拍摄CT还可以降低打乱女性生理周期、改变组织性能的风险(Malini, et al, 1985; Fowler, et al, 1990; Graham, et al, 1995; Kato, et al, 1995; White, et al, 1998; Hussain, et al, 1999)和组织特性(Ferguson, Anderson, 1981; Vogel, et al, 1981; Nelson, et al, 1985; Malberger, et al, 1987; Going, et al, 1988; Ferguson, et al, 1990, 1992; Graham, et al, 1995; Simpson, et al, 1996; Dabrosin, et al, 1997; Dzendrowskyj, et al, 1997; Zarghami, et al, 1997; Cubeddu, et al, 2000)。

10.14 聚焦乳腺癌检查

我记不清最初是什么原因促使我将CT技术应用于乳腺摄影,但我记得我在NIH听证会上向大概500位听众介绍我的观点,我建议女性拍摄CT影像以探查乳腺小肿瘤,每次检查计算只需要花费大约1周的时间。当时在场的人都觉得我是异想天开,发出阵阵嘲笑声(Gordon, 1976a)。做人就需要厚脸皮,我用自己的方式进行了有力的还击[正如多年后我冒着风险计算了(Gordon, 1989)使用避孕套减少HIV病毒/艾滋病传播的有效率(Gordon, 1987)]。我率先研究了一种直接解决乳腺CT扫描所需高分辨率的算法,并将计算机处理时间压缩到可以接受的范围内(Gordon, 1977)。我又首先向医学界提出减少CT剂量(Gordon, 1976b)。在CT分辨率可以达到的水平方面,我与物理学家们进行了激烈的辩论。早期乳腺癌不易被检测的事实令我心痛,后来我越发确定如果人们能听信我的建议,可以拯救更多的生命!这对我来说简直就是一种折磨,人的脸皮一定不能太厚。

很不幸,从长远角度看,乳腺X线检查给女性健康带来的危害远大于好处,这确实是一种头脑发热的做法:

"在陈述过程中,我描述了乳腺X线检查的一些好处以及它带来的众多危害,并且尝试在两者之间寻找平衡。同时,我认为对于绝经前的女性来说,乳腺X线扫描没有任何好处。虽然1988年时,我以伦敦大学国王学院院长的身份参与国家筛查项目,但是我的论点却遭到非议,很多听众愤然离场。我得到了深刻的教训,很多观点,特别是关于乳腺癌筛查方面的,没有得到听众们的认可,甚至没能引起一场理性的辩论"(Baum, 2004)。

我在1978年时转战到了Manitoba大学，在当地的活动中重新振奋起来，通过远程放射学提供服务。在发展中国家也是这样，放射学家往往在城市中心工作，通过远程放射学来服务于住在偏远地区及乡村的居民。那时没有互联网，只能利用声音耦合器通过电话线传输图像，这还真不是一件容易的事情。我对远程放射学提出了更高的要求，建议通过仅传输投影数据来进行远程CT检测（Rangayyan，Gordon，1982a），包括乳腺癌检测，然后集中进行图像重建和诊断。我们建立了从布兰登（Brandon）到温尼伯（Winnipeg）的传输渠道（大约200km），并进行了实验（Gordon，Rangaraj，1982）。后来，虽然没能得到当地政府的进一步支持，但我仍将实验的范围扩大到了中国。然而，天安门事件迫使我在中国的同事分散开，使得项目研究无法继续进行。当时，由于经济条件所限，我们只能提供光导摄像管摄影机及分辨率为512×512、灰度为8bit的数字化图像（当时，数字照相机约需5万美元），所以该项目绝对称不上是临床学上的重大科研成果。就在因特网诞生前，我们的研究项目终止了（Gordon，1990）。回想起来，是我自己走了回头路，在没有足够技术支持的条件下却企图进行原理求证来使人信服。

10.15 显像模式结合

还处于"悬而未决"的下一步是考虑在一个扫描仪中整合多种显像模式。起初，人们研究叠合，比如说在一个断层上显示一副CT图像和一副MRI图像，但是共轴或实时扫描仪的机械钢性显然是超凡的。当我在NIH工作时，曾向一个由PET/核医学临床医生组成的参观小组介绍了这种想法，如今我们已经有了PET/CT扫描仪。

之后，我又提议通过机械手段在"更多维的空间"中处理数据（Gordon，Coumans，1984）。我举了双能量CT的例子，每个像素点得到两个吸收系数（X1，X2），与MRI相结合，即得到两个弛豫时间（T1，T2）。观察者们完全可以通过每种模式下显现出的组织特征辨别出组织结构或者肿瘤形状。然而，两个2D空间交错的产物就是一个4D空间（X1，X2，T1，T2），在这种情况下，我们可以从中找到特殊的联系，做出更精准的判断。通过将2D与3D乳腺X线摄影技术进行类比，2D数据空间得到的是来自4D数据空间的投影，这些投影中存在聚类重叠部分，使得一些细节区域难以分辨。这种关联需要凭借经验来解答。这个研究项目旨在将成像病理学的研究提上一个新的台阶。

10.16 CT成像中去卷积算法及自适应邻域

我和我从事远程放射学研究的博士后学生Rangaraj Rangayyan一起进行了另外两项大胆而富有创意的尝试。首先，我们通过去卷积算法解决有限角度范围内CT扫描的各向异性问题（Gordon，Rangayyan，1983；Gordon，et al，1985；Soble，et al，1985）；其次，我们发明了自适应邻域图像处理法，抑制CT图像中因高对比度对象（金属植入物，骨骼或微钙化物质）（Rangayyan，Gordon，1982b）产生的条纹伪影，并提出一个类似的方法以数字化乳房X线摄影图像模拟高剂量乳房干板摄影术，也就是说，不额外加量（Gordon，Rangayyan，1984a、b；Dhawan，et al，1986a、b；Dhawan，Gordon，1986）。自适应邻域成为了图像处理中的一个子分支（Jiang，et al，1992；Sivaramakrishna，et al，2000；Rangayyan，et al，2001；Vasile，et al，2004）。

10.17 维纳去卷积技术（Wiener Deconvolution）

埃塔·达万（Atam Dhawan）将去卷积方法运用到了极致，他解决了一个CT算法自身的点扩散函数（PSF）去卷积问题。魏因施泰因曾将其阐释为模糊函数（Vainshtein, 1971）（图10.4），但现在，对于手边的算法和几何学来说，它是特定的。比如说，一个容易被看成圆形的圆盘，通过在有限角度范围内拍摄的几个图像重建，得到的圆盘影像呈现出椭圆形。我们做出大胆猜想（也就是数学上的错误），将由一个CT算法重建得到的图像，看作是一个由于真实图像受到单一PSF影响而产生的具有各向异性的模糊像。因此，我们采用维纳滤波恢复未受点扩散函数影响的图像。实验结果令人惊讶，在采取维纳滤波技术后（Dhawan, et al, 1984a, 1985），我们得到了达万妻子脸部的影像（图10.4A）。之前，我们运用有限范围内的ART重建算法也不能清晰地分辨脸部图像（图10.4B），在维纳去卷积后图像会凸出变形（图10.4C）（Dhawan, et al, 1985）。ART算法本身就在FBP算法的基础上取得了巨大的进展，而现在维纳滤波技术的运用又在ART算法的基础上更进一步，并且没有增加CT剂量。这个算法适用于投影数据非常有限的光学显微镜，用于估计痣的厚度（Gordon,

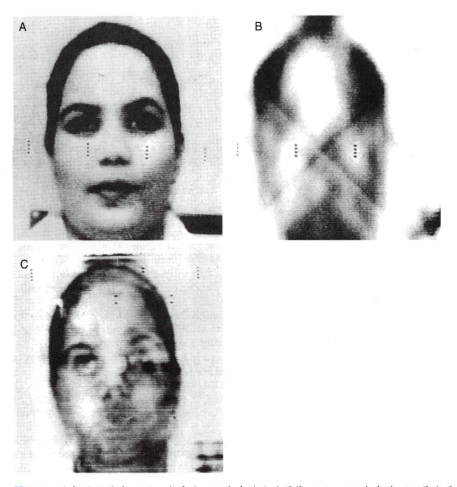

图10.4 脸部原始图片（A），由乘法ART重建的脸的图像（B），从5个角度（0°是水平度，45°，67.5°，90°，112.5°和135°）。维纳滤波后，点扩散函数去卷积后的图像（C）（Dhawan, 1985）

1983b；Dhawan，et al，1984a、b、c）。在那之后，就再也没有人研究过这个算法了。我仍在等待有人研发一种机器人皮肤扫描仪，用于筛查早期黑色素瘤。因为转移前的肿瘤没有受到外层组织的掩盖，所以这种检测相较于乳腺检测更加简单。

维纳滤波技术的应有还存在3个问题有待进一步研究。第一，点扩散函数并不像我们假设的那样是空间不变的，托普利兹矩阵（Toeplitz matrix）可以解决这个问题（Nagy，1993）。托普利兹矩阵是为纠正光学色差而设计的，比如在哈勃天文望远镜一个零件放反了或者其他一些错误操作时，会产生色差（Baker，et al，1992；Beekman，et al，1996）。第二，图像中引入了边缘振荡效应，可能会被抑制（Ruttimann，et al，1989；Hu，et al，1991；Zhou，et al，1993；Schlueter，et al，1994；Sijbers，Postnov，2004）。第三，去卷积图像并不是投影方程式的答案，但是也许可以作为如ART这样的迭代CT算法的起始图像，最后可能会聚于一副既去卷积又满足方程式的图像（Gordon，1973）。

根据经验，所有基于解决联立方程式的CT算法得到的图像都是相似的。而维纳去卷积技术却惊人的不同。ART算法曾被证实可将未知图像与重建图像之间的欧几里得（Euclidean）距离最小化（Kaipio，Somersalo，2004），而乘法ART（MART）算法则得到熵值最大化的图像（Lent，1977；Dusaussoy，Abdou，1991；Lent，Censor，1991）。因此，它们被归类为数学家们所说的正则化算法（Bertero，Boccacci，1998；Engl，et al，2000）。但是维纳去卷积法则证明正则化算法实际上得出的是错误的结论。因此，CT反过来带给数学家们一些新的见解。

10.18 纵向图像的配准

我在一场由我组织的工业CT研讨会（Gordon，1985a）上向大家介绍了维纳过滤法（Dhawan，et al，1985），我借此机会总结了自己关于有限视图CT的几点思考（Rangayyan，et al，1985），并谈及怎样检测小型乳腺肿瘤（Gordon，1985b）。3D乳腺成像可能会显示很多假阳性"病变"，而且之后我们了解到一些小型肿瘤会退化（Nielsen，et al，1987；Nielsen，1989）。此外，特别是因为很多小肿瘤还没有血管化，它们的特征与邻近的正常组织并无太大差异。所以，我们唯一可以确定为小肿瘤病变的一个征象就是不断生长。为了观测到这个特征，我们必须精确配准两幅乳腺纵向图像（以"筛查间隔"为基点，拍摄于不同的时间）。由于乳房是一种"柔软的物体"，它每次不可能以同一状态被置于精确的扫描仪之下，也不可能将两幅图像以数字化的方式直接相减，进行对比。我基于硬件几何整经机的迭代法运用提出了一种复杂的配准算法。硬件几何整经机是一种具有特殊用途的电脑，最近开始投入市场（Gordon，1985b）。

我开始寻找一种稳健的3D图像配准算法，通过每个体素邻域内独特的内部结构、局部肌理及3D纹理进行图像配准。我连续3位学生的博士论文都围绕这个研究课题展开。我和周晓华（Xiaohua Zhou）讨论了这个领域的相关问题（Zhou，Gordon 1989），并进一步提出了一种用泽尔尼克（Zernicke）多项式制订框标的方法。这种方法可以为一组3D乳腺图像从多个基点生成几何扭曲（Zhou，1991）。Andrzej Mazur越过晓华的研究，他认为自己可以不用框标、而用模拟退火算法处理这个问题（Mazur，1992；Mazur，et al，1993）。Radhika Sivaramakrishna采用一种名为starbyte转型的算法将乳腺图像分成几个区域，可以将纵向图像通过这几个区域进行对比（Sivaramakrishna，Gordon，1997b；Sivaramakrishna，1998）。我们运用卡通人物Waldo的形象制作了一个生动的展示片，讲述怎样配准和比对图片能够比较容易发现肿瘤。但是只有当我们采用3D成像技术取代2D乳腺X线摄影时，这些规则才有效（Gordon, Sivaramakrishna, 1999）。有一部分研究工作是由我和Anthony Miller共同完成的。这也是我唯一一个得到资金资助的乳腺癌方面的研究项目，由我和米勒共同担任项目研究员。如果没有高层的支持，乳腺癌研究方面的同行评审给我的印象就是："先向我们展示得到的图像，然后我们会给予你资金支持来获得这些图像"，这就是一种类似第22条军规一样的自相矛盾的困境（Heller, 1961）。国会证词（Gordon, 1992）对这种尴尬的处境并没有什么影响。

3D乳腺纵向图像配准具有了实用价值，令我非常满意。但是在那时，我们的项目仍然是"落选之马"（Sivaramakrishna, et al, 1999; Sivaramakrishna, 2005a; Guo, et al, 2006）。此外，还有一些配准工作有待进一步研究。"在数据收集期间比对两幅图像的做法貌似是可信的，这样做可以使用相较于获得原始图像所需更低的剂量，获得差别图像。如果患者的数字图像记录得以保存，那么从今往后患者便可以接受这样的增量放射学检测"（Gordon, 1979b）。这就好比对视频进行高效传输（Burg, 2003）或是说对串行部分进行压缩（Lee, et al, 1993），只传输一帧到下一帧之间图像发生改变的部分。在增量放射学中，应重视研究减少不同图像的结构性配准噪声的方法（Knoll, Delp, 1986; Gong, et al, 1992; Bruzzone, Cossu, 2003）。

零对比肿瘤会导致正常乳房组织结构局部变形（Chang, et al, 1982; Shaw de Paredes, 1994; Stomper, et al, 1994; Goldberg, Dwyer, 1995; Maes, et al, 1997），纵向配准可以此现象为依据（Mazur, et al, 1993; Liu, et al, 2006），检测零对比肿瘤。这种4D（3D加时间维度）的方法也可以用来检测结构扭曲。在运用未经配准的二维乳腺X线摄影纵向图像进行早期乳腺癌检测时，这种结构扭曲的征象常常被忽略（Ayres, Rangayyan, 2007; Rangayyan, et al, 2007; Banik, et al, 2009）。

在1990年代初期，出现了一种很奇怪的现象：标准乳房X线摄影检查领域的领军人物们都极力抵制乳腺3D成像。从他们的出版物记录中可以看出，他们对3D有关的新发明比较感兴趣，在后期才认可了3D技术。但是，大多数乳腺成像研究者们还是把标准乳房X线摄影检查奉为"黄金标准"。我将其称为铅标准（排在银和铜之后）。这些研究者们对标准乳腺X线摄影检查过分执著，直接导致数十年来乳腺3D成像研究缺乏资金支持。不仅仅是我的研究工作遇到了这样的问题，很多与我的研究毫无干系的项目也遭遇了这样的困境。因此，乳腺影像与3D技术的结合仍处于萌芽状态，进度远晚于其他任何一种放射学成像技术。比如说，尽管乳腺2D数字摄影或者3D MRI技术"已经得到了广泛的应用"（Nelson, et al, 2009），"却没有针对一般罹患乳腺癌风险的女性进行试验，评估这些技术的有效性"，更不用说3D X线CT摄影技术。研究者们在标准2D乳腺摄影技术的基础上停滞不前（Abbott, 1899），女性乳腺癌防治小组对3D乳腺成像工作的延迟不管不问，这是当前乳腺癌研究工作面临的两大误区。科学社会学家们应该好好研究一下这个问题：

"从现有的乳腺癌检测、治疗手段的失败案例或短缺程度来看，这些误区直接导致美国乳腺癌发病率大幅上升。医学家和研究工作者们对乳腺癌的死亡率轻描淡写，却大肆宣扬那些幸存者的事例，虽然他们很清楚那些医学协议会限制治疗效果，却还是推崇遵守这些协议。"（Ehrenreich, 2001）

标准乳房X线检查的图像质量已经饱和，显然达到了它的极限（Spelic, 2009）（图10.5）。因此，我们只能期待通过转向3D CT技术，来进一步提高单位X线剂量的图片质量。

我曾经一直支持并资助"为治愈而奔跑（runs for the cure）"公益活动，但是后来我发现这个活动所筹集的大部分资金都用来维持现状，而且它是在告诫女性，她们得亲自进

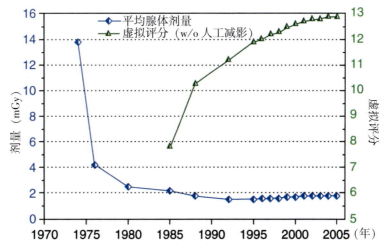

图10.5 "这张图显示了1970年代至2005年,平均腺体剂量(下降曲线)和标准乳腺X线摄影的图像质量(上升曲线)"(Spelic,2009)(经美国FDA授权)

行这方面的研究,所以我不再支持这个活动。极少数理解我意图的人,很快就死于乳腺癌。这个活动存在的另一个问题就是,它将重点放在乳腺癌晚期患者身上。在癌症早期,患者往往不会表现出症状,她们也不清楚正确应对乳腺癌的方法。所以很少有患者能及时预防乳腺癌,或者在早期接受筛查。其实真正的"治愈方法(the cure)"应该关注那些没有症状的早期患者。

10.19 更快更好的ART算法

我们已经知道了如何加速ART算法,使它收敛于三次左右迭代(Guan, Gordon 1994, 1996; Guan, et al, 1998; Colquhoun, Gordon, 2005b)。因为速度是ART算法无法克服的瓶颈,所以FBP算法数十年来在速度方面一直处于领先地位。ART算法研究者们花费了这么长的时间,终于发现只要采取对投影进行重新排序的小技巧,而不是按照角度顺序进行处理,就可以保持投影过程中彼此相邻的超平面尽可能的正交,进而加快收敛速度。如今,尽管绕了一段弯路,我的同事格伦·柯恩宽(Glen Colquhoun)已经初步掌握了证据,证明完全3D ART算法并不需要采取类似的技巧。

艾姿碧塔·玛祖尔(Elzbieta Mazur)发现,旋转每个像素,使其投影呈矩形而不是梯形,这样可以大幅提升ART重建算法的性能。当然,前提是每幅投影需从不同的角度进行拍摄(Mazur, Gordon, 1995)。我们全然不顾像素刚性的影响,认为如点画法(Düchting, 2001),当从足够远的距离观察图片时,每个像素的精确形状、大小、方向及位置的影响不大。我们计划将这种概念应用于实践工作。

我们还发现由乘法迭代算法MART重建得到的图像可以通过修正值自乘进行锐化(PMART=Power MART)。令我们惊讶的是,这种算法存在一个临界值,超过这个临界值后,计算就会变得混乱(Badea, Gordon, 2004)。这个问题后来得到了解决,并进一步形成了"改进PMART"算法(Yoshinaga, et al, 2008)。

10.20 以小乳腺癌为目标进行流行病学推断

Miller一直在为加拿大国家乳腺普查研究得出的结果进行辩护,他的行动使我意识到流行病学在解决乳腺癌问题上的重要性（Baines, et al, 1986; Burhenne, Burhenne, 1993; Mettlin, Smart, 1993; Miller, 1993; Baines, 1994; Tarone, 1995; Bailar, MacMahon, 1997）。流行病学家约翰·贝勒（John Bailar）在1970年左右进行了标准乳腺X线检查试验（Bailar, 1976; Lerner, 2001），将放射剂量减少了7倍（Spelic, 2009）（图10.6），这更加坚定了我的想法。因此，我开始通过分析流行病学的数据，推测有影像上不可见的小尺寸肿瘤的存在，并且，我试着去思索，我们究竟需要对多大尺寸的肿瘤成像，才能够对疾病的治疗产生影响。结果令人震惊：在当时，如果能以100%的效率检测出4mm的肿瘤并进行摧毁，那么抑制乳腺癌的成功率将高达99.6%（Sivaramakrishna, Gordon, 1997a）。随着商业X线CT逐渐达到0.5mm的分辨率、数字化X线摄影分辨率为0.05~0.1mm的检测仪愈发普及，这个目标是可以实现的。数据推断必然存在风险，为了确定结论的有效性，我与流行病学家们进行了合作，考察不同的数据集是否能推断出相同的结论（Sun, et al, 1998; Chapman, et al, 1999; Sun, et al, 2002; Verschraegen, et al, 2005; Vinh-Hung, Gordon, 2005）。结果证明这个结论是可靠的：如果我们可以检测并摧毁2~4mm大小的肿瘤，那么实际上，我们便可以遏制癌症的发生。大多数这样的肿瘤都没有或未能成功转移。

10.21 开展各种成像模式之间的竞争

我设想，多种成像模式之间展开一场竞争，筛查转移前肿瘤，要包括MRI（Tomanek, et al, 2000）和EIT（电阻抗断层成像）（Murugan, 2000）。乳腺MRI检查费用太高，乳腺EIT检查分辨率太低（我认为原因在于使用的电极数量级太少，现在在128（Ye, et al, 2008）至256（Cherepenin, et al, 2002）之间，使得这些技术难以用于乳腺3D X线筛查。然而，与X线CT相比，这些技术都是无害的。我认为这些技术在达到物理极限之前，都具备研究价值。以下是我最近参考的一份不完全目录的截取部分（cf. Suri, et al, 2006），记载了乳腺成像领域所应用的多种物理技术：

- CT激光乳房X线检查（Yee, 2009）
- EIT（电阻抗断层成像）（Cherepeninetal, 2002; PrasadandHouserkova, 2007; Chen, et al, 2008; Halter, et al, 2008; Steiner, et al, 2008; Ye, et al, 2008），包括最新的重建磁共振EIT（Gao, He, 2008; Ng, et al, 2008）和EIT光谱仪（EIS）（Choi, et al, 2007; Kim, et al, 2007a; Poplack, et al, 2007; Karellas, Vedantham, 2008）
- 微波成像（Fang, et al, 2004; Chen, et al, 2007, 2008; Hand, 2008; Kanj, Popovic, 2008; Karellas, Vedantham, 2008; Pramanik, et al, 2008），雷达（Poyvasi, et al, 2005; Flores-Tapia, et al, 2008），微波成像光谱仪（MIS）（Poplack, et al, 2007; Lazebnik, et al, 2008）和双极化法（Woten, El-Shenawee, 2008）
- 微波热声扫描CT（Nie, et al, 2008）
- 分子和纳米粒子成像（Rayavarapu, et al, 2007），包括量子点（Park, Ikeda, 2006; Chang, et al, 2008）
- MRI（Kuhl, et al, 2005; Park, Ikeda, 2006; Brenner, Parisky, 2007; Kim, et al, 2007b; Hand, 2008; Karellas, Vedantham, 2008; Yee, 2009）和MRS（Smith, Andreopoulou, 2004）
- 多频互导纳扫描（TAS）（Oh, et al, 2007）
- 近红外光谱成像（NIR）（Poplack, et al, 2007）
- 中子受激发射计算机断层扫描（Bender, et al, 2007）
- 光学成像（Huang, Zhu, 2004; Park, Ikeda,

2006; Karellas, Vedantham, 2008; Konovalov, et al, 2008; Lazebnik, et al, 2008; Fang, et al, 2009),包括透照法（Blyschak, et al, 2004; Simick, et al, 2004）

- PET或正电子发射乳腺X线检查（PEM）和PET/CT（Pawlak, Gordon, 2005; Jan, et al, 2006; Park, Ikeda, 2006; Aliaga, et al, 2007; Brenner, Parisky, 2007; Prasad, Houserkova, 2007; Shibata, et al, 2007; Tafra, 2007; Thie, 2007; Yang, et al, 2007; Zhang, et al, 2007; Karellas, Vedantham, 2008; Bowen, et al, 2009; Wu, et al, 2009; Yee, 2009），可能与强磁场相结合成为Mag PET，在正电子湮灭前限制其范围（Iida, et al, 1986; Rickey, et al, 1992; Hammer, et al, 1994; Burdette, et al, 2009），从而提高PET/MRI的分辨率（Cherry, et al, 2008; Judenhofer, et al, 2008）
- 光声层析成像（Pramanik, et al, 2008）
- 质子和重离子CT（IonCT）（Holley, et al, 1981a、b; Muraishi, et al, 2009）
- 单光子发射CT（SPECT）（More, et al, 2007; Karellas, Vedantham, 2008）和乳腺核素成像（McKinley, et al, 2006; Li, et al, 2007; Prasad, Houserkova, 2007; Spanu, et al, 2007; Thie, 2007）
- 超导量子干涉器件（SQUID）（Anninos, et al, 2000）和SQUID MRI（Clarke, et al, 2007）
- 热声学断层扫描（Pramanik, et al, 2008）
- 层析X射线照相组合（Karellas, et al, 2008; Karellas, Vedantham, 2008; Dobbins, 2009; Gur, et al, 2009; Yee, 2009）
- 超声波（US）（Huang, Zhu, 2004; Brenner, Parisky, 2007; Karellas, Vedantham, 2008; Yee, 2009）
- 超声弹性成像（Bagchi, 2007; Garra, 2007）和振动声成像（Alizad, et al,

2005; Silva, et al, 2006）
- 超声波反射成像（Steiner, et al, 2008）
- X线衍射增强成像CT或X线相敏成像CT（Bravin, et al, 2007; Karellas, Vedantham, 2008; Zhou, Brahme, 2008; Kao, et al, 2009; Parham, et al, 2009）
- X线散射光子能量鉴别CT（Van Uytven, et al, 2007, 2008）
- 单能或双能X射线成像CT（Chen, Ning, 2003; McKinley, et al, 2006; Kalender, Kyriakou, 2007; Kwan, et al, 2007; Li, et al, 2007; Karellas, et al, 2008; Karellas, Vedantham, 2008; Lindfors, et al, 2008; Nelsona, et al, 2008; Yang, et al, 2008; Yee, 2009; McKinley, et al, 2004; Kappadath, Shaw, 2005; Bliznakova, et al, 2006），特别是采用同步加速器辐射（Fabbri, et al, 2002; Pani, et al, 2004）

这些参考中包含很多双能成像技术，其中一些融合了两种成像模式，以提高单一模式下得到的图像的质量。如果将现有的成像方法排列成一个矩阵，不难发现，目前为止人们只考虑到了其中一小部分两种成像模式的组合。虽然有一定难度，但是，一次融合3种或以上的成像模式在技术层面上是可行的（Cherry, 2006）。

因为这些新方法耗资巨大，很多研究者们放弃尝试。从另一方面来说，怀有这样的忧虑是因为他们缺乏远见，实际上所有的高科技技术研发都要花费大额资金，之后单位成本就会下降。但即使是耗资巨大，例如一次MRI筛查仍需花费1000美元之多，但最终的问题是：女性的生命到底值多少钱？

在各种乳腺成像模式之间开展竞争的想法（目的是"为了治愈"）激励我着手举办一系列"乳腺X线检查替代方案（WAM）"讨论会。我本以为在找到对抗乳腺癌的方法后，研讨会才会结束。可惜的是，只有两场研讨会成功举行，一场于2004年在Winnipeg召开（Colquhoun, Gordon, 2005a; Sivaramakrishna，2005b，c），另一场在Tibor Tot的主持下于2005年在哥本哈根召开。也许这个活动应该由一个诊治乳腺癌的专业组织负责，重点筛查并摧毁转移前的肿瘤。

10.22 未来设想0：聚焦像素 (Foxels) 和第七代乳腺筛查CT技术

在第二次WAM讨论会上，Colquhoun和我向大家介绍了我们所谓的"逆向锥束"成像（Colquhoun，et al，2004；Colquhoun，Gordon，2005a）。这个结论是在过去几十年观察的基础上得来的。尽管X射线管的聚焦光斑没有大幅度减小，但是探测仪零件体积却显著减小。因此，从探测仪像素的角度来看，X线成像一般被认为是发自一个点光源的射线束以锥辐射照射患者，它的聚焦光斑宽度是它本身宽度的10倍以上，射线的形状呈逆向锥束的形状。为了充分利用这个特点，我们将聚焦光斑划分为一个由发光像素组成的阵列，每个发光像素的大小与探测仪原件相当，称为聚焦像素（foxels）。我们现在正在研究编写计算机代码，在迭代重建过程中细解卷积，在不增加剂量的前提下不断提高空间分辨率。Michael J. A. Potter加入了我们的行列，一起研究这个问题（Potter，et al，2009）。我们意识到逆向锥束CT与"反几何CT"（Schmidt，et al，2006；Mazin，Pelc，2008；Bhagtani，Schmidt，2009）不同，后者并没有对聚焦光斑图像进行去卷积，而是使用多重、广泛分布的X线束在一组小的探测器阵列上成像。

我们又重新尝试了我以前研究的超平面法（Gordon，1973），并把CT当做一种元启发式算法（meta-algorithm），使标准CT算法（ART，MART，perhaps even FBP，etc.）彼此之间相互辅助交叉，同时又与其他多种图像处理及模式识别技术结合，包括维纳滤波（Wiener filtration）、替代ART和其他一些算法、图像增强、图像分割、聚焦像素去卷积（foxel deconvolution）、确定功能的可靠性等等。通过使用这种元程序法，我们可以更有效地对转移前肿瘤进行筛查，并实施摧毁。最后，为了尽可能达到Vainshtein所提出的均向性成像的目标，并得到$1/r2PSF$（由于胸壁阻挡，对于乳腺摄影来说，这个目标难以达到），我们编写的代码适用于任意位置的X线源及2D探测器阵列。只有确定了定位配置的最优集或程序［包括替代数据空间子集或"分区"（Pan，et al，2009）］，机架才能携带X线源［以动态准直或者编码准直的方式（Pan，et al，2009）］和探测器阵列进行独立运动。齐次坐标的使用大大简化了我们的编码过程（Schaller，et al，1998；Karolczak，et al，2001；Alpuche Avilés，2004）。

很多人推崇将CT检查与工业生产结合，形成一种"即插即用"的效果。这要求算法开发者采用真实CT扫描仪的数据，并生成有用的图像。这也的确是他们追求的目标："……在工程师们具备使用高级图像重建算法的相关经验，就可以运用这些知识设计更高效的CT扫描仪。这些研究在专用CT系统中较易取得突破，如头部或颈部CT，牙科CT及乳腺CT"。显然，上段提到的提升CT成像性能的方法与这种倡议背道而驰。

我们将这种新尝试命名为第七代CT，因为它具有以下4个新特点：①它是一种运用聚焦像素的几何精确算法，可以控制任何3D X线源及探测器阵列的定位，进行3D重建；②在成像计算过程中，采用元编程可以选择不同的CT算法、成像方式及模式识别步骤；③重建算法与扫描系统之间存在互动，反馈信息可以根据目前所得3D图像指导X线源及探测器阵列进行下一步定位；④专供机架进行特别定位的3D计算机存储阵列与包含重建3D图像的主计算机存储阵列内信息的差异，可以在二者间进行合理的3D转换。

我将第七代CT技术标为"未来设想0"，因为现在只需要决心及少量资金，就可以制造它所需要的所有元件或是撰写相关代码。

10.23 未来设想1：智能操控X射线微束

只要能在技术或物理学上取得突破，X线CT就仍有升级的空间。智能操控X射线微束就是其中一种。30年前，理查德·韦伯（Richard L. Webber）成立了一间实验室，专门研究这种技术（Webber，1979）：

"间隔适当的时间，在每个点照射同一定向光束，就能得到相同的信噪比。如果可以根据每一局域光学厚度，动态调节X射线频谱的峰值，以得到最优能量，就可以进一步减小CT剂量"（Gordon，1979b）。

早在1950年，日立公司（Hitachi）就尝试将此技术应用于CT（Moon，1950），通过电子显微技术操控电子束，生成一个移动的X线聚焦光斑（Tateno，Tanaka，1976；Tateno，et al，1976）。通过移动小孔依次屏蔽不能穿过小孔的X线，从而对X线实施操控。

通过智能操控X线微束技术减少剂量的方法之一，就是应用一种特殊的模式识别方式。我一开始总是回避采用这种方式，现在回想起来，我发现自己常常提到它。除了受限于准直仪的光子，如今的X线成像仪器会从各个角度发射X射线光子穿透人体，光子不加选择地撞击所有特征点。设想一下，如果我们只发射少量光子，从而获得一幅3D"侦察"图像，这幅图像中将包含真正的病征以及由噪声波动造成的假象。随后，我们可以将光束锁定在那些可疑的特征点上（通过图像特点或一些先验标准判断得出）。如果这些特征点是由于噪声波动而产生，则它们最终会消失，相反那些真实病征会变得更加明显。这种方法可以"智能地"引导X线微束照射那些需要照射的部位，从而大幅减少总剂量。想要实现这个方法，需先研发一种小型可操控X射线激光器（Fill，1992），或是折射和聚焦X线束（Cederstroem，et al，1999；Jorgensen，et al，1999；Gorenstein，2007），抑或是掠角反射X线束（Signorato，et al，1997；Harvey，et al，2001）。这些X射线极具强度，其中每个辐射光子都具有足够的能量，可以用于乳腺及身体其他部位成像。同步加速器拥有足够的射束强度（Burattini，et al，1995），可以检验这些想法的可行性，它现在用于乳腺X射线衍射成像的实验中（Bravin，et al，2007），然而，它的体积太大（通常有600m），想要通过它完成3D成像，需要环绕患者进行3D双轴旋转。即使正在研发的"小型"同步加速器也有一个"房间大小"（Lyncean Technologies，2009）（cf. Yamada，et al，2004；Hirai，et al，2006）（图10.6），但是考虑到梅奥诊所（Mayo Clinic）曾研发出一款直径为5m的CT扫描仪（Altschuler，et al，1980），那么，在一位女性的乳房周围旋转一整个房间那么大的仪器并不算太荒谬。

10.24 未来设想2：栅门和纠缠光子：乳腺成像如同一盘海战棋

大多数X射线光子都经过两次随机排列，一次是在正极发射时，另一次是在散射或被吸收时，均服从Poisson统计规律。对于可见光光子，已经有方法可以通过改变电压控

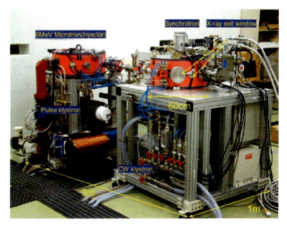

图10.6 一个"小型"的同步X线加速器（From Yamada，et al，2004；Elsevier授权图片）

制它们的发射，以实现量子水平通信及光学计算。这也就是所谓的栅门光子。在光学计算中，每个比特就相当于一个光量子（Imamoglu, Yamamoto, 1994; Law, Kimble, 1997; Kim, et al, 1998, 1999; Benjamin, 2000; Michler, et al, 2000; McKeever, 2004; Oxborrow, Sinclair, 2005; Dayan, et al, 2008），也可以被极化（Lukishova, et al, 2007），还可以使它们瞄准一个特定的方向（Taminiau, et al, 2008）。如果我们能找到方法如此控制X射线光子，光子统计性能将大幅提升，因为我们只用处理一次Poisson过程，而不用解决两个Poisson分布的卷积（Melvin, et al, 2002）。如此，X线成像就好比一盘海战棋（Hasbro, 2004），一方在看不见对方领地（乳腺）的情况下投下一枚"炸弹"（光子），然后被告知是否击中"船只"（肿瘤）（Foo, 1999）。更明晰的统计数据能够有效减少剂量。在这里，我们面临的挑战是如何研发一种可以发射栅门X射线光子的纳米材料。

还有一种选择可以达到和栅门光子一样的效果（Edward H. Sargent, 个人交流）（Sargent, 2005）。有一种叫做参量下转换的方法，它是一种非线性光学过程，可以生成一对时间相关的纠缠光子（Abouraddy, et al, 2001），其中一个为X射线光子，另一个为可见光光子。如果我们检测到了可见光光子，就知道同时有一个X射线光子发射向乳腺了。

10.25 从现在起消灭乳腺癌！

终极乳腺癌筛查扫描仪将通过对比现有图像与该乳腺以前的3D图像，检测出所有的转移前肿瘤，并采用现有任何一种处于研究中的切除技术（Noguchi, 2003; Simmons, 2003; Singletary, 2003; O'Neal, et al, 2004; Roubidoux, et al, 2004; Vargas, et al, 2004; Agnese, Burak, 2005; Glaiberman, et al, 2005; Huston, Simmons, 2005; Lobo, et al, 2005; Morrison, et al, 2005; Nields, 2005; Bao, et al, 2008; Barnett, et al, 2009），根据治疗操作特性（TOC）曲线确定采取切除手段的临界值（Barrett, et al, 2010），自动摧毁所有可疑病变。皮肤科医生就采用我的这种模式来诊治可疑痣：先将它们切除，再提出疑问（如切除边缘是否足够）。这种手段能替代如今2D乳腺X线检查中耗费最大的乳腺活体检查。任何可以自动检测并摧毁微小潜在肿瘤的设备都可以经过设置，更多地关注之前出现过肿瘤的部位，防止复发。这是一种有效的观察等待治疗方式，并且不会耗费太长时间。观察等待治疗取代了病理报告。

我非常清楚，如果我的提议被证实可行，放射学家、放射学技师、外科医生、负责放射治疗的医学物理学家、肿瘤学家、病理学家、乳腺癌分子生物学专家乃至理论生物学家都没有存在的必要了。我们已经受够了与乳腺癌之间的斗争（Lerner, 2001），在我们能够控制乳腺癌之后，所有研究乳腺癌的团队都应该解散。现在，我们已经具备了实践这个方法的所有条件：我们在数量上预测出了欲探测并摧毁的目标肿瘤大小（2~4mm）；研发了多种成像模式，可以单独或者联合工作检测上述目标；掌握了可以在小切缘下摧毁肿瘤的切除技术。根据相同的策略，如果小概率的复发情况出现，在转移前就能被消灭。日后的研究可以重点关注如何遵循标准，能否安全、有效地将该标准用于放射线摄影下乳腺组织致密的年轻女性（Law, et al, 2007），是否采用"外科手术驱动癌细胞转移"（Retsky, et al, 2008）这一情况也存在于不完全切除转移前肿瘤的方法中，不断在实践中完善该方法，检测诱发性肿瘤（Heyes, et al, 2009; Shuryak, et al, 2009），及进一步减少X线剂量。

很多人认为人工环境毒素、生活方式、提高对初生肿瘤的免疫反应或者改变异常的原癌基因和对放射线敏感的基因（如某些女性患有对放射线格外敏感的共济失调毛细血管扩张症）（Hall，et al，1992；Ramsay，et al，1996，1998））是在通向阻止肿瘤萌生道路上的难题。在接下来的几十年里，我们会不断收集通过检测并被摧毁消灭的微小肿瘤的数据，积累得到一个可靠的涉及不同人群的数据库，最终解决上述难题。与此同时，如果找到了对抗乳腺癌的灵丹妙药（Hubbard，1986；Strebhardt，Ullrich，2008），那么我们将放弃这一套检测并摧毁策略。但是，即使真能发现这种灵丹妙药，恐怕也是很久以后的事情了。"…尽管近年来分子生物学研究取得了巨大进展，但是却没能发现任何一种癌细胞表面抗原"（Gonenne，2009），说这句话的学者现在又宣称：

"MabCure公司成功开发了一个杂交瘤细胞库，可以针对3种癌症分别产生抗体，包括黑色素瘤、恶性前列腺癌和卵巢癌。这些抗体对不同的癌症具有针对性，同时又具有'普适性'，适用于不同的个体。从目前为止的实验结果来看，它们不会与任何正常抗原发生反应，并能识别出不同个体体内的每一种肿瘤。这些单克隆抗体为发展治疗相应癌症的新式诊断工具、显像剂和药物奠定了基础。"（Mabcure，2009）

这种寻找治愈药物的方法与我们的检测并摧毁手段存在巨大反差。在实行检测并摧毁操作时，我们不需要关注特异性、进行诊断或是治疗，而是要在早期检测出癌症并摧毁所有可疑病征。在这个过程中，我们无需确认这些病征是否有恶性发展的可能性。虽然如此，但通过分子成像技术，两者之间有望实现互补。

人们会认真对待"从现在起消灭乳腺癌"的提议吗？有些人可能会嘲讽道：研究乳腺癌的学者都不希望真正解决问题，这样他们就可以获得一些既得利益。但是我认为问题并不在这里，而在于科学研究和医学研究的组织方法，以及抑制创新发明的同行评审制度。也许这次，我们需要复活1714年英国国会设立的经度奖的办法（Sobel，1995），激励研究者们一次性彻底解决乳腺癌的问题。尽管这样看上去可能是获胜者独揽所有奖励，但实际上，女性（和少部分男性）才是最大的赢家，她们的生命将不会再受到乳腺癌的威胁。

美国国家航空航天局复兴了这种以奖励取代基金的模式：

"1903年12月，两名自行车修理师，威尔伯（Wilbur）和奥维尔·莱特（Orville Wright），在没有政府支持的条件下于基蒂霍克（Kitty Hawk）成功试飞第一架飞机，开启了动力飞行的新时代。2003年，为了发扬莱特兄弟及其他独立发明者的精神，同时纪念第一架动力飞行器诞生100周年，美国国家航空航天局制订了NASA奖金计划。此外，NASA世纪挑战项目中也开展了多场有奖竞赛，在人类百年飞行史早期促使航天领域研究快速、惊人的发展。"（NASA，2009a）

但是现有的奖金并不丰厚：……在研究与开发过程中所花费的资金一般都是奖金的很多倍"（NASA，2009b）。

10.26 病态乳腺小叶理论："一个似是而非的论点，一个自相矛盾的议题，一个机智的悖论"（Gilbert，Sullivan，1879）

我和Tibor Tot只在寻找乳腺X线检查代替法的第二场研讨会上进行过合作，对他并不了解。所以，当他向我征询我能否在这章内谈谈他所述的病态乳腺小叶假设的意见时，我立马想到了我的合作者Vincent Vinh-Hung提到的悖论：

一方面：据流行病学数据推测结果，杀灭微小的未转移的乳腺病灶可以治愈乳腺癌。

另一方面：转移前肿瘤往往是多病灶的，也许这些病灶都集中在一个病态腺叶上。

正如歌舞剧《屋顶上的小提琴手》所言，这是一个普遍的困境：

"Avram：（朝着Perchik和Mordcha做手势）他是对的，那他也是对的吗？他们不可能都对。

Tevye：你知道……你也是对的"（United Artists Corporation，1971）。

此时此刻，我们只能进行推测。我从我们的邮件中截取了部分对话，谈及我们最初的想法：

Tibor Tot：

用简单的话说，"乳腺病态腺叶"理论是指乳腺癌肿瘤不止在一点、而是同时在一个几厘米大的区域内的几点发展。事实上，根据我们的研究，<10mm的肿瘤有37%的可能性是单病灶的，63%的可能性是多病灶的。在50%的情况下，病灶范围≥40mm（大量病例）。这意味着我们不止需要消灭1个2~3mm大小的病变，而是要切除多个这样的病变及其周围基因变异的部分。我相信应该切掉整个病变腺叶，也可以被称为"癌变区域"。

Richard Gordon：

我想问问你，每一个已发现的病灶的小尺寸与它们彼此之间的距离对于转移可能性的推测。这是对你的病态腺叶假设与我们之前关于获得病灶尺寸的推测之间的关系的一个适当的分析，至少这是我的第一个猜想。

同时，我也希望你也能够提供证据说明多病灶集中于一个病态腺叶之上。尽管我能够理解你的假设，但是我想了解具体的实验过程，以及你是如何得出结论的。

此外，我也不清楚需要找到多少个（和多少处）目标病灶（<4mm）才能够确认整个乳腺腺叶发生了病变。假设判断成功率>99%（预测值），如果乳腺腺叶为病态腺叶，我们是该通过外科手术切除该乳腺病态腺叶还是应该进行观察等待治疗呢？更何况，如今我们没有任何一种成像方法可以可靠地勾勒出乳腺腺叶的轮廓。特别是X线CT，想要得到乳腺腺叶图像，恐怕需要增加剂量，这样做岂不是得不偿失。

Tibor Tot：

虽然"乳腺病态腺叶"假设只是一个假设，但是即使在发病初期，大多数乳腺肿瘤都具有多发性，这是一个形态学事实。我曾多次对此进行研究，并发表相关文章。此外，在我之前，也有人采用细胞组织学技术得出相似的结论。在原位癌阶段，即癌症浸润周围组织并发生远处转移前，其多病灶性就已经呈现出来了。

现在回到我的主题上来。在实际操作中，存在一个困难：如果一名外科医生阅读了本书的前几章，可能会认为在乳腺癌早期，正确的手术方法就是切除范围要大，大到数厘米的患病区域。读到你写的章节，他们会改变想法，认为只用切除一小块，最小仅为4mm的区域，就可以达到目标。我每天都在观察早期乳腺癌肿瘤，因此我坚信，这种方法存在局限性，不足以应对大多数案例，但是对30%~40%的单灶性病症适用。因为很多病灶在放射学检测中容易被忽略，所以我仍觉得即使是对于这些病例，也该切除较大的区域。

Vincent Vinh-Hung：

我不知道怎样就这一问题建模，但是我喜欢悖论。病态腺叶或者区域癌变与早期检测的概念并不是完全互斥的。

Richard Gordon

我认为Vicent把这称之为悖论的说法一针见血：

1. 流行病学数据指出，在肿瘤转移前检测并摧毁单个肿瘤可以治愈乳腺癌。

2. 多病灶数据显示对于一个<4mm的肿瘤，不止需要切除1个组织部位。

所以我们应该想想办法，提出一些同时满足两种结论的假设，并且设计一些方法来验证这些假设。下面是我的一些想法，请你考虑一下：

1. 推断是正确的，但是较大的切缘（也

许是整个乳腺腺叶）将更大程度地降低之后发病（不只指复发）的概率。从逻辑层面分析，它与乳房切除术这种极端做法是保持一致的（Mokbel，2003）（从本质上来说，这就是乳房肿瘤切除术与乳房切除术之间的竞争。）

2. 切除一个转移前肿瘤可以延迟同一乳腺腺叶上其他肿瘤的形成。但是如果不将其去除，就会引发多灶性疾病。

3. 转移前肿瘤既具有多灶性，又与推断保持一致的原因是因为它们可以发生退化（Nielsen，et al，1987；Nielsen，1989）。在这种情况下，因为我们不知道哪些病灶会退化而哪些不会退化，所以我们需要切除所有肿瘤。这也意味着也许在多灶性肿瘤中还存在竞争，大肿瘤会抑制小肿瘤的生长。

我意识到想要解开这个悖论还需要进行很多新研究。也许现在Vicent赞成我的想法。

Vincent Vinh-Hung：

仔细想一下，如果没有宿主的支撑，肿瘤能单独长大吗？我们应该更多地考虑到肿瘤生长的基质或微环境（Hu，Polyak，2008）。乳腺腺叶的概念是合理的，这个说法的确有道理（Ellsworth，et al，2004）。某个腺叶中，当第一个肿瘤生长至数毫米后，该腺叶会更容易成为其他肿瘤的滋生地［肿瘤的瀑布效应和（或）利用宿主资源的募集效应］。尽早切除第一个肿瘤可以降低多灶性发病的概率。这样就又绕回到了你的第2个观点。

这是一个极具挑战性的问题，需要耗费多年时间才能解决。

所以，我们3个人达成了一致意见，接受这个挑战。

10.27 结　论

近百年来，人们都固执地认为能找到一种灵丹妙药应对癌症，实则不然。这种无谓的坚持已经在生物化学、分子生物学、基因组学以及大规模制药行业中形成了一种"霸权"，认定可以为治疗任何一种癌症研制相应的药物。与此同时，在过去的一个世纪中，X线及其他成像方式都取得了卓有成效的发展。现在这些技术已经足以取代药物，因为它们具有普适性，具有检测所有肿瘤的潜力。根据3组相互独立的流行病学数据推断的结果，在转移前，超过99%的乳腺肿瘤目标大小都在2~4mm。高分辨率加上多模式成像，再结合神奇的分子成像技术，使我们可以在乳腺癌早期准确地检测出肿瘤，并且紧接着通过多种模式共同配合，对筛查出的肿瘤进行小切缘切除。我们需要团结起来实现这个目标。乍看之下，病态腺叶假设似乎与这个流行病学推断结论存在矛盾，我们仍需要继续研究以解开这个悖论。

参考文献

[1] Abbott EA. Flatland: a romance of many dimensions. Little, Brown, Boston, 1899.

[2] Abouraddy AF, Saleh BE, Sergienko AV, et al. Role of entanglement in two-photon imaging. Phys Rev Lett, 2001, 87: 123602.

[3] Agnese DM, Burak WE Jr. Ablative approaches to the minimally invasive treatment of breast cancer. Cancer J, 2005, 11: 77–82.

[4] Aliaga A, Rousseau JA, Cadorette J, et al. A small animal positron emis-sion tomography study of the effect of chemotherapy and hormonal therapy on the uptake of 2-deoxy-2-F-18fuoro-d-glucose in murine models of breast cancer. Mol Imaging Biol, 2007, 9: 144–150.

[5] Alizad A, Whaley DH, Greenleaf JF, et al. Potential applications of vibro-acoustography in breast imaging. Technol Cancer Res Treat, 2005, 4: 151–158.

[6] Alpuche Avilés JE. Multiplicative Algebraic Reconstruction Techniques for 3D Cone Beam CT of the Breast Undergraduate Thesis, Supervisor: R. Gordon. Mérida, Yucatán, México: Facultad de Ingeniería de la Universidad Autónoma de Yucatán, 2004.

[7] Alpuche Avilés JE, Pistorius S, Gordon R, et al. A novel hybrid reconstruction algorithm for frst generation incoherent scatter CT (ISCT) of large objects with potential medical imaging applications. J X-ray Sci Technol: in press, 2010.

[8] Altschuler MD, Censor Y, Eggermont PP, et al. Demonstration of a software package for the reconstruction of the dynamically changing structure of the human heart from cone beam X-ray projections. J Med Syst, 1980, 4: 289–304.

[9] Ambrose J. Computerised transverse axial scanning (tomog-raphy). II Clinical application. Br J Radiol, 1973, 46: 1023–1047.

[10] Ambrose J. Computerized x-ray scanning of brain. J Neurosurg, 1974, 40: 679–695.

[11] Andersen AH, Kak AC. Simultaneous algebraic reconstruction technique (SART): a superior implementation of the ART algorithm. Ultrason Imaging, 1984, 6: 81–94.

[12] Anninos PA, Kotini A, Koutlaki N, et al. Differential diagnosis of breast lesions by use of biomagnetic activity and non-linear analysis. Eur J Gynaecol Oncol, 2000, 21: 591–595.

[13] Ayres FJ, Rangayyan RM. Reduction of false positives in the detection of architectural distortion in mammograms by using a geometrically constrained phase portrait model. Int J Comput Assist Radiol Surg, 2007, 1: 361–369.

[14] Badea C, Gordon R. Experiments with the nonlinear and chaotic behaviour of the multiplicative algebraic reconstruc-tion technique (MART) algorithm for computed tomogra-phy. Phys Med Biol, 2004, 49: 1455–1474.

[15] Bagchi S. New technique for detecting breast cancer. Lancet Oncol, 2007, 8: 12.

[16] Bailar JC III. Mammography: a contrary view. Ann Intern Med, 1976, 84: 77–84.

[17] Bailar JC III, MacMahon B. Randomization in the Canadian National Breast Screening Study: a review for evidence of subversion. CMAJ, 1997, 156: 193–199.

[18] Baines CJ. The Canadian National Breast Screening Study: a perspective on criticisms. Ann Intern Med, 1994, 120: 326–334.

[19] Baines CJ, Miller AB, Wall C, et al. Sensitivity and specifcity of frst screen mammography in the Canadian National Breast Screening Study: a preliminary report from fve centers. Radiology, 1986, 160: 295–298.

[20] Baker JR, Budinger TF, Huesman RH. Generalized approach to inverse problems in tomography: image reconstruction for spatially variant systems using natural pixels. Crit Rev Biomed Eng, 1992, 20: 47–71.

[21] Bakic PR, Albert M, Brzakovic D, et al. Mammogram synthesis using a 3D simulation. I. Breast tissue model and image acquisition simulation. Med Phys, 2002a, 29: 2131–2139.

[22] Bakic PR, Albert M, Brzakovic D, et al. Mammogram synthesis using a 3D simulation. II.Evaluation of synthetic mammogram texture. Med Phys, 2002b, 29: 2140–2151.

[23] Bakic PR, Albert M, Brzakovic D, et al. Mammogram synthesis using a three-dimensional simulation. Modeling and evaluation of the breast ductal net-work. Med Phys, 2003, 30: 1914–1925.

[24] Banik S, Rangayyan RM, Desautels JEL. Detection of architectural distortion in prior mammograms of interval-cancer cases with neural networks//31st annual international conference of the IEEE EMBS. Minneapolis, Minnesota: USA, 2009: pp 6667–6670

[25] Bao A, Goins B, Dodd GD, et al. Real-time iterative monitoring of radiofrequency ablation tumor therapy with 15 O-water PET imaging. J Nucl Med, 2008, 49: 1723–1729.

[26] Barbieri M. A criterion to evaluate three dimensional reconstructions from projections of unknown structures. J Theor Biol, 1974, 48: 451–467.

[27] Barbieri M. Co-information: a new concept in theoretical biology. Riv Biol, 1987, 80: 101–126.

[28] Barbieri M, Pettazzoni P, Bersani F, et al. Isolation of ribosome microcrystals. J Mol Biol, 1970, 54: 121–124.

[29] Barnett GH, Sloan AE, Torchia MG. Preliminary results of novel laser interstitial therapy system for treatment of recurrent glioblastoma//American Association of Neurological Surgeons annual meeting, San Diego, 2009: pp 54756.

[30] Barrett HH, Müller S, Wilson DW. Therapy operating characteristic (TOC) curves and their application to the evaluation of segmentation algorithms. Proceedings of SPIE, 2010, 7627: 76270Z.

[31] Baum M. Breast cancer screening comes full circle. J Natl Cancer Inst, 2004, 96: 1490–1491.

[32] Beekman FJ, Kamphuis C, Viergever MA. Improved SPECT quantitation using fully three-dimensional iterative spatially variant scatter response compensation. IEEE Trans Med Imaging, 1996, 15: 491–499.

[33] Bellman SH. A perfect and absolute blank. J Theor Biol, 1970, 29: 482.

[34] Bellman SH, Bender R, Gordon R, et al. ART is science, being a defense of Algebraic Reconstruction Techniques for three-dimensional electron microscopy. J Theor Biol, 1971, 32: 205–216.

[35] Bender R, Duck PD. Chemical synthesis apparatus for preparation of polynucleotides. US Patent, 1982, 4: 353, 989.

[36] Bender R, Bellman SH, Gordon R. ART and the ribosome: a preliminary report on the three-dimensional structure of individual ribosomes determined by an Algebraic Reconstruction Technique. J Theor Biol, 1970, 29: 483–488.

[37] Bender JE, Kapadia AJ, Sharma AC, et al. Breast cancer detection using neutron stimulated emission computed tomography: prominent elements and dose requirements. Med Phys, 2007, 34: 3866–3871.

[38] Benjamin S. Quantum cryptography: single photons "on demand". Science, 2000, 290: 2273–2274.

[39] Berdon WE, Slovis TL. Where we are since ALARA and the series of articles on CT dose in children and risk of long-term cancers: what has changed. Pediatr Radiol, 2002, 32: 699.

[40] Bertell R, Ehrle LH, Schmitz-Feuerhake I. Pediatric CT research elevates public health concerns: low-dose radiation issues are highly politicized. Int J Health Serv, 2007, 37: 419–439.

[41] Bertero M, Boccacci P. Introduction to inverse problems in imaging. Taylor & Francis, Oxford Bhagtani R, Schmidt TG Simulated scatter performance of an inverse-geometry dedicated breast CT system. Med Phys, 1998, 36: 788–796.

[42] Bjarnason GA. Menstrual cycle chronobiology: is it important in breast cancer screening and therapy. Lancet, 1996, 347: 345–346.

[43] Bliznakova K, Bliznakov Z, Pallikarakis N. A 3D breast software phantom for tomosynthetic mammography//Third European symposium on BME and MP. Patras, 2002.

[44] Bliznakova K, Bliznakov Z, Bravou V, et al. A three-dimensional breast software phantom for mammography simulation. Phys Med Biol, 2003, 48: 3699–3719.

[45] Bliznakova K, Kolitsi Z, Pallikarakis N. Dual-energy mam-mography: simulation studies. Phys Med Biol, 2006, 51: 4497–4515.

[46] Blyschak K, Simick M, Jong R, et al. Classifcation of breast tissue density by optical transillumination spectros-copy: optical and physiological effects governing predictive value. Med Phys, 2004, 31: 1398–1414.

[47] Boone JM, Lindfors KK, Seibert JA, et al. Breast cancer screening using a dedicated breast CT scanner: a fea-sibility study//Peitgen H-O (ed) IWDM 2002. Sixth inter-national workshop on digital mammography. Bremen: Germany. New York: Springer, 2003: pp 6–11.

[48] Bowen SL, Wu Y, Chaudhari AJ, et al. Initial characterization of a dedicated breast PET/CT scanner during human imaging. J Nucl Med, 2009, 50: 1401–1408.

[49] Bracewell RN. Correction for collimator width (restoration) in reconstructive X-ray tomography. J Comput Assist Tomogr, 1977, 1: 6–15.

[50] Bradford CD, Peppler WW, Ross RE. Multitapered X-ray capillary optics for mammography. Med Phys, 2002, 29: 1097–1108.

[51] Bravin A, Keyrilainen J, Fernandez M, et al. High-resolution CT by diffraction-enhanced X-ray imaging: mapping of breast tissue samples and comparison with their histo-pathology. Phys Med Biol, 2007, 52: 2197–2211.

[52] Brenner DJ. Estimating cancer risks from pediatric CT: going from the qualitative to the quantitative. Pediatr Radiol, 2002, 32: 228–244.

[53] Brenner RJ, Parisky Y. Alternative breast-imaging

approaches. Radiol Clin North Am, 2007, 45: 907–923.

[54] Brenner D, Elliston C, Hall E, et al. Estimated risks of radiation-induced fatal cancer from pediatric CT. AJR Am J Roentgenol, 2001, 176: 289–296.

[55] Brettle DS, Ward SC, Parkin GJ, et al. A clinical comparison between conventional and digital mammography utilizing computed radiography. Br J Radiol, 1994, 67: 464-468.

[56] Bruzzone L, Cossu R. An adaptive approach to reducing registration noise effects in unsupervised change detection. IEEE Trans Geosci Remote Sens, 2003, 41: 2455–2465.

[57] Burattini E, Cossu E, Di Maggio C, et al. Mammography with synchrotron radiation. Radiology, 1995, 195: 239–244.

[58] Burdette D, Albani D, Chesi E, et al. A device to measure the effects of strong magnetic felds on the image resolution of PET scanners. Nucl Instrum Methods Phys Res A, 2009, 609: 263–271.

[59] Burg A. Image and video compression: the principles behind the technology. Curr Probl Dermatol, 2003, 32: 17–23.

[60] Burhenne LJ, Burhenne HJ. The Canadian National Breast Screening Study: a Canadian critique. AJR Am J Roentgenol, 1993, 161: 761–763.

[61] Byrne CL. Iterative image reconstruction algorithms based on cross-entropy minimization. IEEE Trans Image Process, 1993, 2: 96–103.

[62] Byrne CL. Block-iterative methods for image reconstruction from projections. IEEE Trans Image Process, 1996, 5: 792–794.

[63] Byrne C. A unifed treatment of some iterative algorithms in signal processing and image reconstruction. Inverse Prob, 2004, 20: 103–120.

[64] Candes EJ, Wakin MB. An introduction to compressive sampling. IEEE Signal Process Mag, 2008, 25: 21–30.

[65] Carroll L. The hunting of the snark: an agony in eight fts. New York: Macmillan, 1876.

[66] Carron I. CS: these technologies do not exist: random X-ray collectors in CT, 2009. http://nuit-blanche.blogspo, com/2009/11/cs-these-technologies-do-not-exist_28.html

[67] Cederstroem B, Cahn RN, Danielsson M, et al. Refractive X-ray focusing with modifed phonograph records. Proc SPIE, 1999, 3767: 80–89.

[68] Censor Y, Zenios SA. Parallel optimization: theory, algo-rithms, and applications. New York: Oxford University Press, 1997.

[69] Chan HP, Vyborny CJ, MacMahon H, et al. Digital mammography. ROC studies of the effects of pixel size and unsharp-mask fltering on the detection of subtle microcalcifcations. Invest Radiol, 1987, 22: 581–589.

[70] Chang CH, Sibala JL, Gallagher JH, et al. Computed tomography of the breast. A preliminary report. Radiology, 1977, 124: 827–829.

[71] Chang C, Sibala J, Fritz S, et al. Computed tomographic evaluation of the breast. AJR Am J Roentgenol, 1978, 131: 459–464.

[72] Chang CH, Nesbit DE, Fisher DR, et al. Computed tomo-graphic mammography using a conventional body scanner. AJR Am J Roentgenol, 1982, 138: 553–558.

[73] Chang CF, Chen CY, Chang FH, et al. Cell tracking and detection of molecular expression in live cells using lipid-enclosed CdSe quantum dots as contrast agents for epi-third harmonic generation microscopy. Opt Express, 2008, 16: 9534–9548.

[74] Chapman J-A, Gordon R, Link MA, et al. Infltrating breast carcinoma smaller than 0.5 centimeters. Is lymph node dissection necessary. Cancer, 1999, 86: 2186–2188.

[75] Chen B, Ning R. Cone-beam volume CT breast imaging: feasibility study. Med Phys, 2002, 29: 755–770.

[76] Chen ZK, Ning R. Why should breast tumour detection go three dimensional. Phys Med Biol, 2003, 48: 2217–2228.

[77] Chen YM, Wu SJ, Wang YY. Application of holographic tomography to the measurement of 3D fame temperature feld. J Chin Inst Chem Eng, 1997, 28: 197–203.

[78] Chen YF, Gunawan E, Low KS, et al. Time of arrival data fusion method for two-dimen-sional ultrawideband breast cancer detection. IEEE Trans Antennas Propag, 2007, 55: 2852–2865.

[79] Chen YF, Gunawan E, Low KS, et al. Time-reversal

ultrawideband breast imaging: pulse design criteria considering multiple tumors with unknown tissue properties. IEEE Trans Antennas Propag, 2008, 56: 3073-3077.
[80] Cherepenin VA, Karpov AY, Korjenevsky AV, et al. Three-dimensional EIT imaging of breast tissues: system design and clinical testing. IEEE Trans Med Imaging, 2002, 21: 662-667.
[81] Cherry SR. Multimodality in vivo imaging systems: twice the power or double the trouble. Annu Rev Biomed Eng, 2006, 8: 35-62.
[82] Cherry SR, Louie AY, Jacobs RE. The integration of positron emission tomography with magnetic resonance imaging. Proc IEEE, 2008, 96: 416-438.
[83] Choi MH, Kao TJ, Isaacson D, et al. A reconstruction algorithm for breast cancer imaging with electrical impedance tomography in mammography geometry. IEEE Trans Biomed Eng, 2007, 54: 700-710.
[84] Christ M, Kenig CE, Sadosky C, et al. Alberto Pedro Calderón (1920-1998). Not Amer Math Soc, 1998, 45: 1148-1153.
[85] Clarke J, Hatridge M, Mössle M. SQUID-detected magnetic resonance imaging in microtesla felds. Annu Rev Biomed Eng, 2007, 9: 389-413.
[86] Clarkson E, Barrett H. A bound on null functions for digital imaging systems with positivity constraints. OptLett, 1997, 22: 814-815.
[87] Clarkson E, Barrett H. Bounds on null functions of linear digital imaging systems. J Opt Soc Am A Opt Image Sci Vis, 1998, 15: 1355-1360.
[88] Colang JE, Killion JB, Vano E. Patient dose from CT: a literature review. Radiol Technol, 2007, 79: 17-26.
[89] Colquhoun GD, Gordon R. A superresolution computed tomography algorithm for reverse cone beam 3D X-ray mam-mography// Tot T (ed) Workshop on alternatives to mam-mography. Copenhagen, 2005a: 29-30.
[90] Colquhoun GD, Gordon R. The use of control angles with MART .Multiplicative Algebraic Reconstruction Technique. Technol Cancer Res Treat, 2005b, 4: 183-184.
[91] Colquhoun GD, Gordon R, Elbakri IA. Reversed cone beam coded aperture mammography (Abstract: 4408744). RSNA (rejected), 2004.
[92] Cooley JW, Tukey JW. An algorithm for machine calcula-tion of complex Fourier series. Math Comput, 1965, 19: 297-301.
[93] Cormack AM. Representation of a function by its line integrals, with some radiological applications. J Appl Phys, 1963, 34: 2722-2727.
[94] Cormack AM. Representation of a function by its line integrals, with some radiological applications. II. J Appl Phys, 1964, 35: 2908-2913.
[95] Cormack AM. Nobel Award address. Early two-dimensional reconstruction and recent topics stemming from it. Med Phys, 1980, 7: 277-282.
[96] Cormack AM. EMI patent litigation in the US. Br J Radiol, 1994, 67: 316-317.
[97] Cornely PRJ. Flexible prior models: three-dimensional ionospheric tomography. Radio Sci 38. Article Number: 1087, 2003.
[98] Crewe AV, Crewe DA. Inexact reconstructions from projections. Ultramicroscopy, 1984, 12: 293-298.
[99] Crowther RA, Klug A. ART and science or conditions for three-dimensional reconstruction from electron microscope images. J Theor Biol, 1971, 32: 199-203.
[100] Crowther RA, Klug A. Three dimensional image recon-struction on an extended feld: fast, stable algorithm. Nature, 1974, 251: 490-492.
[101] Cubeddu R, D'Andrea C, Pifferi A, et al. Effects of the menstrual cycle on the red and near-infrared optical properties of the human breast. Photochem Photobiol, 2000, 72: 383-391.
[102] Dabrosin C, Hallstrom A, Ungerstedt U, et al. Microdialysis of human breast tissue during the menstrual cycle. Clin Sci, 1997, 92: 493-496.
[103] Danielli JF. Preface. J Theor Biol 1: I, 1961.
[104] Daun KJ, Thomson KA, Liu F, et al. Deconvolution of axisymmetric fame properties using.Tikhonov regularization. Appl Opt, 2006, 45: 4638-4646.
[105] Dawson P. Patient dose in multislice CT: why is it increasing and does it matter. Br J Radiol, 2004, 77 (Spec No 1): S10-S13.
[106] Dayan B, Parkins AS, Aoki T, et al. A photon turnstile dynamically regulated by one atom. Science, 2008, 319: 1062-1065.

[107] De Rosier DJ, Klug A. Reconstruction of three dimensional structures from electron micrographs. Nature, 1968, 217: 130.

[108] Dhawan AP. Nevoscopy: three-dimensional computed tomography of nevi and melanomas in situ by transillumination to detect early cutaneous malignant melanomas. Ph.D. thesis, Supervisor: R. Gordon, Department of Electrical Engineering, University of Manitoba, Winnipeg, 1985.

[109] Dhawan AP, Gordon R. Reply to comments on "Enhancement of mammographic features by optimal adap-tive neighborhood image processing". IEEE Trans Med Imaging, 1986, MI-6: 82-83.

[110] Dhawan AP, Rangayyan RM, Gordon R. Wiener fltering for deconvolution of geometric artifacts in limited-view image reconstruction. Proc SPIE, 1984a, 515: 168-172.

[111] Dhawan AP, Gordon R, Rangayyan RM. Computed tomography by transillumination to detect early melanoma. IEEE Trans Biomed Eng BME, 1984b, 31: 574.

[112] Dhawan AP, Gordon R, Rangayyan RM. Nevoscopy: three-dimensional computed tomography for nevi and mela-nomas in situ by transillumination. IEEE Trans Med Imaging MI, 1984c, 3 (2): 54-61.

[113] Dhawan AP, Rangayyan RM, Gordon R. Image restoration by Wiener deconvolution in limited-view computed tomography. Appl Opt, 1985, 24: 4013-4020.

[114] Dhawan AP, Buelloni G, Gordon R. Enhancement of mammographic features by optimal adaptive neighborhood image processing. IEEE Trans Med Imaging MI, 1986a, 5: 8-15.

[115] Dhawan AP, Buelloni G, Gordon R. Errata: enhancement of mammographic features by optimal adaptive neigh-borhood image processing. IEEE Trans Med Imaging, 1986b, MI-5: 120.

[116] Dobbins JT. Tomosynthesis imaging: at a translational crossroads. Med Phys, 2009, 36: 1956-1967.

[117] Donaire JG, Garcia I. On improving the performance of ART in 3D cone beam transmission tomography//Proceedings of the 1999 international meeting on fully 3D image reconstruc-tion in radiology and nuclear medicine, 1999: pp 73-76.

[118] Donaire JG, Garcia I. On using global optimization to obtain a better performance of a MART algorithm in 3D X-ray tomography. J Imaging Sci Technol, 2002, 46: 247-256.

[119] Donnelly LF, Frush DP. Fallout from recent articles on radiation dose and pediatric CT. Pediatr Radiol, 2001, 31: 388-391.

[120] Düchting H. Georges Seurat (1859-1891): the master of pointillism. Koln: Taschen, 2001.

[121] Duclaux é. Pasteur, the history of a mind. W.B. Philadelphia: Saunders, 1920.

[122] Dusaussoy NJ, Abdou IE. The extended MENT algorithm: a maximum-entropy type algorithm using prior knowledge for computerized-tomography. IEEE Trans Signal Process, 1991, 39: 1164-1180.

[123] Dzendrowskyj TE, Noyszewski EA, Beers J, et al. Lipid composition changes in normal breast throughout the menstrual cycle. Magn Reson Mater Phys, Biol Med, 1997, 5: 105-110.

[124] Eggermont PPB, Herman GT, Lent A. Iterative algorithms for large partitioned linear systems. with applications to image reconstruction. Linear Algebra Appl, 1981, 40: 37-67.

[125] Ehrenreich B. Welcome to Cancerland. Harper's Magazine November, 2001.http://www.barbaraehrenreich.com/cancerland.htm.

[126] Ellsworth DL, Ellsworth RE, Love B, et al. Genomic patterns of allelic imbalance in disease free tissue adjacent to primary breast carcinomas. Breast Cancer Res Treat, 2004, 88: 131-139.

[127] Engl HW, Hanke M, Neubauer A. Regularization of inverse problems. Dordrecht: Springer, 2000.

[128] Fabbri S, Taibi A, Longo R, et al. Signal-to-noise ratio evaluation in dual-energy radiography with synchrotron radiation. Phys Med Biol, 2002, 47: 4093-4105.

[129] Fang Q, Meaney PM, Geimer SD, et al. Microwave image reconstruction from 3-D felds coupled to 2-D parameter estimation. IEEE Trans Med Imaging, 2004, 23: 475-484.

[130] Fang QQ, Carp SA, Selb J, et al. Combined optical imaging and mammography of the healthy breast:

optical contrast derived from breast structure and compression. IEEE Trans Med Imaging, 2009, 28: 30–42.

[131] Feldkamp LA, Davis LC, Kress JW. Practical cone-beam algorithm. J Opt Soc Am A, 1984, 1: 612–619.

[132] Fellholter A, Mewes D. Mixing of large-volume gas-fows in pipes and ducts: visualization of concentration profles. Chem Eng Technol, 1994, 17: 227–234.

[133] Ferguson DJ, Anderson TJ. Morphological evaluation of cell turnover in relation to the menstrual cycle in the "rest-ing" human breast. Br J Cancer, 1981, 44: 177–181.

[134] Ferguson JE, Schor AM, Howell A, et al. Tenascin distribution in the normal human breast is altered during the menstrual cycle and in carcinoma. Differentiation, 1990, 42: 199–207.

[135] Ferguson JE, Schor AM, Howell A, et al. Changes in the extracellular matrix of the normal human breast during the menstrual cycle. Cell Tissue Res, 1992, 268: 167–177.

[136] Fiedler S, Bravin A, Keyrilainen J, et al. Imaging lobular breast carcinoma: comparison of synchrotron radiation DEI-CT technique with clinical CT, mammography and histology. Phys Med Biol, 2004, 49: 175–188.

[137] Fill EE (ed). X-ray lasers 1992: proceedings of the third international colloquium on X-ray lasers held at Schliersee. London: IOP, 1992.

[138] Fitchett JW. A locally synchronous globally asynchronous vertex-8 processing element for image reconstruction on a mesh. Masters thesis. Department of Electrical and Computer Engineering. Winnipeg: University of Manitoba, 1993.

[139] Flores-Tapia D, Thomas G, Pistorius S. A wavefront reconstruction method for 3-D cylindrical subsurface radar imaging. IEEE Trans Image Process, 2008, 17: 1908–1925.

[140] Foo C. X-ray imaging via intelligently steered X-ray micro-beams. B.Sc. thesis, Supervisor: R. Gordon. Department of Electrical & Computer Engineering. Winnipeg: University of Manitoba, 1999.

[141] Forsdyke DR. Canadian Association for Responsible Research Funding, 2009. http://post.queensu.ca/~forsdyke/peer-rev.htm#PEER%20REVIEW

[142] Fowler PA, Casey CE, Cameron GG, et al. Cyclic changes in composition and volume of the breast during the menstrual cycle, measured by magnetic resonance imaging. Br J Obstet Gynaecol, 1990, 97: 595–602.

[143] Gamow G. My world line: an informal autobiography. New York: Viking Adult, 1970.

[144] Gao N, He B. Noninvasive imaging of bioimpedance distribution by means of current reconstruction magnetic resonance electrical impedance tomography. IEEE Trans Biomed Eng, 2008, 55: 1530–1538.

[145] Garcia I, Roca J, Sanjurjo J, et al. Implementation and experimental evaluation of the constrained ART algorithm on a multicomputer system. Signal Process, 1996, 51: 69–76.

[146] Garmire GP, Bautz MW, Ford PG, et al. Advanced CCD imaging spectrometer (ACIS) instrument on the Chandra X-ray Observatory//Proceedings of SPIE, 2003, vol 4851: pp 28–44.

[147] Garra BS. Imaging and estimation of tissue elasticity by ultrasound. Ultrasound, 2007, 23: 255–268.

[148] Gavrielides MA, Lo JY, Floyd CE Jr. Parameter optimization of a computer-aided diagnosis scheme for the segmentation of microcalcifcation clusters in mammograms. Med Phys, 2002, 29: 475–483.

[149] Gilbert WS, Sullivan A. The pirates of Penzance, or the slave of duty, 1879. http://math.boisestate.edu/GaS/pirates/web_op/pirates18.html

[150] Glaiberman CB, Pilgram TK, Brown DB. Patient factors affecting thermal lesion size with an impedance-based radiofrequency ablation system. J Vasc Interv Radiol, 2005, 16: 1341–1348.

[151] Gmitro AF, Greivenkamp JE, Swindell W, et al. Optical computers for reconstructing objects from their X-ray projections. Opt Eng, 1980, 19: 260–272.

[152] Goel NS, Campbell RD, Gordon R, et al. Self-sorting of isotropic cells. J Theor Biol, 1970, 28: 423–468.

[153] Going JJ, Anderson TJ, Battersby S, et al. Proliferative and secretory activity in human breast during nat-ural and artifcial menstrual cycles. Am J Pathol, 1988, 130: 193–204.

[154] Goldberg MA, Dwyer SJ 3rd. Telemammography: imple-mentation issues. Telemed J, 1995, 1: 215-226.

[155] Gonenne A. Tumour-specifc markers: the holy grail of cancer diagnostics. Biotechnol Focus, 2009, 12: 17-18, 27.

[156] Gong P, Ledrew EF, Miller JR. Registration noise reduction in difference images for change detection. Int J Remote Sens, 1992, 13: 773-779.

[157] Gordon R. Oh Dear What Can the Matter Be. Oh dear what can the matter be. University of Chicago Laboratory School: Chicago, 1960.

[158] Gordon R. On stochastic growth and form. Proc Natl Acad Sci USA, 1966, 56: 1497-1504.

[159] Gordon R. Polyribosome dynamics at steady state. J Theor Biol, 1969, 22: 515-532.

[160] Gordon R. Steps in performing a 3-dimensional reconstruction of single asymmetric particles from a tilt series of electron micrographs// Workshop on information treatment in electron microscopy, Basel, 1972.

[161] Gordon R. Artifacts in reconstructions made from a few projections//Fu KS (ed) Proceedings of the frst international joint conference on pattern recognition, Washington, D.C. Northridge: IEEE Computer Society, 1973: pp 275-285.

[162] Gordon R. A tutorial on ART (Algebraic Reconstruction Techniques). IEEE Trans Nucl Sci, 1974, NS-21: 78-93, 95.

[163] Gordon R. A bibliography on reconstruction from pro-jections. In: Digest of technical papers. Topical meeting on image processing for 2-D and 3-D reconstruction from projections: theory and practice in medicine and the physical sciences, Stanford University. Washington, D.C: Optical Society of America, 1975a.

[164] Gordon R. Digest of technical papers. Topical meeting on image processing for 2-D and 3-D reconstruction from projections: theory and practice in medicine and the physical sciences. Washington, D.C: Optical Society of America, 1975b.

[165] Gordon R. Maximal use of single photons and particles in reconstruction from projections by ARTIST, Algebraic Reconstruction Techniques Intended for Storage Tubes// Gordon R (ed) Technical digest. Topical meeting on image processing for 2-D and 3-D reconstruction from pro-jections: theory and practice in medicine and the physical sciences. Washington, D.C: Optical Society of America, 1975c: pp paper TuC4.

[166] Gordon R. Dose reduction in computed tomography //Di Chiro G, Brooks RA (eds) Book of abstracts of the international symposium on computer assisted tomography in nontumoral diseases of the brain, spinal cord and eye. National Institutes of Health: Bethesda, 1976a: 2 pp.

[167] Gordon R. Dose reduction in computerized tomography. Guest Editorial. Invest Radiol, 1976b, 111: 508-517.

[168] Gordon R. High-speed reconstruction of the fnest details available in X-ray projections// Ter-Pogossian MM, Phelps ME, Brownell GL, Cox JR Jr, et al. Reconstruction tomography in diagnostic radiology and nuclear medicine. University Park Press: Baltimore, 1977: pp 77-83.

[169] Gordon R. Higher-resolution tomography. Phys Today, 1978a, 31: 46.

[170] Gordon R. Reconstruction from projections in medicine and astronomy//van Schoonveld C, Holland D (eds) Image formation from coherence functions in astronomy. Reidel, Dordrecht, 1978b: pp 317-325.

[171] Gordon D. Spring linocut//Yochim LD (ed) Role and impact: the Chicago Society of Artists. Chicago: Chicago Society of Artists, 1979a, 138, 240-241.

[172] Gordon R. Feedback control of exposure geometry in dental radiography workshop, University of Connecticut.Appl Opt, 1979b, 18: 1769, 1834

[173] Gordon R. Questions of uniqueness and resolution in reconstruction from projections Book Review. Phys Today, 1979c, 32: 52-56.

[174] Gordon R. One man's noise is another man's data: the ARTIST algorithm for positron tomography post-deadline paper, 2 pp//Topical meeting on signal recovery and synthesis with incomplete information and partial con-straints. Optical Society of America: Washington, D.C, 1983a.

[175] Gordon R. Three dimensional computed tomography

of nevi in situ by transillumination. Anal Quant Cytol, 1983b, 5: 208.

[176] Gordon R. Industrial applications of computed tomography and NMR imaging: an OSA topical meeting. (Invited). Appl Opt, 1985a, 24: 3948–3949.

[177] Gordon R. Toward robotic X-ray vision: new directions for computed tomography. Appl Opt, 1985b, 24: 4124–4133.

[178] Gordon R. There is no such thing as safe sex: chance of AIDS infection increases with time. Winnipeg Free Press, 1987, 7: 7.

[179] Gordon R. A critical review of the physics and statistics of condoms and their role in individual versus societal sur-vival of the AIDS epidemic. J Sex Marital Ther, 1989, 15: 5–30.

[180] Gordon R. Inexpensive computed tomography for remote areas//SPIE Proceedings, 1990, vol 1355: pp184–188.

[181] Gordon R. Testimony on breast cancer and mammography. Canadian House of Commons Proceedings, Sub-Committee on the Status of Women, 1992, 21: 1–23.

[182] Gordon R. Grant agencies versus the search for truth. Accountability Res: Policies Qual Assur, 1993, 2 (4): 297–301.

[183] Gordon R. Epilogue: the diseased breast lobe in the context of X-chromosome inactivation and differentiation waves//Tot T (ed) Breast cancer: a lobar disease. Springer, 2011: pp205–210.

[184] Gordon R, Bender R. New three-dimensional algebraic reconstruction techniques (ART) //Proceedings of 29th annual meeting of the Electron Microscopy Society of America, Boston, 1971a: pp 82–83.

[185] Gordon R, Bender R . The ART of sectioning without cutting//Third international congress for stereology, Berne. Abstracts, 1971b: 17 pp.

[186] Gordon R, Bender R. Three-dimensional algebraic reconstruction techniques: a preliminary course. J Theor Biol, 1971c, 32: 217.

[187] Gordon R, Coumans J. Combining multiple imaging techniques for in vivo pathology: a quantitative method for coupling new imaging modalities. Med Phys, 1984, 11 (1): 79–80.

[188] Gordon R, Herman GT. Reconstruction of pictures from their projections. Commun ACM, 1971, 14: 759–768.

[189] Gordon R, Herman GT. Three dimensional reconstruction from projections: a review of algorithms. Int Rev Cytol, 1974, 38: 111–151.

[190] Gordon R, Hirsch HVB. Vision begins with direct recon-struction of the retinal image, how the brain sees and stores pictures. In: Schallenberger H, Schrey H (eds) Gegenstrom, Für Helmut Hirsch zum Siebzigsten Against the stream, for Helmut Hirsch on his 70th birthday. Wuppertal: Peter Hammer, 1977: pp 201–214.

[191] Gordon R, Kane J. Three-dimensional reconstruction: the state of the "ART" // Fourth international biophysics congress, Moscow. Abstracts of Contributed Papers, 1972: 2, 37.

[192] Gordon R, Lauterbur PC. Introduction to the session on experimental aspects of reconstruction from projections//Marr RB (ed) Techniques of three-dimensional reconstruction. Proceedings of an international workshop. Brookhaven National Laboratory, Upton, 1974: pp 17–19.

[193] Gordon R, Poulin BJ. Cost of the NSERC science grant peer review system exceeds the cost of giving every quali-fed researcher a baseline grant. Accountability Res: Policies Qual Assur, 2009a, 16: 1–28.

[194] Gordon R, Poulin BJ . Indeed: cost of the NSERC science grant peer review system exceeds the cost of giving every qualifed researcher a baseline grant. Accountability Res: Policies Qual Assur, 2009b, 16: 232–233.

[195] Gordon R, Rangaraj MR. The need for cross-fertilization between the felds of profle inversion and computedtomography//BestWG, WeselakeSA(eds) Proceedings of the seventh Canadian symposium on remote sensing. Canadian Aeronautics and Space Institute, Ottawa, 1981: pp 538–540.

[196] Gordon R, Rangaraj MR. Computed tomography from a few ordinary radiographs//Proceedings of IEEE, COMPMED–82, 1982: pp 54–58.

[197] Gordon R, Rangayyan RM. Geometric deconvolution: a meta-algorithm for limited view computed tomog-

[198] Gordon R, Rangayyan RM. Correction: feature enhancement of flm mammograms using fxed and adaptive neigh-borhoods. Appl Opt, 1984a, 23: 2055.

[199] Gordon R, Rangayyan RM. Feature enhancement of flm mammograms using fxed and adaptive neighborhoods. Appl Opt, 1984b, 23: 560-564.

[200] Gordon R, Sivaramakrishna R. Mammograms are waldograms: why we need 3D longitudinal breast screening Guest Editorial. Appl Radio, 1999, 28: 12-25.

[201] Gordon R, Tweed D. Quantitative reconstruction of visual cortex receptive felds. Univ Manit Med J, 1983, 53 (2): 75.

[202] Gordon R, Bender R, Herman GT. Algebraic reconstruction techniques (ART) for three-dimensional electron microscopy and X-ray photography. J Theor Biol, 1970, 29: 471-481.

[203] Gordon R, Rowe JE Jr, Bender R. ART: a possible replacement for X-ray crystallography at moderate resolution//Broda E, Locker A, Springer-Lederer H (eds) Proceedings of the frst European biophysics congress, vol.VI: Theoretical molecular biology, biomechanics, biomath-ematics, environmental biophysics, techniques, education. Vienna: Verlag der Wiener Medizinischer Akademie, 1971: pp 441-445.

[204] Gordon R, Carmichael JB, Isackson FJ. Saltation of plastic balls in a 'one-dimensional' fume. Water Resour Res, 1972, 8: 444-459.

[205] Gordon R, Herman GT, Johnson SA. Image reconstruction from projections. Sci Am, 1975, 233: 56-61, 64-68.

[206] Gordon R, Silver L, Rigel DS. Halftone graphics on computer terminals with storage display tubes. Proc Soc Inf Disp, 1976, 17: 78-84.

[207] Gordon R, Dhawan AP, Rangayyan RM. Reply to "Comments on geometric deconvolution: a meta-algorithm for limited view computed tomography". IEEE Trans Biomed Eng BME, 1985, 32 (3): 242-244.

[208] Gorenfo R, Vessella S. Abel integral equations: analysis and applications. Springer, Berlin, 1991.

[209] Gorenstein P. Diffractive-refractive X-ray optics for very high angular resolution X-ray astronomy. Adv SpaceRes, 2007, 40: 1276-1280.

[210] Graham SJ, Stanchev PL, Lloydsmith JOA, et al. Changes in fbroglandular volume and water content of breast tissue during the menstrual cycle observed by MR imaging at 1.5 T. J Magn Reson Imaging, 1995, 5: 695-701.

[211] Grant CS, Ingle JN, Suman VJ, et al. Menstrual cycle and surgical treatment of breast cancer: fndings from the NCCTG N9431 study. J Clin Oncol, 2009, 27: 3620-3626.

[212] Groetsch CW. Inverse problems, activities for under-graduates. Washington D.C: The Mathematical Association of America, 1999.

[213] Guan H, Gordon R. A projection access order for speedy convergence of ART (Algebraic Reconstruction Technique): a multilevel scheme for computed tomography. Phys Med Biol, 1994, 39: 2005-2022.

[214] Guan H, Gordon R. Computed tomography using Algebraic Reconstruction Techniques (ARTs) with different projection access schemes: a comparison study under practical situations. Phys Med Biol, 1996, 41: 1727-1743.

[215] Guan H, Gordon R, Zhu Y. Combining various projection access schemes with the Algebraic Reconstruction Technique for low-contrast detection in computed tomography. Phys Med Biol, 1998, 43: 2413-2421.

[216] Guan H, Gaber MW, DiBianca FA, et al. CT recon-struction by using the MLS-ART technique and the KCD imaging system-I: low-energy X-ray studies. IEEE Trans Med Imaging, 1999, 18: 355-358.

[217] Guo YJ, Sivaramakrishna R, Lu CC, et al. Breast image registration techniques: a survey. Med Biol Eng Comput, 2006, 44: 15-26.

[218] Gur D, Abrams GS, Chough DM, et al. Digital breast tomosynthesis: observer performance study. AJR Am J Roentgenol, 2009, 193: 586-591.

[219] Hall EJ, Geard CR, Brenner DJ. Risk of breast cancer in ataxia-telangiectasia. N Engl J Med,

1992, 326: 1358–1361.

[220] Hallégot P, Audinot JN, Migeon HN. Direct Nano SIMS imaging of diffusible elements in surfaced block of cryo-processed biological samples. Appl Surf Sci, 2006, 252: 6706–6708.

[221] Halter RJ, Hartov A, Paulsen KD. A broadband high-frequency electrical impedance tomography system for breast imaging. IEEE Trans Biomed Eng, 2008, 55: 650–659.

[222] Hamaker C, Smith KT, Solmon DC, et al. The divergent beam X-ray transform. Rocky Mountain J Math, 1980, 10: 253–283.

[223] Hammer BE, Christensen NL, Heil BG. Use of a magnetic feld to increase the spatial resolution of positron emission tomography. Med Phys, 1994, 21: 1917–1920.

[224] Han T, Shaw CC, Chen L, et al. Simulation of mammograms and tomosynthesis imaging with cone beam breast CT images. Proc SPIE, 2008, 6913: 1711–1717.

[225] Hand JW. Modelling the interaction of electromagnetic felds (10MHz-10GHz) with the human body: methods and applications. Phys Med Biol, 2008, 53: R243–R286.

[226] Hardin P. To be honest, I would have never invented the wheel if not for Urg's ground breaking theoretical work with the circle. Artist: Hardin, Patrick, Catalogue Ref, 2003: pha0045. http: //www.cartoonstock.com/

[227] Harvey JE, Krywonos A, Thompson PL, et al. Grazing-incidence hyperboloid-hyperboloid designs for wide-feld X-ray imaging applications. Appl Opt 200140: 136–144.

[228] Hasbro. Battleship Game, 2004.http: //www.hasbro.com

[229] Haselkorn R, Fried VA. Cell-free protein synthesis: messenger competition for ribosomes. Proc Natl Acad Sci USA, 1964, 51: 1001–1007.

[230] Hatziioannou K, Papanastassiou E, Delichas M, et al. A contribution to the establishment of diagnostic reference levels in CT. Br J Radiol, 2003, 76: 541–545.

[231] Heller J. Catch-22: a novel. Simon and Schuster: New York, 1961.

[232] Herman GT. Image reconstruction from projections: the fundamentals of computerized tomography. Academic, San Francisco, 1980.

[233] Herman GT. SNARK09-a programming system for the reconstruction of 2D images from 1D projections, 2009.http: //www.snark09.com/

[234] Herman GT, Davidi R. Image reconstruction from a small number of projections. Inverse Prob, 2008, 24: 17.

[235] Herman GT, Rowland S. Three methods for reconstruct-ing objects from X-rays: a comparative study. Comput Graphics Image Process, 1973, 2: 151–178.

[236] Heyes GJ, Mill AJ, Charles MW. Mammography-oncogenecity at low doses. J Radiol Prot, 2009, 29: A123–A132.

[237] Hirai T, Yamada H, Sasaki M, et al. Refraction contrast 11×-magnifed X-ray imaging of large objects by MIRRORCLE-type table-top synchrotron. J Synchrotron Radiat, 2006, 13: 397–402.

[238] Hoeschen C, Fill U, Zankl M, et al. A high-resolution voxel phantom of the breast for dose calculations in mammography. Radiat Prot Dosimetry, 2005, 114: 406–409.

[239] Holley WR, Tobias CA, Fabrikant JI, et al. Computerized heavyion tomography: phantom and tissue specimen studies. AJR Am J Roentgenol, 1981a, 136: 1278.

[240] Holley WR, Tobias CA, Fabrikant JI, et al. Computerized heavyion tomography. Proc SPIE, 1981b, 273: 283–293.

[241] Hounsfeld GN. Computerized transverse axial scanning (tomography). 1. Description of system. Br J Radiol, 1973, 46: 1016–1022.

[242] Hounsfeld GN. Method of and apparatus for examining a body by radiation such as X or gamma radiation. US Patent 3, 924, 131. United States Patent Offce: Washington, D.C, 1975.

[243] Hounsfeld GN. Historical notes on computerized axial tomography. J Can Assoc Radiol, 1976, 27: 135–142.

[244] Hounsfeld GN. Nobel lecture, 8 December 1979. Computed medical imaging. J Radiol, 1980, 61: 459–468.

[245] Houzel C. The work of Niels Henrik Abel. Springer: New York, 2004.

[246] Hu M, Polyak K. Molecular characterisation of the tumour microenvironment in breast cancer. Eur J Cancer, 2008, 44: 2760-2765.

[247] Hu XP, Johnson V, Wong WH, et al. Bayesian image processing in magnetic resonance imaging. Magn Reson Imaging, 1991, 9: 611-620.

[248] Huang M, Zhu Q. Dual-mesh optical tomography recon-struction method with a depth correction that uses a priori ultrasound information. Appl Opt, 2004, 43: 1654-1662.

[249] Hubbard D. A magic bullet for breast cancer.J Nucl Med, 1986, 27: 305.

[250] Huda W. Dose and image quality in CT. Pediatr Radiol, 2002, 32: 709-713, discussion 751-754.

[251] Hussain Z, Roberts N, Whitehouse GH, et al. Estimation of breast volume and its variation during the menstrual cycle using MRI and stereology. Br J Radiol, 1999, 72: 236-245.

[252] Huston TL, Simmons RM. Ablative therapies for the treatment of malignant diseases of the breast. Am J Surg, 2005, 189: 694-701.

[253] Iida H, Kanno I, Miura S, et al. A simulation study of a method to reduce positron annihilation spread distributions using a strong magnetic feld in positron emission tomography. IEEE Trans Nucl Sci, 1986, 33: 597-599.

[254] Imamoglu A, Yamamoto Y. Turnstile device for heralded single photons: Coulomb blockade of electron and hole tunneling in quantum confned p-i-n heterojunctions.Phys Rev Lett, 1994, 72: 210-213.

[255] Imhof H, Schibany N, Ba-Ssalamah A, et al. Spiral CT and radiation dose. Eur J Radiol, 2003, 47: 29-37.

[256] Inoué S, Walter RJ Jr, Berns MW, et al. Video microscopy. New York: Plenum, 1986.

[257] Isaacson M, Kopf D, Utlaut M, et al. Direct observations of atomic diffusion by scanning transmission electron microscopy. Proc Natl Acad Sci: USA, 1977, 74: 1802-1806.

[258] Jan ML, Ni YC, Chuang KS, et al. Detection-ability evaluation of the PEImager for positron emission applications. Phys Med, 2006, 21 (Suppl 1): 109-113.

[259] Jansson P. Deconvolution, with applications in spectroscopy. Academic, Orlando, 1984.

[260] Jansson PA. Deconvolution of images and spectra. Academic, San Diego, 1997.

[261] Jia X, Lou Y, Lewis J, et al. GPU-based cone beam CT reconstruction via total variation regu-larization, 2010. http://arxiv.org/ftp/arxiv/papers/1001/1001.0599.pdf

[262] Jiang X, Guan H, Gordon R. Contrast enhancement using "feature pixels" or "fxels" for pixel independent image processing. Radiology, 1992, 185, (Suppl): 391.

[263] Jonges R, Boon PNM, van Marle J, et al. CART: a controlled algebraic reconstruction technique for electron microscope tomography of embed-ded, sectioned specimen. Ultramicroscopy, 1999, 76: 203-219.

[264] Jorgensen SM, Reyes DA, MacDonald CA, et al. Micro-CT scanner with a focusing polycapillary X-ray optic.Proc SPIE, 1999, 3772: 158-166.

[265] Judenhofer MS, Wehrl HF, Newport DF, et al. Simultaneous PET-MRI: a new approach for functional and morphological imaging. Nat Med 2008, 14: 459-465.

[266] Kaczmarz S. Angenäherte Aufösung von Systemen lin-earer Gleichungen. Bull Int Acad Pol Sci Let A, 1937, 35: 335-357.

[267] Kaipio J, Somersalo E. Statistical and computational inverse problems. New York: Springer, 2004.

[268] Kak AC, Slaney M. Principles of computerized tomo-graphic imaging. Society of Industrial and Applied Mathematics. Philadelphia, 2001.

[269] Kalender W. Computed tomography: fundamentals, system technology, image quality, applications. Publicis MCD, Munich, 2000.

[270] Kalender WA, Kyriakou Y. Flat-detector computed tomography (FD-CT). Eur Radiol, 2007, 17: 2767-2779.

[271] Kalender WA, Deak P, Kellermeier M, et al. Application-and patient size-dependent optimization of X-ray spectra for CT. Med Phys, 2009, 36: 993-1007.

[272] Kalos MH, Davis DSA, Mittelman MPS, et al.

[272] Conceptual design of a vapor fraction instrument. Nuclear. Development Corporation of America, White Plains, 1961.http://www.osti.gov/energy-citations/product.biblio.jsp? query_id =0&page = 0&osti_id=4837780

[273] Kane IJ. Section radiography of the chest. Springer, New York Kanj H, Popovic M (2008) Two-element T-array for cross-polarized breast tumor detection. Appl Computat Electromagnetics Soc, 1953, 23: 249-254.

[274] Kao T, Connor D, Dilmanian FA, et al. Characterization of diffraction-enhanced imaging contrast in breast cancer. Phys Med Biol, 2009, 54: 3247-3256.

[275] Kappadath SC, Shaw CC. Dual-energy digital mammography for calcifcation imaging: scatter and nonuniformity corrections. Med Phys, 2005, 32: 3395-3408.

[276] Karellas A, Vedantham S. Breast cancer imaging: a per-spective for the next decade. Med Phys, 2008, 35: 4878-4897.

[277] Karellas A, Lo JY, Orton CG. Cone beam X-ray CT will be superior to digital X-ray tomosynthesis in imaging the breast and delineating cancer. Med Phys, 2008, 35: 409-411.

[278] Karolczak M, Schaller S, Engelke K, et al. Implementation of a conebeam reconstruction algorithm for the single-circle source orbit with embedded misalignment correction using homo-geneous coordinates. Med Phys, 2001, 28: 2050-2069.

[279] Karssemeijer N, Frieling JT, Hendriks JH. Spatial resolution in digital mammography. Invest Radiol, 1993, 28: 413-419.

[280] Kato I, Beinart C, Bleich A, et al. A nested case-control study of mammographic patterns, breast volume, and breast cancer (New York City, NY, United States). Cancer Causes Control, 1995, 6: 431-438.

[281] Kazantsev IG, Pickalov VV. On the accuracy of line, strip-and fan-based algebraic reconstruction from few projections. Signal Process, 1999, 78: 117-126.

[282] Kim J, Benson O, Kan H, et al. Single-photon turnstile device: simultaneous Coulomb blockade for electrons and holes. Semicond Sci Technol, 1998, 13 (8A Suppl S): A127-A129.

[283] Kim J, Benson O, Kan H, et al. A single-photon turnstile device. Nature, 1999, 397: 500-503.

[284] Kim BS, Isaacson D, Xia HJ, et al. A method for analyzing electrical impedance spec-troscopy data from breast cancer patients. Physiol Meas, 2007a, 28: S237-S246.

[285] Kim DY, Moon WK, Cho N, et al. MRI of the breast for the detection and assessment of the size of ductal carcinoma in situ. Korean J Radiol, 2007b, 8: 32-39.

[286] Klug A. From macromolecules to biological assemblies. Nobel lecture. Biosci Rep, 1983, 3: 395-430.

[287] Knoll TF, Delp EJ. Adaptive gray scale mapping to reduce registration noise in difference images. Comp Vis Graphics Image Proc, 1986, 33: 129-137.

[288] Konovalov AB, Vlasov VV, Mogilenskikh DV, et al. Algebraic reconstruction and postpro-cessing in one-step diffuse optical tomography. Quantum Electron, 2008, 38: 588-596.

[289] Kroman N. Timing of breast cancer surgery in relation to the menstrual cycle-the rise and fall of a hypothesis. Acta Oncol, 2008, 47: 576-579.

[290] Krotz D.U.S. watches efforts in Europe to slash CT radia-tion load. Diagn Imaging (San Franc), 1999, 21: 47-49.

[291] Kuhl CK, Schild HH, Morakkabati N. Dynamic bilateral contrast-enhanced MR imaging of the breast: trade-offbetween spatial and temporal resolution. Radiology, 2005, 236: 789-800.

[292] Kuzmiak CM, Pisano ED, Cole EB, et al. Comparison of full-feld digital mammography to screen-flm mammography with respect to contrast and spatial resolution in tissue equivalent breast phantoms. Med Phys, 2005, 32: 3144-3150.

[293] Kwan ALC, Boone JM, Yang K, et al. Evaluation of the spatial resolution characteristics of a cone-beam breast CT scanner. Med Phys, 2007, 34: 275-281.

[294] Ladas KT, Devaney AJ. Generalized ART algorithm for diffraction tomography. Inverse Prob, 1991, 7: 109-125.

[295] Ladas KT, Devaney AJ. Application of an ART algorithm in an experimental study of ultrasonic diffraction tomography. Ultrason Imaging, 1993, 15: 48-58.

[296] Lauterbur PC. Image formation by induced interactions: examples employing nuclear magnetic resonance. Nature, 1973, 242: 191-192.

[297] Law CK, Kimble HJ. Deterministic generation of a bit-stream of single-photon pulses. J Mod Opt, 1997, 44: 2067-2074.

[298] Law J, Faulkner K, Young KC. Risk factors for induction of breast cancer by X-rays and their implications for breast screening. Br J Radiol, 2007, 80: 261-266.

[299] Lazebnik M, Zhu CF, Palmer GM, et al. Electromagnetic spectroscopy of normal breast tissue specimens obtained from reduction surgeries: comparison of optical and microwave properties. IEEE Trans Biomed Eng, 2008, 55: 2444-2451.

[300] Leahy JV, Smith KT, Solmon DC. Uniqueness, nonu-niqueness, and inversion in the X-ray and Radon problems//Proceedings of the international symposium on ill-posed problems. Newark: University of Delaware, 1979.

[301] Lee H, Frank MS, Rowberg AH, et al. A new method for computed tomography image compression using adjacent slice data. Invest Radiol, 1993, 28: 678-685.

[302] Lee NY, Jung SH, Kim JB. Evaluation of the measurement geometries and data processing algorithms for industrial gamma tomography technology. Appl Radiat Isot, 2009, 67: 1441-1444.

[303] Lent A. A convergent algorithm for maximum entropy image restoration, with a medical X-ray application// Shaw R (ed) Image analysis and evaluation. Washington, D.C.: Society of Photographic Scientists and Engineers, 1977: pp 249-257.

[304] Lent A, Censor Y. The primal-dual algorithm as a constraint-set-manipulation device. Math Program, 1991, 50: 343-357.

[305] Lerner BH. Breast cancer wars: hope, fear, and the pursuit of a cure in twentieth-century America. New York: Oxford University Press, 2001.

[306] Levinthal C. Are there pathways for protein folding. J Chim Phys, 1968, 65: 44-45.

[307] Li FP, Corkery J, Vawter G, et al. Breast carcinoma after cancer therapy in childhood. Cancer, 1983, 51: 521-523.

[308] Li T, Liang Z, Singanallur JV, et al. Reconstruction for proton computed tomogra-phy by tracing proton trajectories: a Monte Carlo study. Med Phys, 2006, 33: 699-706.

[309] Li H, Zheng YB, More MJ, et al. Lesion quantifcation in dual-modality mammotomography. IEEE Trans Nucl Sci, 2007, 54: 107-115.

[310] Li CM, Segars WP, Tourassi GD, et al. Methodology for generating a 3D computerized breast phantom from empirical data. Med Phys, 2009, 36: 3122-3131.

[311] Lindfors KK, Boone JM, Nelson TR, et al. Dedicated breast CT: initial clinical experience. Radiology, 2008, 246: 725-733.

[312] Linton OW, Mettler FA Jr. National conference on dose reduction in CT, with an emphasis on pediatric patients. AJR Am J Roentgenol, 2003, 181: 321-329.

[313] Liu DS, Gong P, Kelly M, et al. Automatic registration of airborne images with complex local distortion. Photogramm Eng Remote Sens, 2006, 72: 1049-1059.

[314] Lobo SM, Liu ZJ, Yu NC, et al. RF tumour ablation: computer simulation and mathematical modelling of the effects of electrical and thermal conductivity. Int J Hyperthermia, 2005, 21: 199-213.

[315] Lukishova SG, Schmid AW, Knox R, et al. Room temperature source of single photons of defnite polarization. J Mod Opt, 2007, 54: 417-429.

[316] Lyncean Technologies. Illuminating X-ray science. The technology, 2009. http://www.lynceantech.com/Mabcure.http://www.mabcure.com/technology.html

[317] Machlin ES, Freilich A, Agrawal DC, et al. Field ion microscopy of biomolecules. J Microsc, 1975, 104: 127-168.

[318] Maes RM, Dronkers DJ, Hendriks JH, et al. Do non-specifc minimal signs in a biennial mam-mographic breast cancer screening programme need further diagnostic assessment. Br J Radiol,

1997, 70: 34-38.

[319] Maganti SS, Dhawan AP. Three-dimensional Nevoscope image reconstruction using diverging ray ART. Proc SPIE, 1997, 3032: 340-348.

[320] Malberger E, Gutterman E, Bartfeld E, et al. Cellular changes in the mammary gland epithelium during the menstrual cycle. A computer image analysis study. Acta Cytol, 1987, 31: 305-308.

[321] Malini S, Smith EO, Goldzieher JW. Measurement of breast volume by ultrasound during normal menstrual cycles and with oral contraceptive use. Obstet Gynecol, 1985, 66: 538-541.

[322] Marabini R, Herman GT, Carazo JM. 3D reconstruction in electron microscopy using ART with smooth spherically symmetric volume elements (blobs). Ultramicroscopy, 1998, 72: 53-65.

[323] March DE, Wechsler RJ, Kurtz AB, et al. CT-pathologic correlation of axillary lymph nodes in breast carcinoma. J Comput Assist Tomogr, 1991, 15: 440-444.

[324] Markussen T, Fu XW, Margulies L, et al. An algebraic algorithm for generation of three-dimensional grain maps based on diffraction with a wide beam of hard X-rays. J Appl Crystallogr, 2004, 37: 96-102.

[325] Marti JT. Convergence of the discrete ART algorithm for the reconstruction of digital pictures from their projections. Computing, 1979, 21: 105-111.

[326] Martin D, Thulasiraman P, Gordon R. Local independence in computed tomography as a basis for parallel computing. Technol Cancer Res Treat, 2005, 4: 187-188.

[327] Matej S, Herman GT, Narayan TK, et al. Evaluation of task-oriented performance of several fully 3D PET reconstruction algorithms. Phys Med Biol, 1994, 39: 355-367.

[328] Mazin SR, Pelc NJ. Fourier rebinning algorithm for inverse geometry CT. Med Phys, 2008, 35: 4857-4862.

[329] Mazur AK. Image correlation technique for recovering deformation felds from pictures. Ph.D. thesis, Supervisor: R. Gordon. Department of Electrical & Computer Engineering. University of Manitoba: Winnipeg, 1992.

[330] Mazur EJ, Gordon R. Interpolative algebraic reconstruction techniques without beam partitioning for computed tomography. Med Biol Eng Comput, 1995, 33: 82-86.

[331] Mazur AK, Mazur EJ, Gordon R. Digital differential radi-ography (DDR): a new diagnostic procedure for locating neoplasms, such as breast cancers, in soft, deformable tissues. SPIE, 1993, 1905: 443-455.

[332] McKeever WF. An X-linked three allele model of hand preference and hand posture for writing. Laterality, 2004, 9: 149-173.

[333] McKinley RL, Tornai MP, Samei E, et al. Simulation study of a quasi-monochromatic beam for X-ray computed mammotomography. Med Phys, 2004, 31 (4): 800-813.

[334] McKinley RL, Tornai MP, Brzymialkiewicz C, et al. Analysis of a novel offset cone-beam computed mammotomography system geometry for accommodating various breast sizes. Phys Med, 2006, 21 (Suppl 1): 48-55.

[335] Melvin C, Abdel-Hadi K, Cenzano S, et al. A simulated comparison of turnstile and Poisson photons for X-ray imaging// Canadian conference on electrical and computer engineering, 2002. IEEE CCECE 2002, 2002, vol 2. IEEE: pp 1165-1170.

[336] Mettlin CJ, Smart CR. The Canadian National Breast Screening Study. An appraisal and implications for early detection policy. Cancer, 1993, 72 (4 Suppl): 1461-1465.

[337] Michler P, Kiraz A, Becher C, et al. A quantum dot single-photon turnstile device. Science, 2000, 290: 2282-2285.

[338] Miller AB. Canadian National Breast Screening Study: response. Can Med Assoc J, 1993, 149: 1374-1375.

[339] Mishra D, Muralidhar K, Munshi P. A robust MART algorithm for tomographic applications. Num Heat Transf B-Fund, 1999, 35: 485-506.

[340] Mokbel K. Risk-reducing strategies for breast cancer-a review of recent literature. Int J Fertil Womens Med, 2003, 48: 274-277.

[341] Moon RJ. Amplifying and intensifying the fuoroscopic image by means of a scanning X-ray tube.

Science, 1950, 112: 389-395.

[342] More MJ, Li H, Goodale PJ, et al. Limited angle dual modality breast imaging. IEEE Trans Nucl Sci, 2007, 54: 504-513.

[343] Morrison PR, vanSonnenberg E, Shankar S, et al. Radiofrequency ablation of thoracic lesions: part 1, experiments in the normal porcine thorax. AJR Am J Roentgenol, 2005, 184: 375-380.

[344] Mueller K, Yagel R, Cornhill JF. The weighted-distance scheme: a globally optimizing projection ordering method for ART. IEEE Trans Med Imaging, 1997, 16: 223-230.

[345] Mueller K, Yagel R, Wheller JJ. A fast and accurate projection algorithm for the Algebraic Reconstruction Technique (ART). Proc SPIE, 1998, 3336: 724-732.

[346] Muraishi H, Nishimura K, Abe S, et al. Evaluation of spatial resolution for heavy ion CT system based on the measurement of residual range distribution with HIMAC. IEEE Trans Nucl Sci, 2009, 56: 2714-2721.

[347] Murata K, Takahashi M, Mori M, et al. Pulmonary metastatic nodules: CT-pathologic correlation. Radiology, 1992, 182: 331-335.

[348] Murugan RM. An improved electrical impedance tomography (EIT) algorithm for the detection of early stages of breast cancer. Ph.D. thesis, Supervisors: A. Wexler & R. Gordon. Department of Electrical & Computer Engineering, University of Manitoba: Winnipeg, 2000.

[349] Nab HW, Karssemeijer N, Van Erning LJ, et al. Comparison of digital and conventional mammography: a ROC study of 270 mammograms. Med Inform (Lond), 1992, 17: 125-131.

[350] Nagy JG. Fast inverse QR factorization for Toeplitz matrices. SIAM J Sci Stat Comput, 1993, 14: 1174-1193.

[351] Nandi RJ, Nandi AK, Rangayyan RM, et al. Classifcation of breast masses in mammograms using genetic programming and feature selection. Med Biol Eng Comput, 2006, 44: 683-694.

[352] NASA. Innovative Partnerships Program, 2009a. http://www.nasa.gov/offces/ipp/innovation_incubator/cc_home.html

[353] NASA. New NASA prize challenges: an opportunity to shape the prize challenges that NASA will offer to America's citizen inventors. External call for prize concepts. Innovative. Partnerships Program.National Aeronautics and Space Administration: Washington, D.C, 2009b.

[354] Nelson TR, Pretorius DH, Schiffer LM. Menstrual variation of normal breast NMR relaxation parameters. J Comput Assist Tomogr, 1985, 9: 875-879.

[355] Nelson HD, Tyne K, Naik A, et al. Screening for breast cancer: systematic evidence review update for the U. S. Preventive Services Task Force. Evidence Review Update No. 74. AHRQ Publication No. 10-05142-EF-1. Agency for Healthcare Research and Quality, Rockville, 2009.

[356] Nelsona TR, Cervino LI, Boone JM, et al. Classifcation of breast computed tomography data. Med Phys, 2008, 35: 1078-1086.

[357] Ng EY, Sree SV, Ng KH, et al. The use of tissue electrical characteristics for breast cancer detection: a perspective review. Technol Cancer Res Treat, 2008, 7: 295-308.

[358] Nickoloff EL, Donnelly E, Eve L, et al. Mammographic resolution: infuence of focal spot intensity distribution and geometry. Med Phys, 1990, 17: 436-447.

[359] Nie LM, Xing D, Zhou Q, et al. Microwave-induced thermoacoustic scanning CT for high-contrast and noninvasive breast cancer imaging. Med Phys, 2008, 35: 4026-4032.

[360] Nields M. Industry perspective: maximizing the benefit of improved detection with guided and monitored thermal ablation of small tumors. Technol Cancer Res Treat, 2005, 4: 123-130.

[361] Nielsen M. Autopsy studies of the occurrence of cancerous, atypical and benign epithelial lesions in the female breast. APMIS, 1989, 10 (Suppl): 1-56.

[362] Nielsen M, Thomsen JL, Primdahl S, et al. Breast cancer and atypia among young and middle-aged women: a study of 110 medicolegal autopsies. Br J Cancer, 1987, 56: 814-819.

[363] Nielsen T, Manzke R, Proksa R, et al. Cardiac

[363] cone-beam CT volume reconstruction using ART. Med Phys, 2005, 32: 851-860.

[364] Noguchi M. Radiofrequency ablation treatment for breast cancer to meet the next challenge: how to treat primary breast tumor without surgery. Breast Cancer, 2003, 10: 1-3.

[365] Nomura M. The role of RNA and protein in ribosome function: a review of early reconstitution studies and prospects for future studies. Cold Spring Harb Symp Quant Biol, 1987, 52: 653-663.

[366] Novick A, Szilard L. Experiments with the chemostat on spontaneous mutations of bacteria. Proc Natl Acad Sci USA, 1950, 36: 708-719.

[367] O'Connor JM, Das M, Didier C, et al. Using mastectomy specimens to develop breast models for breast tomosynthesis and CT breast imaging. Proc SPIE, 2008, 6913: 15.11-15.16.

[368] Oh TI, Lee J, Seo JK, Kim SW, et al. Feasibility of breast cancer lesion detection using a multi-frequency trans-admittance scanner (TAS) with 10 Hz to 500 kHz bandwidth. Physiol Meas, 2007, 28: S71-S84.

[369] O'Neal DP, Hirsch LR, Halas NJ, et al. Photothermal tumor ablation in mice using near infrared-absorbing nanoparticles. Cancer Lett, 2004, 209: 171-176.

[370] Ortega JK, Harris JF, Gamow RI. The analysis of spiral growth in Phycomyces using a novel optical method. Plant Physiol, 1974, 53: 485-490.

[371] Oxborrow M, Sinclair AG. Single-photon sources. Contemp Phys 2005, 46: 173-206.

[372] Pachoud M, Lepori D, Valley JF, et al. Objective assessment of image quality in conventional and digital mammography taking into account dynamic range. Radiat Prot Dosimetry, 2005, 114: 380-382.

[373] Pan X, Sidky EY, Vannier M. Why do commercial CT scanners still employ traditional, fltered back-projection for image reconstruction. Inverse Prob, 2009, 25: 1-36, #123009.

[374] Pani S, Longo R, Dreossi D, et al. Breast tomography with synchrotron radiation: preliminary results. Phys Med Biol, 2004, 49: 1739-1754.

[375] Parham C, Zhong Z, Connor DM, et al. Design and implementation of a compact low-dose diffraction enhanced medical imaging system. Acad Radiol, 2009, 16: 911-917.

[376] Park JM, Ikeda DM. Promising techniques for breast cancer detection, diagnosis, and staging using nonionizing radiation imaging techniques. Phys Med, 2006, 21 (Suppl 1): 7-10.

[377] Park DY, Fessler JA, Yost MG, et al. Tomographic reconstruction of tracer gas concentration profles in a room with the use of a single OP-FTIR and two iterative algo-rithms: ART and PWLS. J Air Waste Manag Assoc, 2000, 50: 357-370.

[378] Pawlak B. Density estimation for positron emission tomog-raphy. Masters thesis, Supervisor: R. Gordon. Department of Electrical & Computer Engineering, University of Manitoba, Winnipeg, 2007.

[379] Pawlak B, Gordon R. Density estimation for positron emission tomography. Technol Cancer Res Treat, 2005, 4: 131-142.

[380] Pawlak B, Gordon R. Low dose positron emission tomography algorithm: kernel density estimation, in preparation Perutz MF (1990) Haemoglobin. Nature, 2010, 348: 583-584.

[381] Perutz MF. I wish I'd made you angry earlier. Essays on science, scientists and humanity. New York: Cold Spring Harbor Laboratory Press, 1998.

[382] Poplack SP, Tosteson TD, Wells WA, et al. Electromagnetic breast imaging: results of a pilot study in women with abnormal mammograms. Radiology, 2007, 243: 350-359.

[383] Porter FS. Low-temperature detectors in X-ray astronomy. Nucl Instrum Methods A, 2004, 520: 354-358.

[384] Potter MJA, Colquhoun G, Gordon R. Design of a 3D microtumour breast scanner using 7th-generation CT (Computed Tomography) // PowerPoint presentation, Department of Cell Biology & Anatomy/Faculty of Medicine, University of Calgary, 10 September 2009. Department of Radiology. Winnipeg: University of Manitoba, 2009.

[385] Poulin BJ, Gordon R. How to organize science

funding: the new Canadian Institutes for Health Research (CIHR), an opportunity to vastly increase innovation. Can Public Policy, 2001, 27: 95-112.

[386] Poyvasi M, Noghanian S, Thomas G, et al. Ultra-wide-band radar for early breast tumor detection. Technol Cancer Res Treat, 2005, 4: 190-191.

[387] Pramanik M, Ku G, Li CH, et al. Design and evaluation of a novel breast cancer detection system combining both thermoacoustic (TA) and photoacoustic (PA) tomogra-phy. Med Phys, 2008, 35: 2218-2223.

[388] Prasad SN, Houserkova D. The role of various modalities in breast imaging. Biomed Pap Med Fac Univ Palacky Olomouc Czech Repub, 2007, 151: 209-218.

[389] Prokop M. Cancer screening with CT: dose controversy. Eur Radiol, 2005, 15 (Suppl 4): D55-D61.

[390] Qian X, Rajaram R, Calderon-Colon X, et al. Design and characterization of a spatially distributed multibeam feld emission X-ray source for stationary digital breast tomosynthesis. Med Phys, 2009, 36: 4389-4399.

[391] Radon J .über die Bestimmung von Funktionen durch ihre integralwerte langs gewisser Mannigfaltigkeiten. On the determination of functions from their integrals along certain manifolds German. Ber Sachs Akad Wiss Leipzig, Math-Phys Kl, 1917, 69: 262-277.

[392] Rajan K, Patnaik LM. CBP and ART image reconstruction algorithms on media and DSP processors. Microprocess Microsyst, 2001, 25: 233-238.

[393] Ramachandran GN, Lakshminarayanan AV. Three-dimensional reconstruction from radiographs and electron micrographs: application of convolutions instead of Fourier transforms. Proc Natl Acad Sci USA, 1971, 68: 2236-2240.

[394] Ramlau R, Teschke G, Zhariy M. A compressive Landweber iteration for solving ill-posed inverse problems. Inverse Prob 24. Article Number 065013, 2008.

[395] Ramsay J, Birrell G, Lavin M. Breast cancer and radiother-apy in ataxia-telangiectasia heterozygote. Lancet, 1996, 347: 1627.

[396] Ramsay J, Birrell G, Lavin M. Testing for mutations of the ataxia telangiectasia gene in radiosensitive breast cancer patients. Radiother Oncol, 1998, 47: 125-128.

[397] Rangayyan RM, Gordon R. Computed tomography for remote areas via teleradiology. Proc SPIE, 1982a, 318: 182-185.

[398] Rangayyan RM, Gordon R. Streak preventive image reconstruction with ART and adaptive fltering. IEEE Trans Med Imaging, 1982b, MI-1: 173-178.

[399] Rangayyan RM, Dhawan AP, Gordon R. Algorithms for limited-view computed tomography: an annotated bibliogra-phy and a challenge. Appl Opt, 1985, 24: 4000-4012.

[400] Rangayyan RM, Alto H, Gavrilov D. Parallel implementation of the adaptive neighborhood contrast enhancement technique using histogram-based image partitioning. J Electron Imaging, 2001, 10: 804-813.

[401] Rangayyan RM, Ayres FJ, Desautels JEL. A review of computer-aided diagnosis of breast cancer: toward the detec-tion of subtle signs. J Franklin Inst, 2007, 344: 312-348.

[402] Rayavarapu RG, Petersen W, Ungureanu C, et al. Synthesis and bioconjuga-tion of gold nanoparticles as potential molecular probes for light-based imaging techniques. Int J Biomed Imaging, 2007: 1-10, Article Number29817

[403] Rehani MM. CT: caution on radiation dose. Indian J Radiol Imaging, 2000, 10: 19-20.

[404] Reiser I, Sidky EY, Nishikawa RM, et al. Development of an analytic breast phantom for quantitative comparison of reconstruction algorithms for digital breast tomosynthesis//Astley SM, Brady M, Rose C, Zwiggelaar R (eds) Proceedings, digital mammography, 8th international workshop, IWDM 2006, Manchester, UK, 18-21 June 2006. Berlin: Springer, 2006: pp 190-196.

[405] Retsky MW, Demicheli R, Hrushesky WJ, et al. Dormancy and surgery-driven escape from dor-

mancy help explain some clinical features of breast cancer. AP MIS, 2008, 116: 730-741.

[406] Rickey DW, Gordon R, Huda W. On lifting the inherent limitations of positron emission tomography by using mag-netic felds (MagPET). Automedica, 1992, 14: 355-369.

[407] Romberg J. Imaging via compressive sampling. IEEE Signal Process Mag, 2008, 25: 14-20.

[408] Ron E. Cancer risks from medical radiation. Health Phys, 2003, 85: 47-59.

[409] Rosen R. James F. Danielli: 1911-1984. J Soc Biol Struct, 1985, 8: 1-11.

[410] Rosenfeld NS, Haller JO, Berdon WE. Failure of development of the growing breast after radiation therapy. Pediatr Radiol, 1989, 19: 124-127.

[411] oubidoux MA, Sabel MS, Bailey JE, et al. Small (<2.0cm) breast cancers: mam-mographic and US fndings at US-guided cryoablation-initial experience. Radiology, 2004, 233: 857-867.

[412] Ruttimann UE, Qi XL, Webber RL. An optimal synthetic aperture for circular tomosynthesis. Med Phys, 1989, 16: 398-405.

[413] Sabatini DD. In awe of subcellular complexity: 50 years of trespassing boundaries within the cell. Annu Rev Cell Dev Biol, 2005, 21: 1-33.

[414] Saez F, Llebaria A, Lamy P, et al. Three-dimensional reconstruction of the streamer belt and other large-scale structures of the solar corona. Astron Astrophys, 2007, 473: 265-277.

[415] Sargent EH. The dance of molecules: how nanotechnology is changing our lives. Viking Canada: Toronto, 2005.

[416] Schaller S, Karolczak M, Engelke K, et al. Implementation of a fast cone-beam backprojection algorithm for microcomputed tomography (HCT) using homogeneous coordinates. Radiology, 1998, 209P: 433-434.

[417] Schlueter FJ, Wang G, Hsieh PS, et al. Longitudinal image deblurring in spiral CT. Radiology, 1994, 193: 413-418.

[418] Schmidt TG, Star-Lack J, Bennett NR, et al. A prototype table-top inverse-geometry volumetric CT system. Med Phys, 2006, 33: 1867-1878.

[419] Shao YP, Yao RT, Ma TY. A novel method to calibrate DOI function of a PET detector with a dual-ended-scintillator readout. Med Phys, 2008, 35: 5829-5840.

[420] Shaw de Paredes E. Evaluation of abnormal screening mammograms. Cancer, 1994, 74 (1 Suppl): 342-349.

[421] Shibata K, Uno K, Wu J, et al. Imaging of cancer activity and range of tumor involvement-applying to cancer. Rinsho Byori, 2007, 55: 648-655.

[422] Shorey J. Stochastic simulations for the detection of objects in three dimensional volumes: applications in medical imaging and ocean acoustics. Ph. D. thesis, Duke University, Durham, 2007.

[423] Shuryak I, Hahnfeldt P, Hlatky L, et al. A new view of radiation-induced cancer: integrating short-and long-term processes. Part II: second cancer risk estimation. Radiat Environ Biophys, 2009, 48: 275-286.

[424] Sidky EY, Pan XC. Image reconstruction in circular cone-beam computed tomography by constrained, total-variation minimization. Phys Med Biol, 2008, 53: 4777-4807.

[425] Sidky EY, Kao CM, Pan XH. Accurate image reconstruction from few-views and limited-angle data in divergent-beam CT. J Xray Sci Technol, 2006, 14: 119-139.

[426] Signorato R, Susini J, Goulon J, et al. Refective optics for the ESRF beamline ID 26. J Phys IV, 1997, 7 (C2): 331-332.

[427] Sijbers J, Postnov A. Reduction of ring artefacts in high resolution micro-CT reconstructions. Phys Med Biol, 2004, 49: N247-N253.

[428] Silva GT, Frery AC, Fatemi M. Image formation in vibro-acoustography with depth-of-feld effects. Comput Med Imaging Graph, 2006, 30: 321-327.

[429] Simick MK, Jong R, Wilson B, et al. Non-ionizing near-infrared radiation transillumination spectroscopy for breast tissue density and assessment of breast cancer risk. J Biomed Opt, 2004, 9: 794-803.

[430] Simmons RM. Ablative techniques in the treatment of benign and malignant breast disease. J

Am Coll Surg, 2003, 197: 334-338.

[431] Simpson HW, Griffths K, McArdle C, et al. The luteal heat cycle of the breast in disease. Breast Cancer Res Treat, 1996, 37: 169-178.

[432] Singletary SE. Radiofrequency ablation of breast cancer. Am Surg, 2003, 69: 37-40.

[433] Sivaramakrishna R. Breast image registration using a textural transformation. Med Phys, 1998, 25: 2249.

[434] Sivaramakrishna R. 3D breast image registration-a review. Technol Cancer Res Treat, 2005a, 4: 39-48.

[435] Sivaramakrishna R. Foreword: imaging techniques alter-native to mammography for early detection of breast cancer. Technol Cancer Res Treat, 2005b, 4: 1-4.

[436] Sivaramakrishna R. Foreword: workshop on alternatives to mammography II. Technol Cancer Res Treat, 2005c, 4: 121-122.

[437] Sivaramakrishna R, Gordon R. Detection of breast cancer at a smaller size can reduce the likelihood of metastatic spread: a quantitative analysis. Acad Radiol, 1997a, 4: 8-12.

[438] Sivaramakrishna R, Gordon R. Mammographic image registration using the Starbyte transformation//McLaren PG, Kinsner W (eds) WESCSAN-EX'97. IEEE, Winnipeg, 1997b: pp 144-149.

[439] Sivaramakrishna R, Powell KA, Chilcote WA, et al. Comparing the performance of image enhancement algorithms utilizing different method-ologies in visualizing known lesions in digitized mammo-grams in a soft-copy display setting. Radiology, 1999, 213P: 969.

[440] Sivaramakrishna R, Obuchowski NA, Chilcote WA, et al. Comparing the performance of mammographic enhancement algorithms: a preference study. AJR Am J Roentgenol, 2000, 175: 45-51.

[441] Smith JA, Andreopoulou E. An overview of the status of imaging screening technology for breast cancer. Ann Oncol, 2004, 15 (Suppl 1): 118-126.

[442] Smith KT, Solmon DC, Wagner SL. Practical and math-ematical aspects of the problem of reconstructing objects from radiographs. Bull Am Math Soc, 1977, 83: 1227-1270.

[443] Smith KT, Solmon DC, Wagner SL, et al. Mathematical aspects of divergent beam radiography. Proc Natl Acad Sci USA, 1978, 75: 2055-2058.

[444] Sobel D. Longitude: the true story of a lone genius who solved the greatest scientifc problem of his time. New York: Walker, 1995.

[445] Soble P, Rangayyan RM, Gordon R. Quantitative and qualitative evaluation of geometric deconvolution of distortion in limited-view computed tomography. IEEE Trans Biomed Eng BME, 1985, 32: 330-335.

[446] Song YZ, Hu GY, He AZ. Simple self-correlative alge-braic reconstruction technique. Spectroscop Spectral Anal, 2006a, 26: 2364-2367.

[447] Song YZ, Sun T, Hu GY, et al. Analyzing the methods to smooth feld reconstructed by algebraic reconstruction technique with spectroscopy. Spectroscop Spectral Anal, 2006b, 26: 1411-1415.

[448] Spanu A, Cottu P, Manca A, et al. Scintimammography with dedicated breast camera in unifocal and multifocal/multicentric primary breast cancer detection: a comparative study with SPECT. Int J Oncol, 2007, 31: 369-377.

[449] Spelic DC. Updated trends in mammography dose and image quality, 2009. http://www.fda.gov/Radiation-EmittingProducts/MammographyQualityStandardsActandProgram/FacilityScorecard/ucm113352.htm

[450] Stein WD. James Frederic Danielli, 1911-1984, Elected F.R.S. 1957. Biogr Mem Fellows R Soc, 1986, 32: 115-135.

[451] Steiner G, Soleimani M, Watzenig D. A bio-electrome-chanical imaging technique with combined electrical impedance and ultrasound tomography. Physiol Meas, 2008, 29: S63-S75.

[452] Stomper PC, Mazurchuk RV, Tsangaris TN. Breast MRI as an adjunct in the diagnosis of a carcinoma partially obscured on mammography. Clin Imaging, 1994, 18: 195-198.

[453] Strebhardt K, Ullrich A. Paul Ehrlich's magic bullet concept: 100 years of progress. Nat Rev Cancer, 2008, 8: 473-480.

[454] Strong AB, Hurst RA. EMI patents on computed

[455] Subbarao PMV, Munshi P, Muralidhar K. Performance evaluation of iterative tomographic algorithms applied to reconstruction of a three-dimensional temperature feld. Num Heat Transf B-Fund, 1997a, 31: 347-372.

[456] Subbarao PMV, Munshi P, Muralidhar K. Performance of iterative tomographic algorithms applied to non-destructive evaluation with limited data. NDT and E Int, 1997b, 30: 359-370.

[457] Subramanian E. G.N. Ramachandran Obituary. Nat Struct Biol, 2001, 8: 489-491.

[458] Sun J, Chapman JA, Gordon R, et al. Survival from primary breast cancer by tumour size for the age groups with different screening guidelines. Breast Cancer Res Treat, 1998, 50: 281.

[459] Sun J, Chapman JA, Gordon R, et al. Survival from primary breast cancer after routine clinical use of mammography. Breast J, 2002, 8: 199-208.

[460] Suri JS, Rangayyan R, Laxminarayan S. Emerging technologies in breast and mammography imaging and its applications. ASP, Stevenson Ranch, 2006.

[461] Szent-Gyorgyi A. Introduction to a submolecular biology. New York: Academic, 1960.

[462] Szent-Gyorgyi A. The living state, with observations on cancer. New York: Academic, 1972.

[463] Tafra L. Positron emission tomography (PET) and mam-mography (PEM) for breast cancer: importance to surgeons. Ann Surg Oncol, 2007, 14: 3-13.

[464] Takahashi S. An atlas of axial transverse tomography and its clinical application. New York: Springer, 1969.

[465] Taminiau TH, Stefani FD, Segerink FB, et al. Optical antennas direct single-molecule emission. Nat Photonics, 2008, 2: 234-237.

[466] Tarone RE. The excess of patients with advanced breast cancer in young women screened with mammography in the Canadian National Breast Screening Study. Cancer, 1995, 75: 997-1003.

[467] Tateno Y, Tanaka H. Low-dosage X-ray imaging system employing fying spot X-ray microbeam (dynamic scanner). Radiology, 1976, 121: 189-195.

[468] Tateno Y, Tanaka H, Watanabe E. Dynamic scanner, an imaging system employing fying spot X-ray microbeam. J Nucl Med, 1976, 17: 551-552.

[469] Taylor PHS. Computational physiology of the human breast. Ph.D. thesis. Department of Computer Science.University of Western Australia: Australia, 2002.

[470] Taylor P, Owens R .Simulated mammography of a three-dimensional breast model//Astley S, Fujita H, Gale A, Giger M, Karssemeijer N, Peitgen HO, Pisano E, Williams M, Yaffe M (eds) IWDM 2000. Abstracts of the 5th interna-tional conference on digital mammography, Toronto. Medical Physics, Madison, 2001: 138.

[471] Thie JA. Optimizing dual-time and serial positron emission tomography and single photon emission computed tomography scans for diagnoses and therapy monitoring. Mol Imaging Biol, 2007, 9: 348-356.

[472] Thorpe H, Brown SR, Sainsbury JR, et al. Timing of breast cancer sur-gery in relation to menstrual cycle phase: no effect on 3-year prognosis: the ITS Study. Br J Cancer, 2008, 98: 39-44.

[473] Tomanek B, Hoult DI, Chen X, et al. A probe with chest shielding for improved breast MR imaging. Magn Reson Med, 2000, 43: 917-920.

[474] Trummer MR. Reconstructing pictures from projections: on the convergence of the ART algorithm with relaxation. Computing, 1981, 26 (3): 189-195.

[475] Trummer MR. SMART: an algorithm for reconstructing pictures from projections. Z Angew Math Physik, 1983, 34: 743-753.

[476] Turunen MJ, Huikuri K, Lempinen M. Results of 32 major hepatic resections for primary and secondary malig-nancies of the liver. Ann Chir Gynaecol, 1986, 75: 209-214.

[477] United Artists Corporation. Fiddler on the roof Video Vainshtein BK (1971) The synthesis of

projecting functions. Sov Physics Dokl, 1971, 16: 66-99.

[478] Van Uytven E, Pistorius S, Gordon R. An iterative three-dimensional electron density imaging algorithm using uncol-limated Compton scattered X-rays from a polyenergetic primary pencil beam. Med Phys, 2007, 34: 256-274.

[479] Van Uytven E, Pistorius S, Gordon R. A method for 3D electron density imaging using single scattered X rays with application to mammographic screening. Phys Med Biol, 2008, 53: 5445-5459.

[480] Vargas HI, Dooley WC, Gardner RA, et al. Focused micro-wave phased array thermotherapy for ablation of early-stage breast cancer: results of thermal dose escalation. Ann Surg Oncol, 2004, 11: 139-146.

[481] Vasile G, Trouve E, Ciuc M, et al. General adaptive-neighborhood technique for improving synthetic aperture radar interferometric coherence estimation. J Opt Soc Am A Opt Image Sci Vis, 2004, 21: 1455-1464.

[482] Verschraegen C, Vinh-Hung V, Cserni G, et al. Modeling the effect of tumor size in early breast cancer. Ann Surg, 2005, 241: 309-318.

[483] Vinh-Hung V, Gordon R. Quantitative target sizes for breast tumor detection prior to metastasis: a prerequisite to rational design of 4D scanners for breast screening. Technol Cancer Res Treat, 2005, 4: 11-21.

[484] Vinh-Hung V, Tot T, Gordon R. One or many targets.Towards resolving the paradox of single versus multifocal breast cancer from epidemiological data, in preparation, 2010.

[485] Vock P. CT dose reduction in children. Eur Radiol, 2005, 15: 2330-2340.

[486] Vogel PM, Georgiade NG, Fetter BF, et al. The correlation of histologic changes in the human breast with the menstrual cycle. Am J Pathol, 1981, 104: 23-34.

[487] Wade N. Maurice H. F. Wilkins, 87, a DNA Nobelist, Dies. NY Times, 2004.

[488] Wall J, Langmore J, Isaacson M, et al. Scanning transmission electron microscopy at high resolution. Proc Natl Acad Sci USA, 1974, 71: 1-5.

[489] Wan X, Gao YQ, Wang Q, et al. Limited-angle optical computed tomography algorithms. Opt Eng, 2003, 42: 2659-2669.

[490] Wang G, Snyder DL, O'Sullivan JA, et al. Iterative deblurring for CT metal artifact reduction. IEEE Trans Med Imaging, 1996, 15: 657-664.

[491] Wang G, Vannier MW, Cheng PC. Iterative X-ray cone-beam tomography for metal artifact reduction and local region reconstruction. Microsc Microanal, 1999, 5: 58-65.

[492] Watt DW. Column relaxed algebraic reconstruction algorithm for tomography with noisy data. Appl Opt, 1994, 33: 4420-4427.

[493] Webber RL. Feedback control of exposure geometry in dental radiography. Publication No. 80-1954. National Institutes of Health: Bethesda, 1979.

[494] Wen DB, Yuan YB, Ou JK, et al. A hybrid reconstruction algorithm for 3-D ionospheric tomography. IEEE Trans Geosci Remote Sens, 2008, 46: 1733-1739.

[495] White E, Velentgas P, Mandelson MT, et al. Variation in mammo-graphic breast density by time in menstrual cycle among women aged 40-49 years. J Natl Cancer Inst, 1998, 90: 906-910.

[496] Wiest PW, Locken JA, Heintz PH, et al. CT scanning: a major source of radiation exposure. Semin Ultrasound CT MR, 2002, 23: 402-410.

[497] Wikipedia Contributors. Japanese rock garden. Wikipedia, the free encyclopedia. Wikimedia Foundation: San Francisco, 2009.http://en.wikipedia.org/wiki/Japanese_rock_garden

[498] Woten DA, El-Shenawee M. Broadband dual linear polarized antenna for statistical detection of breast cancer. IEEE Trans Antennas Propag, 2008, 56: 3576-3580.

[499] Wu T, Stewart A, Stanton M, et al. Tomographic mammography using a limited number of low-dose cone-beam projection images. Med Phys, 2003, 30: 365-380.

[500] Wu YB, Bowen SL, Yang K, et al. PET characteristics of a dedicated breast PET/CT scanner prototype. Phys Med Biol, 2009, 54: 4273-4287.

[501] Yaffe MJ, Mainprize JG, Jong RA. Technical developments in mammography. Health Phys, 2008, 95: 599-611.

[502] Yamada H, Saisho H, Hirai T, et al. X-ray fuorescence analysis of heavy elements with a portable synchrotron. Spectrochim Acta B, 2004, 59: 1323-1328.

[503] Yang SK, Cho N, Moon WK. The role of PET/CT for evaluating breast cancer. Korean J Radiol, 2007, 8: 429-437.

[504] Yang K, Kwan ALC, Huang SY, et al. Noise power properties of a cone-beam CT system for breast cancer detection. Med Phys, 2008, 35: 5317-5327.

[505] Ye G, Lim KH, George RT, et al. 3D EIT for breast cancer imaging: system, measurements, and reconstruction. Microwave Opt Technol Lett, 2008, 50: 3261-3271.

[506] Yee KM. Breast imaging: new technologies emerge, 2009. http://medicalphysicsweb.org/cws/article/research/40184.

[507] Yoshinaga T, Imakura Y, Fujimoto K, et al. Bifurcation analysis of iterative image reconstruction method for computed tomography. Int J Bifurcation Chaos, 2008, 18: 1219-1225.

[508] Yu HY, Cao GH, Burk L, Lee Y, et al. Compressive sampling based interior reconstruction for dynamic carbon nanotube micro-CT. J Xray Sci Technol, 2009, 17: 295-303.

[509] Zarghami N, Grass L, Sauter ER, et al. Prostate-specifc antigen in serum during the menstrual cycle. Clin Chem, 1997, 43: 1862-1867.

[510] Zhang J, Olcott PD, Chinn G, et al. Study of the performance of a novel 1 mm resolution dual-panel PET camera design dedicated to breast cancer imaging using Monte Carlo simulation. Med Phys, 2007, 34: 689-702.

[511] Zhang B, He Y, Song Y, et al. Defection tomographic reconstruction of a complex fow feld from incomplete projection data. Opt Lasers Eng, 2009, 47: 1183-1188.

[512] Zhou X. Digital subtraction mammography via geometric unwarping for detection of early breast cancer. Ph.D. thesis, Supervisor: R. Gordon. Department of Electrical & Computer Engineering, University of Manitoba, Winnipeg, 1991.

[513] Zhou SA, Brahme A. Development of phase-contrast X-ray imaging techniques and potential medical applications. Phys Med, 2008, 24: 129-148.

[514] Zhou XH, Gordon R. Detection of early breast cancer: an overview and future prospects. Crit Rev Biomed Eng, 1989, 17: 203-255.

[515] Zhou X, Liang ZP, Cofer GP, et al. Reduction of ringing and blurring artifacts in fast spinecho imaging. J Magn Reson Imaging, 1993, 3: 803-807.

[516] Zhou L, Oldan J, Fisher P, et al. Low-contrast lesion detection in tomosynthetic breast imaging using a realistic breast phantom. Proc SPIE, 2006, 6142: 5A.1-5A.12.

[517] Zwirewich CV, Miller RR, Muller NL. Multicentric adenocarcinoma of the lung: CT-pathologic correlation. Radiology, 1990, 176: 185-190.

第11章 结语：X染色体失活和分化波与病变的乳腺腺叶

Richard Gordon

关于癌症是始于一个单细胞的病变（Hahn, Weinberg, 2002），还是始于多灶性病变（多指多细胞模型病变）（或场理论）的辩论持续了很长时间。《乳腺癌：腺叶疾病》一书可能是试图解决这个问题的一块敲门砖。我自己开展的乳腺癌检测工作基于以下的假设，虽然第一眼的印象似乎是与Tibor Tot的病态腺叶假说相悖，即控制某一个局限性病灶就可以控制乳腺癌，这个假说看起来也得到了流行病学证据的支持。然而，通过去年我与Tot和Vincent Vinh-Hung的对话（Gordon, 2010）可以看出，通过更加微妙的角度思考能够让我们同时从两个视角观察乳腺癌，它们并不互相矛盾，具体的内容将在本章的末尾呈现。对于乳腺癌患者，切除局部的肿瘤可以在一定时间内阻止疾病复发，或者切除整个病态的腺体可以使患者的余生避免疾病复发，预后孰优孰劣难分高下。正如乳腺癌改良根治术与保乳手术的争议一样（Lerner, 2001），这两种术式均能改善乳腺癌患者的预后，在延长生存期方面近乎相同。尽管腺叶切除手术略逊于乳腺癌改良根治术，但差异不大。虽然我们可以挑出回顾性的流行病学数据的很多问题，但是，要回答这个争议，仍有许多工作要做（Vinh-Hung, et al, 2010）。

我的芝加哥大学附属John Dewey实验中学的物理老师曾经教育过我，关于科学观点的争论就像让一个人去骑对方的马，这个过程艰难无比，因为有太多与我们类似的人将自己包裹在自我的想法中，当现实情况与我们的想法相悖时，思维便开始陷入混乱。幸运的是，此次此时，我抛开了胚胎学工作的背景，开始了一种新的看待疾病组织的思维（Glrdon, 1999）。Tibor Tot要求我写这篇结语就是要我坐着自己的马鞍，但是要骑他的马。

如果我们观察一下同时拥有绿色和白色的杂色植物，就会发现不同的细胞克隆，某些能合成功能性叶绿素，某些不能合成功能性叶绿素（Yu, et al, 2007）。这些细胞都来自于一个单一的接合子，所以在植物生长发育（Linn, et al, 1990; Hoekenga, et al, 2000; Iida, et al, 2004）过程中发生一些表观遗传学的变化。对于植物，缺乏叶绿素通常会降低其生长速度（香蕉可能除外），因此可能减弱了适应性（Funayama, et al, 1997; Funayama-Noguchi, 2001），所以，我们可以把这些白色区域看成"病态腺叶"。的确，在自然界中，杂色植物罕见，只有在人类培育下才能长期生存，由于与人类的共生关系，它们才能适应自然。

在杂色表型的小鼠（Lyon, 1961, 2003）和三花猫（Davidson, 1964; Osgood, 1994），也有导致其色素斑点分布的表观遗传因素。这几乎（Lyon, 2003）只发生在雌性，是由于一条X染色体"随机"失活。现在我们知

R. Gordon
Department of Radiology, University of Manitoba,
Winnipeg, MB, Canada
e-mail: gordonr@cc.umanitoba.ca

第11章　结语：X染色体失活和分化波与病变的乳腺腺叶

道，所有基因型为XX的妇女都是镶嵌生物体，身体内包含了来自一个或另一个激活的X染色体的细胞克隆，这个激活的过程发生在胚胎的4~20个细胞的阶段（Puck，et al，1992；Monteiro，et al，1998；Chitnis，et al，1999；Brown，Robinson，2000）。

Tot假设，胚胎发育的第8~25周这个阶段，一个细胞发育成为一个乳腺小叶（Tot，2010），这个阶段正是X染色体刚刚失活以后。所以，通过检测同一个乳腺小叶是否具有相同的失活X染色体，即可以印证这一理论（Brown，Robinson，2000）。至少那些细胞还没有形成肿瘤，因为肿瘤细胞可以选择让哪个X染色体失活（Viiicent-Salomon，et al，2007）。在这样的试验中，我们还需要寻找一种可能性，即同一个乳腺中存在另一个X染色体激活的健康小叶（Kristiansen，et al，2005）。

X染色体的选择性失活（存在偏度）已经被许多人证实。一个组织中67%~90%的细胞有相同的X染色体被失活，而不是50%（Buller，et al，1999；Lose，et al，2008）。在乳腺小叶中，这一数值的中位数为27（Going，Moffat，2004）。假设我们接受这个假说，即便没有年龄的对照，在X染色体上，某未知基因的一个等位基因的异常参与到了乳腺癌的发病原因中，正如一些作者声称的那样（Lose，et al.，2008）[cf.（Kristiansen，et al，2005）]。然后，我们可以预见，平均而言，病态小叶的数量应该接近50%，或者说大约14个，而不是1或2个，这里需要注意的是，通过类比观察白色三花猫（比玳瑁猫体型小一点）的皮肤大块色斑（Vella，Robinson，1999），我们可以预见局部组织（例如乳腺）中偏度呈双峰分布。并且，组织间偏态一致性的初步证据已在人类中得到证实（Buller，et al，1999）。这3个假说支持了X染色体的选择性失活：X染色体连锁的等位基因赋予了细胞增殖优势；它是由遗传易感性决定的；它是一种保护机制，以减少有害的X连锁基因的表达（Lose，et al，2008）。X染色体选择性失活的未知机制可能在胚胎发育的过程中以一种组织特异的方式在特定时间发生，从50:50的比例开始（Muers，et al，2007），通过随机效应的积累，导致随着时间的延长，从50：50之后的指数偏差（Vickers，et al，2001；Kristiansen，et al，2003）。我们需要密切关注病态小叶学说与X染色体选择性失活之间联系的可能性，直到X染色体选择性失活在空间、统计、时间和流行病学方面被较好地阐明。

病态乳腺小叶是由一个细胞克隆出来的假说与单细胞以及多灶性的观点是兼容的。实际上，我们可以把整个病变的乳腺小叶看做是形成肿瘤前的一种状态。肿瘤细胞整合到正常的胚胎发育过程中，导致看起来完全正常的组织均被变异的细胞占据，这种处于稳态的病例是存在的（Mintz，Illmensee，1975；Pierce，et al，1982；Kulesa，et al，2006；Hendrix，et al，2007；Kasemeier-Kulesa，et al，2008），因此，这是一种合理的场景。

高度克隆化和嵌合式发育存在于如蜗牛发育的早期阶段（Raven，1966），海鞘（Nishida，2005）以及线虫（Sulston，et al，1983）的胚胎。其他种类的机体存在一种被称为"调控式发育"的体系。这会形成这样一种后果：一个给定克隆类别的细胞通常最后分化成不同的细胞类型。很少有人提问这是如何发生的，难道那些克隆能够自身分裂？在胚胎发育过程中，发生了一些其他的事情，例如"表观遗传"改变，这使得同一种克隆细胞具有了不同的命运。

我曾就这个问题写过一本内容洋洋洒洒、霸气侧漏的书（Gordon，1999）。该书的内容根据来自于我当年关于分化波（differentiation wave）的推测（Gordon，Brodland，1987），即胚胎上皮细胞扩张与收缩形成的可见的波形，这个波横跨胚胎的各个胚区（无论它们的细胞克隆起源），并随着波的传递引起下一步的分化。后来这一理论经过Natalie K. Bjorkiund的验证（Brodland，et al，1994），而且这个波形很容易被观察到（Gordon，Bjorklund，1996)。遗憾的是，有些分子发育生物学家并不接受这一理论，几十年来，物理因素触发并组织基因表达这一理论一直被他们唾弃。他们认为基因的"控制"元件理所当然地存在于细胞核中，而不在别处。例如下面的这本教科书所言：

一些研究者提出，在一个胚胎中，所有细胞的初始状态均表达相同的基因，直到它们受到物理因素的影响（例如分化波）后，产生了不同机械状态的细胞群，在此之后，不同的细胞群开始复合表达特异的基因（Gordon，Brodland，1987)。但是，现在大部分研究人员都认同这样一种假设，即细胞在最初时就被编程好表达特定的主控基因，之后主控基因与其他基因一起实现特定的功能……我们将在本文后半段探讨这个话题（kalthoff，2001)。

这种形势正在被扭转："生物力学是最新被发现的胚胎细胞发育系统调节的关键因素…"（Adamo, et al, 2009）[cf.（Beloussov, Gordon, 2006)]，除此之外，它还在细胞分化以及肿瘤形成中发挥了重要作用（Lopez, et al, 2008：Tenney, Discho, 2009：Wang, et al, 2009)。尽管如此，由于上述原因，在对细胞分化的研究中，与所谓的细胞分化决定因素的这些波有关的研究从来就没有得到过资助，这些课题被遗留给了下一代研究者。在虚拟世界中，一个在线的胚胎物理学的课题慢慢地吸引了一些研究者的加入（Gordon, Buckley, 2010)。就这样，将分化波与分化[或许还有去分化（Rossant, 2009)]有关的分子表观遗传学联系起来的研究终于艰难地起步了（Björklund, Gordon, 2006)。

分化波向我们展现一个更简单清晰的进化过程：一个胚胎组织通过两种波分裂成两个新的组织，一种是收缩波，另一种是扩张波。在上皮细胞，这些波似乎通过每个细胞顶端表面的细胞骨架装置传播，我们称其为"细胞状态分裂器"（Gordon, Brodland, 1987；Bjorklund, Gordon, 1993；Martin, Gordon, 1997)。从这个装置在微丝与微管之间产生的机械拮抗作用来看，它有点类似于纺锤体。该装置处于一个亚稳状态中，随时准备在顶端的微管或者顶端的微丝小环之间引发一场径向的"拔河比赛"（Gordon, Brcclmd, 1987)。这种不稳定状态很快会由细胞状态分裂器决出胜负：要么微丝小环获胜，细胞的顶端会剧烈地收缩；要么微管获胜，使细胞变得扁平（Gordon, Brodland, 1987)。我们假设一比特的信号通过一种信号转导的方式进入细胞核，导致两套已经备好的基因瀑布中的一套被级联触发（Bjorklund, Gordon, 1993)。因此，细胞分化被视为一个二进制的分叉过程，即每个胚胎发育过程中的中间型细胞都能够产生两种新类型的细胞。

目前为止，关于分化波的形成以及消减的机制依然处于推测阶段，我们急需在活体胚胎的研究中投入精力，进行定量的、针对所有细胞的全面的、细节的观察（Gordon, Westfall, 2009；Gordon, 2009)。

也许，乳腺小叶是由一个分化波造就出现的，而不是来自一个单个细胞的克隆？如果这个假设成立的话，之后我们必须追问造成乳腺小叶健康抑或是患病的初始事件是什么？有3个方面的因素需要考虑：①细胞状态分裂器；②从细胞状态分裂器到细胞核之间的信号传导；③基因表达的变化。分化波并不能解答这一疑问，只有合理的假设才能引导我们思考。所以，如果分化波产生了乳腺小叶，那么乳腺小叶内应该有不止一个克隆产生，这至少给了我们一个衡量标准来分辨我们的假设与Tot的克隆假说（Tot, 2010)。

如果我们从一个细胞生长发育成为一个完整机体内的角度来考虑，那这个过程中的中间细胞自然有它的来源。我们认为机体内所有的细胞都符合"细胞谱系树"的原则。这种概念上的细胞树互相不交叉，并因细胞分裂以一种严格的二进制形式分叉。除了横纹肌细胞，横纹肌细胞由于肌母细胞的融合形成了多核细胞，不符合细胞谱系树的分裂规则。

分化波为我们提供了另一种目录树——"组织谱系树"。在"组织谱系树"中，所有经历相同顺序收缩波（C）和舒张波（E）的细胞被定义为组织。这意味着，如果分化波是细胞分化初始的触发因素，那么所有细胞在它每一个发育阶段都会被指定一个二进制代码，例如CEECECCEEE等，这些代码代表了细胞参与分化波的历史。这种"分化代码"（Björklund，Gordon，1994）在细胞中可能具有某种表象，这种表象是细胞过去和现在的"记忆"。每一个胚胎组织在进一步的发育中精确地产生了两种组织，这个概念仅仅在文献中有所提及（Gordon，1999），还需进一步研究。因此，"组织谱系树"是否以严格的二进制方式进行分支的观点还有待证明。

在分化波中有一个重要的例外，这个例外导致了另一种看待病态小叶起源的方式。在介于舒张波和收缩波之间的分界线上，有一种既定的胚胎组织，它们有可能是一些从没参与过任何一种分化波的细胞。这也许是干细胞的起源，停留在胚胎阶段的细胞或许能够无限期地等待某种因素触发，向下一阶段分化（Gordon，2006）。这些干细胞的分化代码会限制细胞分化的种类，这或许与某些细胞在过去与其作用有关，或者是过去储存的记忆所致。这也许能解释为什么干细胞通常是多能性的而不是全能性的。因此，分化波理论也许能够解释在近年来已经发现的各种多能干细胞的起源。一些肿瘤干细胞也许来自正常的干细胞（Vermeulen，et al, 2008）。这些肿瘤干细胞在乳腺小叶中的细胞克隆（Howard，Ashworth，2006）也许就产生了病态的乳腺小叶：

流行病学现已发现乳腺癌和前列腺癌与胚胎阶段的关系（Fackelmann，1997）(Trichopoulos，1990；Ekbom，et al，1992）。有人可能会问是不是那些有活性的细胞不知何故错过了分化波，而成为了后来肿瘤发生的"候选人"（Gordon，1999）。

细胞谱系树是组织谱系树的一个亚型，干细胞是细胞谱系树在停滞状态的末端。为了阐明这一关系，我画了一个组织谱系树的分支图［即"分化树"（Gordon，1999）］，其中用少数细胞的分支来表示细胞谱系树（图11.1）。

X染色体失活、细胞、克隆、组织以及分化波之间的相互作用蕴含了许多启示，可以让我们解开癌症的单细胞学说与多灶性学说之间的关系之谜。在这些启示中，我们也许能找到病态乳腺小叶以及在其内形成的异常细胞的基本依据。例如，形态发生场（Waddington，1934；Beloussov，et al，1997）是从致癌和成瘤的组织发生场理论衍生出来的名字（Soto，et al，2008），这个模糊的概念正被具体的、可观察到的分化波（Gordon，1999）所替换。在成年人体内，是什么将类似细胞聚集在一

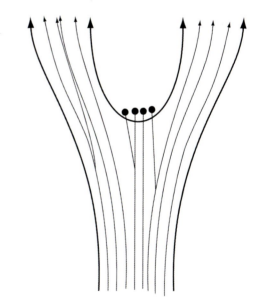

图11.1 粗箭头代表一个组织谱系树或者说"分化树"的分支（Gordon，1999）；纵向代表发育时间的延长。里面是细胞系，细线表示单个细胞。左边的这些细胞经历了一个收缩波，而右边的这些细胞经历了一个舒张波。因此，底部的处于早期发育阶段的细胞开始由一种类型变为两种类型。然而，有些细胞被这两种波同时忽略了，变成了干细胞，这些细胞用离开分化树的点表示。细胞分裂用细胞谱系树上的分支点来表示。遵循时间上的回推法，这两个目录树将会汇聚到胚胎期一个细胞的阶段，即合子

起形成组织（Soto, et al, 2008）是一个谜，也许同样涉及了一些存在于它们之间的持续作用的波（Gordon, 1999）。关于这些还有许多工作要做，但是通过结合细胞遗传学、胚胎学、病理学、分子生物学以及4D显微镜的现代方法，我们也许能够解开这个谜题。

致谢 我要感谢 William R. Buckley, Stephen A. Krawetz 和 Natalie K. Björklund 提出的意见以及 Stephen P. McGrew（New Light Industries, Spokane）和曼尼托巴大学放射科的器官成像基金会提供的支持。

参考文献

[1] Adamo L, Naveiras O, Wenzel PL, et al. Biomechanical forces promote embryonic haematopoiesis. Nature, 2009, 459: 1131-1135.

[2] Attolini CS, Michor F. Evolutionary theory of cancer. Ann NY Acad Sci, 2009, 1168: 23-51.

[3] Beloussov LV, Gordon R. Preface. Morphodynamics: bridging the gap between the genome and embryo physics. Int J Dev Biol, 2006, 50: 79-80.

[4] Beloussov LV, Opitz JM, Gilbert SF. Life of Alexander G. Gurwitsch and his relevant contribution to the theory of morphogenetic felds. Int J Dev Biol, 1997, 41: 771-779.

[5] Bjorklund NK, Gordon R. Nuclear state splitting: a working model for the mechanochemical coupling of differentiation waves to master genes. Russian J Dev Biol, 1993, 24: 79-95.

[6] Bjorklund NK, Gordon R. Surface contraction and expansion waves correlated with differentiation in axolotl embryos. I. Prolegomenon and differentiation during the plunge through the blastopore, as shown by the fate map. Comput Chem, 1994, 18: 333-345.

[7] Bjorklund NK, Gordon R. A hypothesis linking low folate intake to neural tube defects due to failure of post-translation methylations of the cytoskeleton. Int J Dev Biol, 2006, 50: 135-141.

[8] Brodland GW, Gordon R, Scott MJ, et al. Furrowing surface contraction wave coincident with primary neural induction in amphibian embryos. J Morphol, 1994, 219: 131-142.

[9] Brown CJ, Robinson WP. The causes and consequences of random and non-random X chromosome inactivation in humans. Clin Genet, 2000, 58: 353-363.

[10] Buller RE, Sood AK, Lallas T, et al. Association between nonrandom X-chromosome inactivation and *BRCA*1 mutation in germline DNA of patients with ovarian cancer. J Natl Cancer Inst, 1999, 91: 339-346.

[11] Chitnis S, Derom C, Vlietinck R, et al. X chromosome-inactivation patterns confrm the late timing of monoamniotic-MZ twinning. Am J Hum Genet, 1999, 65: 570-571.

[12] Davidson RG. The Lyon hypothesis. J Pediatr, 1964, 65: 765-775.

[13] Ekbom A, Trichopoulos D, Adami HO, et al. Evidence of prenatal infuences on breast cancer risk. Lancet, 1992, 340: 1015-1018.

[14] Fackelmann KA. The birth of a breast cancer: do adult diseases start in the womb. Sci News, 1997, 151: 108-109.

[15] Funayama S, Hikosaka K, Yahara T. Effects of virus infection and growth irradiance on ftness components and photo-synthetic properties of Eupatorium makinoi (Compositae). Am J Bot, 1997, 84: 823-829.

[16] Funayama-Noguchi S. Ecophysiology of virus-infected plants: a case study of Eupatorium makinoi infected by gem-inivirus. Plant Biol, 2001, 3: 251-262.

[17] Going JJ, Moffat DF. Escaping from Flatland: clinical and biological aspects of human mammary duct anatomy in three dimensions. J Pathol, 2004, 203: 538-544.

[18] Gordon R. The hierarchical genome and differentiation waves: novel unifcation of development, genetics and evolution. London: World Scientifc & Imperial College Press, 1999.

[19] Gordon R. Mechanics in embryogenesis and embryonics: prime mover or epiphenomenon. Int J Dev Biol, 2006, 50: 245-253.

[20] Gordon R. Google embryo for building quantitative under-standing of an embryo as it builds itself: II. Progress towards an embryo surface microscope. Biol Theory, 2009, 4: 396-412.

[21] Gordon R. Stop breast cancer now. Imagining imaging pathways towards search, destroy, cure and watchful waiting of premetastasis breast cancer invited//Tot T (ed) Breast cancer-a lobar disease. London: Springer, 2010: pp. 167-203.

[22] Gordon R, Bjorklund NK. How to observe surface contraction waves on axolotl embryos. Int J Dev Biol, 1996, 40: 913-914.

[23] Gordon R, Brodland GW. The cytoskeletal mechanics of brain morphogenesis. Cell state splitters cause primary neural induction. Cell Biophys, 1987, 11: 177-238.

[24] Gordon R, Westfall JE. Google embryo for building quantitative understanding of an embryo as it builds itself: I. Lessons from Ganymede and Google earth. Biol Theory, 2009, 4: 390-395.

[25] Gordon R, Buckley WR. International Embryo Physics Course-An Effort in Reverse Engineering, 2010. http://embryophysics.org/

[26] Hahn WC, Weinberg RA. Modelling the molecular circuitry of cancer. Nat Rev Cancer, 2002, 2: 331-341.

[27] Hendrix MJC, Seftor EA, Seftor REB, et al. Re programming metastatic tumour cells with embryonic microenvironments. Nat Rev Cancer, 2007, 7: 246-255.

[28] Hoekenga OA, Muszynski MG, Cone KC. Developmental patterns of chromatin structure and DNA methylation responsible for epigenetic expression of a maize regulatory gene. Genetics, 2000, 155: 1889-1902.

[29] Howard B, Ashworth A. Signalling pathways implicated in early mammary gland morphogenesis and breast cancer. PLoS Genet, 2006, 2 (e112): 1121-1130.

[30] Iida S, Morita Y, Choi JD, et al. Genetics and epigenetics in fower pigmentation associated with transposable elements in morning glories. Adv Biophys, 2004, 38: 141-159.

[31] Kalthoff KO. Analysis of biological development. McGraw-Hill Higher Education, Columbus, 2001.

[32] Kasemeier-Kulesa JC, Teddy JM, Postovit LM, et al. Reprogramming mul-tipotent tumor cells with the embryonic neural crest microen-vironment. Dev Dyn, 2008, 237: 2657-2666.

[33] Kristiansen M, Helland A, Kristensen GB, et al. X chromosome inactivation in cervical cancer patients. Cancer Genet Cytogenet, 2003, 146: 73-76.

[34] Kristiansen M, Knudsen GP, Maguire P, et al. High incidence of skewed X chromosome inactivation in young patients with familial non-*BRCA*1/*BRCA*2 breast cancer. J Med Genet, 2005, 42: 877-880.

[35] Kulesa PM, Kasemeier-Kulesa JC, Teddy JM, et al. Reprogramming metastatic melanoma cells to assume a neural crest cell-like phenotype in an embryonic microenvironment. Proc Natl Acad Sci USA, 2006, 103: 3752-3757.

[36] Lerner BH. breast cancer wars: hope, fear, and the pursuit of a cure in twentieth-century America. Oxford University Press: New York, 2001.

[37] Linn F, Heidmann I, Saedler H, et al. Epigenetic changes in the expression of the maize A1 gene in Petunia hybrida: role of numbers of integrated gene copies and state of methylation. Mol Gen Genet, 1990, 222: 329-336.

[38] Lopez JI, Mouw JK, Weaver VM. Biomechanical regulation of cell orientation and fate. Oncogene, 2008, 27: 6981-6993.

[39] Lose F, Duffy DL, Kay GF, et al. Skewed X chromosome inactivation and breast and ovarian cancer status: evidence for X-linked modifers of *BRCA*1. J Natl Cancer Inst, 2008, 100: 1519-1529.

[40] Lyon MF. Gene action in the X-chromosome of the mouse (Mus musculus L.). Nature, 1961, 190: 372-373.

[41] Lyon MF. The Lyon and the LINE hypothesis. Semin Cell Dev Biol, 2003, 14: 313-318.

[42] Martin CC, Gordon R. Ultrastructural analysis of the cell state splitter in ectoderm cells differentiating to neural plate and epidermis during gastrulation in embryos of the axolotl Ambystoma mexicanum. Russian J Dev Biol, 1997, 28: 71-80.

[43] Mintz B, Illmensee K. Normal genetically mosaic mice produced from malignant teratocarcinoma cells. Proc Natl Acad Sci USA, 1975, 72: 3585-3589.

[44] Monteiro J, Derom C, Vlietinck R, et al. Commitment to X inactivation precedes the twinning event in monochorionic MZ twins. Am J Hum Genet, 1998, 63: 339-346.

[45] Muers MR, Sharpe JA, Garrick D, et al. Defning the cause of skewed X-chromosome inactivation in X-linked mental retardation by use of a mouse model. Am J Hum Genet, 2007, 80: 1138-1149.

[46] Nishida H. Specifcation of embryonic axis and mosaic development in ascidians. Dev Dyn, 2005, 233: 1177-1193.

[47] Osgood MP. X-chromosome inactivation: the case of the calico cat. Am J Pharm Educ, 1994, 58: 204-205.

[48] Pierce GB, Pantazis CG, Caldwell JE, et al. Specifcity of the control of tumor formation by the blastocyst. Cancer Res, 1982, 42: 1082-1087.

[49] Puck JM, Stewart CC, Nussbaum RL. Maximum-likelihood analysis of human T-cell X chromosome inactivation patterns: normal women versus carriers of X-linked severe combined immunodefciency. Am J Hum Genet, 1992, 50: 742-748.

[50] Raven CP. An outline of development physiology. Pergamon, Oxford, 1966.

[51] Rossant J. Reprogramming to pluripotency: from frogs to stem cells. Cell, 2009, 138: 1047-1050.

[52] Soto AM, Maffni MV, Sonnenschein C. Neoplasia as development gone awry: the role of endocrine disruptors. Int J Androl, 2008, 31: 288-293.

[53] Sulston JE, Schierenberg E, White JG, et al. The embryonic cell lineage of the nematode Caenorhabditis elegans. Dev Biol, 1983, 100: 64-119.

[54] Tenney RM, Discher DE. Stem cells, microenvironment mechanics, and growth factor activation. Curr Opin Cell Biol, 2009, 21: 630-635.

[55] Tot T. The theory of the sick lobe//Tot T (ed) Breast cancera lobar disease. London: Springer, 2011: pp. 1-17.

[56] Trichopoulos D. Hypothesis: does breast cancer originate in utero. Lancet, 1990, 335: 939-940.

[57] TyTy Nursery. Variegated Banana Tree Musa aeae: the fast growth of this remarkable variegated plant ironically grows faster than most pure-green leafed banana plants, which is a shocking inconsistency to normally accepted biological principals, 2010. http://www.tytyga.com/product/Variegated+Banana+Tree.

[58] Vella CM, Robinson R. Robinson's genetics for cat breeders and veterinarians, 4th edn. Amsterdam, Elsevier Health SciencesVermeulen L, Sprick MR, Kemper K, Stassi G, Medema JP (2008) Cancer stem cells-old concepts, new insights. Cell Death Differ, 1999, 15: 947-958.

[59] Vickers MA, McLeod E, Spector TD, et al. Assessment of mechanism of acquired skewed X inactivation by analysis of twins. Blood, 2001, 97: 1274-1281.

[60] Vincent-Salomon A, Ganem-Elbaz C, Manié E, et al. X inactive-specifc transcript RNA coating and genetic instability of the X chromosome in BRCA1 breast tumors. Cancer Res, 2007, 67: 5134-5140.

[61] Vinh-Hung V, Tot T, Gordon R. One or many targets. Towards resolving the paradox of single versus multifocal breast cancer from epidemiological data. In preparation Waddington CH (1934) Morphogenetic felds. Sci Prog (Lond), 2010, 29: 336-346.

[62] Wang N, Tytell JD, Ingber DE. Mechanotransduction at a distance: mechanically coupling the sextracellular matrix with the nucleus. Nat Rev Mol Cell Biol, 2009, 10: 75-82.

[63] Yu F, Fu A, Aluru M, Park S, et al. Variegation mutants and mechanisms of chloroplast biogenesis. Plant Cell Environ, 2007, 30: 350-365.

[64] Zaffari GR, Peres LEP, Kerbauy GB. Endogenous levels of cytokinins, indoleacetic acid, abscisic acid, and pigments in variegated somaclones of micropropagated banana leaves. J Plant Growth Regul, 1998, 17: 59-61.